Of Life and Limb

Rochester Studies in Medical History

Series Editor: Christopher Crenner
Robert Hudson and Ralph Major Professor and Chair
Department of History and Philosophy of Medicine
University of Kansas School of Medicine

Additional Titles of Interest

The Hidden Affliction: Sexually Transmitted Infections and Infertility in History
Edited by Simon Szreter

China and the Globalization of Biomedicine
Edited by David Luesink, William H. Schneider, and Zhang Daqing

Explorations in Baltic Medical History, 1850–2015
Edited by Nils Hansson and Jonatan Wistrand

Health Education Films in the Twentieth Century
Edited by Christian Bonah, David Cantor, and Anja Laukötter

The History of the Brain and Mind Sciences: Technique, Technology, Therapy
Edited by Stephen T. Casper and Delia Gavrus

Technological Change in Modern Surgery:
Historical Perspectives on Innovation
Edited by Thomas Schlich and Christopher Crenner

Setting Nutritional Standards: Theory, Policies, Practices
Edited by Elizabeth Neswald, David F. Smith, and Ulrike Thoms

Fit to Practice:
Empire, Race, Gender, and the Making of British Medicine, 1850–1980
Douglas M. Haynes

Reasoning against Madness: Psychiatry and the State in Rio de Janeiro, 1830–1944
Manuella Meyer

Psychiatry and Racial Liberalism in Harlem, 1936–1968
Dennis A. Doyle

A complete list of titles in the Rochester Studies in Medical History series
may be found on our website, www.urpress.com.

Of Life and Limb

Surgical Repair of the Arteries in War and Peace, 1880–1960

Justin Barr

UNIVERSITY OF ROCHESTER PRESS

First published 2019

University of Rochester Press
668 Mt. Hope Avenue, Rochester, NY 14620, USA
www.urpress.com
and Boydell & Brewer Limited
PO Box 9, Woodbridge, Suffolk IP12 3DF, UK
www.boydellandbrewer.com

ISBN-13: 978-1-58046-966-1
ISSN: 1526-2715

Library of Congress Cataloging-in-Publication Data

Names: Barr, Justin, 1984– author.
Title: Of life and limb : surgical repair of the arteries in war and peace, 1880–1960 / Justin Barr.
Other titles: Rochester studies in medical history ; v. 47.
Description: Rochester : University of Rochester Press, 2019. | Series: Rochester studies in medical history, 1526–2715 ; v. 47 | Includes bibliographical references and index.
Identifiers: LCCN 2019026434 | ISBN 9781580469661 (hardcover) | ISBN 9781787445833 (pdf) | ISBN 9781787446519 (epub)
Subjects: LCSH: Arteries—Surgery—History—20th century. | Arteries—Surgery—History—19th century. | Arteries—Surgery—United States—History—20th century. | Surgery, Military—United States—History—20th century.
Classification: LCC RD598.6 .B37 2019 | DDC 617.4/13—dc23
LC record available at https://lccn.loc.gov/2019026434

This publication is printed on acid-free paper.
Printed in the United States of America.

Contents

Acknowledgments

It is with great pleasure, enormous gratitude, and deep humility that I start by recognizing those who helped me on this journey. Walt Schalick and Ken Ludmerer took an undergraduate pre-med student interested in history and opened his eyes to the possibilities of a dual career as a clinician-historian; over the past fifteen years, they have continued to help me navigate this trajectory. Bob Joy and Dale Smith at Uniformed Services University (USU) introduced me to the still-understudied field of military medical history and demonstrated its academic potential. At Yale, Sue Lederer, Bruno Strasser, Frank Snowden, Dan Kevles, and John Harley Warner worked to turn an enthusiastic amateur into a professional historian—a transformation still ongoing. I am especially grateful for the guidance and mentorship that Dale Smith and John Harley Warner have continued to provide over the years. Both have read multiple drafts of this book and other writings as they selflessly spend their time and energy to nurture my career.

Debbie Doroshow, Todd Olszewski, and Richard Sosa graciously read and improved multiple chapters of this book, aided me through the publication process, and have been stalwart companions since meeting in New Haven. They, along with Paul Shin, Mary Brazelton, Robin Schmitz, and Shuqi Thng, greatly enlivened graduate school. Luke Demaitre, Kris Heitman, Sanders Marble, Walt Schalick, Ken Ludmerer, and Margaret Humphreys helpfully edited portions of the manuscript. Chris Crenner, at KUMC and the University of Rochester Press, has supported me from my earliest days of graduate school. He shepherded this manuscript through to press, sharpening it greatly along the way. Two anonymous reviewers provided insightful feedback that enabled me to improve the book. Carrie Watterson's careful copyediting emended and acuminated the text. Scott Behm, Megan Llewellyn, and the Publications Office of Duke Surgery provided invaluable assistance with the figures, cover image, and title.

Friends graciously opened their homes and provided me a place to stay on my research trips, making such ventures possible: Dr. Robert and Janet Joy, Dr. Stephen and Carolyn Craig, the Herman family, Christine Dang-Vu,

Katie McIntyre and Steve King, Sanders Marble, Sheena Chew, Catherine Kelly, Sara DuBois, and Wennie Huang. They also tolerated absences, silences, and frustrations as I labored over this manuscript, and their humor, support, and encouragement helped see me through the process.

Librarians and archivists held the actual keys to the kingdom and repeatedly went out of their way to direct me to resources, help me find recondite documents, and congenially respond to my innumerable inquiries. A huge thank you to Toby Apel, Melissa Grafe, Flo Gillich, Melanie Norton, and Vermetha Polite at Yale; the late Joan Klein, Janet Pearson, Dan Cavanaugh, Jeri Davis, and Shelby Miller at UVA; Jessica Murphy and Jack Eckert at Countway; Susan Rishworth and Dolores Barber at the American College of Surgeons; Sanders Marble at the Army Medical Department; Amber Dushman at the American Medical Association; Frank Lewis at the American Board of Surgery; Renee Ziemer at Mayo Clinic; Stephen Logsdon at Washington University; Laura Cutter and Trenton Streck-Havill at the National Museum of Health and Medicine; and Rachel Ingold, Brooke Guthrie, and Louis Wiethe III at Duke.

The general and vascular surgery communities have been unbelievably supportive of a young scholar diving into the history of their profession. They have provided sources, shared their memories, opened doors, and welcomed me into their ORs, not only facilitating this entire process but also encouraging a young surgeon along this unconventional course. I would particularly like to thank Norm Rich, James Yao, Ken Cherry, Cynthia Shortell, Neal Barshes, LaMar McGinnis, Don Nakayama, Ken Brayman, Sara Rasmussen, and Ted Pappas.

Duke has created an incredible environment to develop as a surgeon and a scholar. Margaret Humphreys and Jeff Baker have been extraordinarily welcoming as senior clinician-historians, role-modeling how to succeed in both fields. My coresidents (and especially my classmates Karenia Landa, Whitney Lane, Carrie Moore, Paul Schroder, Josh Watson, and John Yerxa) have been terrific. Thank you for helping cover my call and for putting up with my historical musings at all hours of the day and night. I am especially grateful to Allan Kirk and John Migaly for taking a chance on a nontraditional applicant, providing me the resources to succeed, and fully supporting the development of my career as a surgeon-historian. There are few greater privileges in the world than the opportunity to train as a surgeon, and I owe an unrepayable debt to my attendings and my patients for their forbearance during my education.

I am grateful for the generous funding from a number of sources that allowed me to complete this project: ABC-Clio Research Grant, the Society for the History of Navy Medicine Research Grant, the University of Virginia Raven Society Scholarship, sixty-five unique backers from a Kickstarter project, a Yale Dissertation Fellowship, the Elizabeth S. Stout and A. Varick Stout Graduate Fellowship, the General and Mrs. Matthew B. Ridgeway Military History Research Grant, the Michael E. DeBakey Fellowship in the History of Medicine at the National Library of Medicine, the Bernard Becker Medical Library Travel Scholarship, the Josiah Charles Trent Memorial Foundation Grant, and the W. Bruce Fye Medical History Research Travel Grant. Duke Department of Surgery has generously supported my salary while I completed this book over the past eighteen months.

None of this would be possible without my family. Clay Barr read not only every word but also every footnote, saving me from innumerable errors and poorly parsed phrases. The cards and encouragement from her and Irene Baros provided ongoing support and motivation. My siblings, Shayne and Gabrielle, each helped with crucial components of the manuscript and have cheered me on selflessly in my academic pursuits. My parents, Bruce and Lauren, who also read every word and markedly improved the prose, more importantly created a home that valued learning, scholarship, and hard work, establishing a loving foundation that has enabled me to succeed thus far and inspires me to strive ever further.

Introduction

Of Homer's heroes hit by spears, shot with arrows, or struck by swords in *The Iliad*, 90 percent died, most bleeding to death on the battlefield.[1] Weapons have since grown more powerful, but the importance of saving lives and limbs remains unchanged. From Homer to the present, society has asked medical practitioners to arrest the hemorrhage and restore these individuals to their pre-injured state. As doctors have learned more about blood vessels, they have also identified nontraumatic conditions, like the aortic aneurysm that killed Albert Einstein and the clogging of vessels by cholesterol that causes heart attacks and strokes, which are also amenable to structural repair. While recent pharmaceutical interventions can ameliorate some of these conditions, throughout most of history, surgery provided the only effective therapy.

This book studies the process of how surgery changes. It focuses on operations that repair blood vessels and uses them to explore broader issues such as the relationship between theory and practice; how surgical knowledge is generated, validated, and communicated; the nature of surgical authority; the mechanisms by which a particular operation becomes standard of care; and the sociocultural conditions that promote and determine change. Written to inform both historians and surgeons, *Surgical Repair of the Arteries* examines how doctors took care of patients suffering from vascular trauma and disease and how that management developed over the course of the late nineteenth and twentieth centuries.

At its most fundamental level, repairing arteries restores blood flow through diseased or injured vessels. Your cells need oxygen and nutrients to survive. Blood carries these life-sustaining molecules through an interconnected web of arteries and veins called the vascular system. Arteries carry oxygen-rich, nutrient-filled blood from the heart to the periphery; veins return the depleted blood back to the core for replenishment and recirculation. From superhighways like the aorta to the tortuous back roads of microscopic capillaries, this transport network reaches every corner of the human body. Disruptions to this infrastructure can prove fatal. Trauma in the form of stabbings, shootings, and explosions can sever vessels and cause death from bleeding. Dilations of arteries called aneurysms can burst, draining the entire blood supply within minutes. Less dramatically but no less nefariously, cholesterol can clog arteries from the inside, choking off the oxygen and nutrients cells need to survive, leading to heart attacks, strokes, and the amputation of arms and legs. Vascular surgery, and specifically arterial repair, promised to treat these pathologies, saving lives and limbs by restoring blood flow. Later, the technique of anastomosis, or connecting two blood vessels together, proved foundational for other branches of surgery like solid organ transplantation, advanced tissue grafts, and cardiac bypass procedures.

In 1880, there was no such thing as arterial repair. By 1912, Alexis Carrel had won the Nobel Prize for pioneering a technique to sew blood vessels together, inspiring dreams of organ transplantation and the reattachment of severed limbs. Despite attention garnered by the award, for the next forty years the operation remained confined to textbooks, performed by only a few elite practitioners. Then, in the 1950s, surgeons rapidly adopted it as a standard, common procedure. Hope transformed into reality as ever-increasing numbers of patients benefitted from doctors repairing their vasculature. This trajectory introduces a central paradox that makes arterial repair an especially compelling lens through which to investigate how the *practice* of surgery changes. Why did an operation that everyone theoretically agreed to be the ideal therapy for vascular disease and that experience in the operating room had proven to be feasible, go essentially unused for decades? And what in the 1950s prompted the sudden shift to its widespread implementation?

The book starts by analyzing the pursuit and invention of a technique to sew blood vessels together. This integral development occurred over several decades in the late nineteenth and early twentieth centuries, a particularly fertile time for surgery.[2] Understanding the history of arterial repair, and that of surgical change generally, requires an appreciation of the technical component, which fundamentally determines what operations are possible, when, by whom, and under what conditions. Thus, these chapters prioritize the interrogation of what surgeons actually did and did not do in the operating room, how they performed procedures, and what factors drove or restricted their activities. In shifting attention from theory to execution, it focuses on the average surgeon, not just academic elites and thought leaders, in order to capture what happened to the majority of patients. This emphasis on what Erwin Ackerknecht called "behaviorist history" distinguishes *Surgical Repair of the Arteries* from much of academic surgical scholarship, which, as Thomas Schlich has pointed out, has addressed topics of professionalization, education, patient experience, and biography, but not the actual practice of surgical operations.[3] The book simultaneously places in sharp relief the world in which historical actors functioned. This study of the milieu in which arterial repair was invented and came to flourish presents a departure from preceding accounts written by surgeons, which often elide this broader context.[4]

Bridging these two literatures, this account examines the creation, diffusion, and establishment of the operative techniques to repair arteries as well as the social, cultural, military, and medical forces that influenced the construction and eventual adoption of this operation. John Pickstone has emphasized moving beyond the moment of invention to study when, how, and why the medical community incorporates innovations into routine use.[5] While the creation of a new operation is essential for surgical change, the advent of a procedure marks the beginning of that transformation, not its culmination. Surgeons must take up a given technique and apply it to patients for the new intervention to have any clinical, social, or historical relevance. *Surgical Repair of the Arteries* chiefly explores this process of dissemination and adoption. It builds on the scholarship of Thomas Schlich, who investigated the orthopedic case of osteosynthesis.[6] Whereas Schlich's work highlighted the roles of corporate control and transnational differences, this history emphasizes education, surgical training, and military conflict. It tracks the care of vascular trauma and disease across the twentieth century, paying particular attention to medicine in the world wars and the scientific and social movements during peacetime, especially the emergence of specialty education. While these broader forces shaped the development of the field, it remained for individual surgeons like Carrel, the energetic and influential Michael E. DeBakey, and thousands of anonymous practitioners to perform the actual cutting and stitching. Examining the change in management over time demonstrates a rapid and near-total conversion from tying off arteries to repairing them, with the Korean War as the prime inflection point. Shifting wartime practice subsequently drove the implementation of arterial repair in the civilian world in the 1950s, transforming the procedure into a staple of modern surgery.

Specific features of arterial repair make it a particularly instructive case study. Rather than relying on a novel conceptual understanding of pathophysiology like many new surgeries in the late nineteenth and early twentieth centuries (e.g., appendectomy), leaking or clogged arteries clearly needed repair based on simple plumbing principles.[7] From a technical perspective, while many of the popular operations of the era were relatively simple to perform even by general practitioners, arterial repair required fine, precise sutures and near-perfect technique, focusing increased attention on the capabilities and training of the surgeon.[8] Moreover, most new procedures in the nineteenth and early twentieth centuries invaded the chest, abdomen, or head and in so doing produced severe physiological insults involving blood pressure management, fluid shifts, electrolyte imbalances, digestive malfunctions, and difficulties ventilating patients that were poorly understood at that time. Thus, technically feasible thoracic and abdominal operations proved physiologically impossible, with patients dying postoperatively at unacceptable rates. In contrast, vascular surgery predominantly involved the arms and legs of patients. Avoiding the systemic insults of intracavity operations partially freed early arterial repair from having to wait on developments in other fields of medicine to succeed. Finally, demanding little more than basic instruments, needles, and thread, arterial repair did not depend on advanced technology such as special hardware for bones, articulating artificial joints, immuno-suppressive regimens, a heart-lung machine to provide circulation, artificial organs, or laparoscopic cameras that other surgeries required.[9]

The emergent conditions surrounding most early arterial repairs left little room for patient preference to dictate which surgery one received or in what style. Those affected were often soldiers and desperately wounded, lacking the opportunity or even the legal autonomy under military law to seek one intervention over another.[10] The urgency of trauma cases, both in war and peace, particularly precluded negotiations. These situations contrasted starkly with the later rise of elective procedures like breast, cosmetic, and minimally invasive operations such as the laparoscopic cholecystectomy.[11] In these cases, "consumer" demand largely determined the trajectory and utilization of the surgeries. Dominated instead by what doctors considered appropriate and possible, vascular repair provides unique insight into the development of a procedure more securely in control of the surgeons alone.

These doctors, also often in uniform, had no financial and few professional incentives to favor a certain approach.[12] Hardly any surgeon doubted the superiority of arterial repair in theory, as had been the case for certain cancer operations like the modified radical mastectomy.[13] With no expensive, single-use technologies required for vascular work at that time, industry did not lobby for one intervention over another, as it has for pharmaceuticals and, more recently, surgical robots.[14] Instead, doctors questioned the possibility of sewing vessels consistently and efficaciously, pointing again to this paradox of disuse and the central importance of technique.

Thus, in contrast to histories of many surgical innovations that were profoundly shaped by exterior forces, the story of arterial repair revolves around the operation itself, who could perform it, and under what specific conditions. For anastomoses, technical competence mattered more than prevailing medical theories in determining surgical development.[15] Factors such as new instrumentation, patient preference, and financial incentives had little effect on vascular surgery in the late nineteenth and early twentieth centuries. This relative isolation from social, economic, physiological, and technological variables exemplifies why arterial repair makes such a useful model for examining the dynamics of surgical stasis and change.

This focus on the operation directs attention to the men who performed it and especially their professional training.[16] The highly technical nature of arterial repair demanded a cadre of appropriately schooled surgeons to execute cases safely and successfully; until such a group existed, vascular surgery remained confined to ligation, or tying off the artery with suture to prevent blood flow. Arterial repair, and by extension many of the complex operations that emerged in the mid- to late twentieth century, required a high level of manual ability that most surgeons simply lacked before 1950. Producing thousands of highly skilled operators required a conscious, concerted effort by the American surgical profession to create, expand, and structure a system of education that came to be called residency.[17] Between the 1930s and 1950s, residency transformed from a rare, ad hoc, idiosyncratic experience for elite doctors into standardized, ubiquitous, and mandatory education for all American surgeons. These efforts simultaneously reflected and shaped a broader movement to reform graduate medical education in the United States.[18]

Central to this metamorphosis was the institutionalization of residency nationwide as it spread from academia to community hospitals.[19] The federal government and professional organizations like the American College of Surgeons played critical, complementary roles in establishing the necessity and infrastructure of residencies. The government catalyzed their rapid expansion through military policies in World War II, postwar financial incentives, and especially the Veterans Administration hospital system, while professional associations mandated universal criteria for training. By the 1950s, a multiyear, standardized postgraduate educational experience increasingly determined who was a surgeon in the United States. This system began building a cadre of competent practitioners necessary for implementing surgical change in the mid-twentieth century.

When these residency-trained surgeons deployed to the Korean War, they brought with them the skills, experience, and motivation to start repairing arteries; the war created the conditions that enabled them to change their practice. While many writers comment on the close links between war and surgery, few go on to analyze the connection, and those who do often offer generalizations about all of medicine.[20] Surgical historians like Roger Cooter tend to focus on issues of professionalization rather than clinical advances.[21]

Investigations of the Korean War and medicine are particularly limited.[22] While some literature too glibly touts the medical advances of war, other accounts too critically dismiss the medical benefits of military conflict.[23] Combat rarely spawns entirely new therapies, but scholarship has clearly demonstrated how the particular features of battle can catalyze the application and adoption of previously marginalized interventions.[24]

By contrast, historians of science and technology have scrutinized war in great depth as both a stimulant and impediment to innovation.[25] For instance, scholars have shown how during war the military can determine topics of research, erect security measures that hinder the free exchange of ideas, endow scientists with otherwise unavailable resources, and liberate them from bureaucratic and regulatory constraints. Some of these same elements also characterize the interplay between war and surgery. However, the specifics of surgery make its relationship to armed conflict unique. Examining these features through arterial repair provides insight into what drives surgical change.

Defined by the physical manipulation of tissue on a case-by-case basis, surgery stands apart from applied technologies in its expectation that everyday practitioners command a high level of comprehension of the subject, accept the theoretical rationale underpinning each operation, and master the intricate mechanics imperative for executing them. In contrast, devices like the atomic bomb and radar required the best minds of a generation to conceive, design, and assemble. However, end users, be they the crew of the *Enola Gay* or radar operators, needed effectively no understanding of the theory or science and markedly less technical know-how to deploy these technologies effectively.[26] This relationship facilitated top-down distribution, a model equally applied to many medical interventions, such as penicillin.[27] Scientists struggled for years to mass-produce the drug efficiently and determine its efficacy. Physicians certainly provided their expertise in recognizing diseases curable by penicillin, but once they reached a diagnosis, implementing the therapy involved simply writing a prescription. By comparison, effective arterial repair demanded the same ability from average front-line surgeons as it did from the academics who developed the operation. The level of skill required by all users differentiated arterial repair (and surgery more generally) from these other inventions. Both physical technologies and the *theory* of new operations benefitted from the military's ability to leverage its chain of command to communicate new ideas widely, but changing the actual *practice* of surgery demanded that a critical mass of competent practitioners learn and apply a new technique.[28] This parallel, rather than hierarchical process, partly explains its delayed adoption.

Whereas armaments and other scientific endeavors benefited from the infrastructure of war, profiting from extensive funding, lavish research facilities, and prioritization of specific projects, arterial repair depended on the war itself. With medical tools like scalpels and sutures costing pennies, surgical innovation was less contingent on an influx of financial resources. However, the human cost of combat had the potential to drive change. Specifically, the volume and type of casualties catalyzed the practice of arterial repair in a number of ways. First, unlike their civilian counterparts, injured soldiers constituted a relatively homogenous group of eighteen- to thirty-year-old men who, because of medical screening upon enlistment or being drafted, presented to doctors with few health problems other than their traumatic injuries. This standardized population facilitated the propagation of techniques as doctors presumed what worked for one soldier would prove equally effective for another. The governmental penchant for documentation left particularly robust medical records of these patients at a time when civilian hospitals were just beginning to systemize their files; this practice not only provides useful historical evidence but also created a data set contemporary actors investigated in real time to assess the efficacy of various treatments and modify them accordingly.[29]

Second, the sheer number of cases provided unequaled opportunities for surgeons to practice new techniques. Like any manual skill, operating improves with repetition.[30] Even the busiest civilian trauma centers paled in comparison to front-line military hospitals in the quantity and severity of wounds they treated. With battles causing thousands of casualties, physicians rapidly amassed voluminous autonomous experience. This human carnage and its dehumanizing outcomes also instilled an attitude of experimentalism and risk tolerance among some doctors, enabling their perseverance through the high mortality rates that often occur in the early stages of surgical development. This borderline-callous dedication helped propel heart surgery and hip replacement into becoming viable operations following World War II in addition to routinizing arterial repair after Korea.[31] While distinct groups of practitioners developed these procedures, they shared common wartime experience, usually early in their careers.

Third, the slaughter concentrated casualties with the comparatively rare pathologies of vascular trauma in a single time and place. Just as increased hospitalization expanded medical research generally in the late nineteenth and early twentieth centuries by consolidating disease physically, wartime hospitals similarly provided opportunities to learn about and improve treatment of specific conditions.[32] Whereas in peacetime clinicians might build a case series of dozens of patients suffering vascular trauma over many years, in war they could publish similar studies based on only several months of operating. Frequent exposure sensitized clinicians to trends in patient response by providing immediate feedback, equipping them to adjust their practice agilely, continually reassessing and recalibrating in a dynamic circle toward competence.

The specific nature of surgery differentiated it from purely medical innovations. In cutting through tissue, surgery inherently hurts patients, even when it ultimately cures disease.[33] Drugs and laboratory tests certainly have the potential to cause adverse side effects, but few doctors or patients hesitate to accept the risks of swallowing a pill or having blood drawn. Deciding to operate on someone, and accepting the need to be operated on, requires a much stronger conviction in the benefit of that therapy in order to tolerate the iatrogenic harm. This compromise places a greater burden of proof on surgeries and influences the pace of their adoption.

The diffusion of new technologies, particularly those associated with health care, has attracted considerable attention.[34] While the majority of literature in this field analyzes physical technologies, vascular surgery offers a different perspective by demanding appreciation for the diffusion of the physical ability required by the end user. While arterial repair followed a conventional uptake pattern, with a few first adopters, a period of rapid growth, then latecomers, the shape of the standard S-curve skews right, featuring a prolonged gap separating early and mainstream application that reflects the aforementioned paradox. Other historians such as Joel Howell have analyzed analogous delays for innovations like X-rays and sterile gloves.[35] They showed how clinicians' skepticism of the utility or benefit of such inventions slowed their adoption. But, after acknowledging their theoretical superiority, practitioners had no physical difficulty taking an X-ray, donning gloves, or performing a urinalysis. By contrast, most surgeons at the turn of the century accepted the superiority of arterial repair in theory—they just could not perform the operation physically. It took a national educational effort to instill that competency and a war to create the opportunities to use that skill and collect enough data to judge its merits.

Juxtaposing military and civilian practice, *Surgical Repair of the Arteries* investigates the process of surgical change by focusing on the technical challenge of sewing arteries together and what conditions made such suturing possible. Chapter 1 introduces John Hunter's ligation procedure for aneurysms and demonstrates how it defined modern surgery in the eighteenth and early nineteenth centuries. However, the resulting lack of blood flow left patients at significant risk for subsequent amputation. As part of a surgical renaissance in the late nineteenth century, dozens of innovators worked on animals and humans to develop new techniques to repair and anastomose arteries in order to replace the increasingly inadequate ligation operation. The technical details of this progression may be of greater intrinsic interest to surgeons than historians, but the unpackaging of these efforts exposes key themes unique to surgical culture. Interrogating the process of creation unveils standards of evidence, perceived importance of technology, interpersonal communication of practices, and the nature of authority specific to modern surgery. The experiments culminated in Alexis Carrel's 1912 Nobel Prize–winning triangulation method that remains in use today. Examining this groundswell of innovation within a civilian context, chapter 1 highlights the integration of scientific knowledge, surgical culture, and technical skill to demonstrate how surgeries are invented.

Chapter 2 begins by surveying vascular trauma in the First World War. Even though military medical leaders acknowledged the superiority of arterial repair over ligation, conditions of war, limitations in medical science, and the (in)ability of the average World War I doctor prevented any widespread utilization of the technique. Shortly after the war, prominent American surgeons publicly recognized deficiencies in the training of their community and attempted to institutionalize educational reform through professional organizations like the American College of Surgeons and the American Board of Surgery. During the same period, academic surgical innovators developed the technologies of heparin and arteriography, which would later become crucial to the practice of arterial repair. They also pioneered a completely new, simpler alternative to the technically demanding suturing of arteries called sympathectomy, which dominated practice for the next two decades.

Chapter 3 analyzes the practice of arterial repair in World War II, as the book shifts from a global perspective to concentrate on the United States of America, which had attained worldwide leadership in medicine and science by this point. For reasons analogous to those associated with World War I—combat conditions and limited education of the average uniformed surgeon—ligation remained the predominant vascular operation in the Second World War. Surprisingly, however, a definite pivot to arterial repair had occurred by 1945, evident on both the front lines and in military hospitals in the United States. While this transition did not maintain its momentum in the postwar years, it foreshadowed the sea change that the Korean War would instigate less than a decade later.

Chapter 4, covering 1945–50, focuses on a series of organizational changes outside the operating room that proved critical to the traction of arterial repair. Pioneering heart surgeries incited research on blood vessels while academic leaders founded organizations such as the Society for Vascular

Surgery to support the nascent field. Anesthesia evolved from a largely nurse-administered practice to a modern medical specialty, enabling surgeons to perform increasingly complex operations. Most importantly, formal surgical education via residency programs transformed into a standardized portal for American surgeons, providing the training and experience necessary for them to start repairing arteries.

In the Korean War, arterial repair graduated from exceptional to expected. The fifth chapter shows how the specific conditions of this war such as static lines of engagement, mobile army surgical hospital (MASH) units, and powerful antibiotics combined with the major interwar developments of professionalized anesthesia and modern surgical residencies to create a milieu that fostered the surgical repair of arteries. First performed individually and against military policy, arterial repair matured into the official operation of choice for vascular trauma by 1952, halving amputation rates from World War II.

Once proven in combat abroad, arterial repair subsequently became the standard of care in the United States for vascular trauma and disease. Chapter 6 scrutinizes the widespread expansion and utilization of the technique between 1950 and 1960, an embrace precipitated by the clinical outcomes amassed during the Korean War and spearheaded by veteran surgeons returning home now capable of sewing arteries together. A rise in crime and the creation of a highway system in the 1950s expanded the volume of vascular injuries requiring an operation.[36] Atherosclerotic disease, previously recognized but rarely treated, soon overtook trauma as the most common indication for arterial repair. Its millions of sufferers helped drive the proliferation of the operation in the United States and demonstrated that vascular surgery had significant utility beyond trauma and war.

Surgery has been a common and critically important therapy since at least the era of Hippocrates, and it remains so today: more than 105 million procedures were performed in the United States in 2010—one for every three Americans.[37] Surgery has a history at once linked with medicine while also distinct from it. It is a past curiously neglected by scholars, particularly regarding the operations themselves. The six chapters that follow carefully examine the specific factors—internal and external—that contributed to the development and widespread practice of arterial repair. While every operation, and thus its historical trajectory, is unique, the conclusion draws generalizable tropes from this story to illuminate the process of surgical change and better understand this field of health care.

Chapter One

Technical Change, Practical Stasis

The Development of Arterial Repair through 1914

"My left leg is a great deal weaker than my right," wrote Marvin Rynar, a forty-seven-year-old watchman from Georgia to his surgeon, William Halsted. In 1906, Rynar had been struck in the thigh by a metal hoop and subsequently developed an aneurysm of the femoral artery. Halsted treated it by ligating (tying off) his left iliac artery in 1909. Rynar recovered from the surgery and in 1912 wrote Halsted to tell him how he was feeling: the aneurysm had disappeared, but "I can't walk very much as I have pains in my left leg when I do any walking . . . it gets very cold."[1] Rynar's experience exemplifies the progress surgery made in the early modern era while simultaneously demonstrating its limitations. Rynar benefitted from John Hunter's proximal ligation procedure for aneurysm, a scientifically developed operation from the eighteenth century that saved both the lives and limbs of patients who previously faced amputation or death. This clinical success and its intellectual foundation made proximal ligation a hallmark of modern surgery for the next century.

Yet Rynar also suffered for years with a painful, barely functional leg. In an effort to improve patients' outcomes, surgeons spent the decades between 1880 and 1914 devising new operations to repair and even replace injured blood vessels. They relied on the technologies of anesthesia and asepsis, superior training, and unprecedented global collaboration made possible by journals and international conferences. In 1880, the possibility of arterial repair did not exist; by World War I, surgeons had invented a series of innovative procedures to repair arteries and successfully applied them to a few patients. However, the clinical rarity of arterial repair in the 1910s revealed a gap between invention and widespread application.

Exploring the technical development of arterial repair unpackages how procedures are created, unveiling unique elements of surgical culture. It shows how surgeons operated—both specifically in their physical manipulation of tissue and more generally in how they worked in the laboratory and clinic.[2] While research primarily remained a solitary endeavor, the results and their impact simultaneously created and depended on a sense of authority within this community. Investigating the process of invention and dissemination reveals the priority of practical demonstration over theorizing and the crucial reliance on vivisecting animals in providing compelling evidence. The centrality of zoonotic proof and the relatively few human successes needed for physicians to declare victory exposes the tremendous optimism contemporaries placed in the ability of surgery to treat disease even before broad clinical results could justify such celebration. It thus exposes this paradox of establishing the so-called ideal operation to repair arteries, clearly demonstrating its feasibility in human patients, praising its potential, and yet rarely using it in the operating room to help people suffering from vascular trauma and disease.

Proximal Ligation

Medical texts dating from ancient Egypt onward attempted to map the vasculature and offer instructions on how to control it. The significance of blood as one of the four humors stimulated further investigation in ancient Greece and Rome. In the early modern era, scholars directed their attention to anatomy and physiology. Andreas Vesalius artistically depicted arteries and veins in his *De humani corporis fabrica* (1543), and William Harvey's work on circulation in *De motu cordis* (1628) altered how physicians and natural philosophers understood the flow of blood in the human body.

Efforts to stem bleeding and control aneurysms similarly date to antiquity. While sources like Celsus (c. 50 CE) described ligation, until the seventeenth century clinicians primarily relied on cauterization to control blood loss, applying hot irons to singe blood vessels closed.[3] Aneurysms, also identified in ancient times, are balloon-like dilations of an artery that risk rupturing and causing a patient to bleed to death (figure 1.1a).[4] They likely occurred with some frequency following mishaps phlebotomizing patients and particularly increased after syphilis arrived in Europe, as the disease can weaken the walls of arteries and cause them to expand.[5] Roman surgeon Antyllus

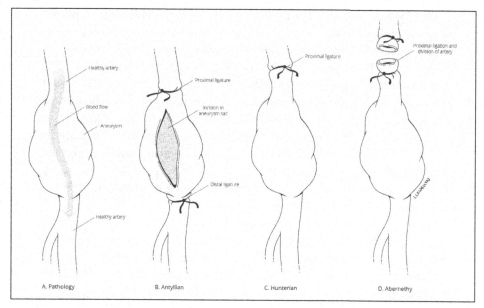

Figure 1.1. Pathology and treatment of arterial aneurysms. (A) Aneurysmal artery, with blood flowing from top to bottom. Note the healthy artery, characterized by its normal diameter, surrounding the dilated aneurysm sac in the middle. (B) Antyllus placed sutures directly above and below the aneurysm sac to control blood flow, then made a longitudinal incision to fillet open the sac and evacuate its contents lest they poison the patient. (C) Relying on the newly discovered principle of circulation, Hunter intentionally placed his suture several centimeters above the aneurysm in healthy tissue to block blood from entering the sac and thus mitigating the risk of rupture. He did not open the sac. (D) Abernethy modified Hunter's operation by dividing the proximal artery between two sutures to guarantee the interruption of blood flow. Drawing rendered by Megan Llewellyn, MSMI.

wrote about a technique in the second century CE to treat aneurysms that involved proximal and distal ligation of the afflicted artery followed by filleting the aneurysm sac open to release the evil humors contained therein (figure 1.1b).[6] While medical literature from ancient Rome through the nineteenth century repeatedly recommended this operation, little evidence substantiates its routine usage.[7] Nonetheless, it remained the theoretical standard of care over a millennium and a half when few new theories or therapies gained prominence. However, the Antyllian operation was so morbid that many surgeons like Percivall Pott (1713–88) preferred to amputate the limb in which the aneurysm occurred rather than risk patient death from the hemorrhage that often followed incision into the sac.[8]

John Hunter (1728–93), a largely self-educated Scottish surgeon practicing in London, published extensively on the anatomy and physiology of the vascular system.[9] Based on his scientific studies, he developed what became known as the Hunterian operation to cure arterial aneurysms.[10] In 1785, he treated a swelling of the popliteal artery behind the knee by tying off its source, the superficial femoral artery, several centimeters above the diseased portion (figure 1.1c).[11] His procedure differed technically from the Antyllian operation in that he never opened the aneurysm, substantially lowering the risk of bleeding to death. Unlike Pott's prophylactic amputation, Hunter's procedure at least gave patients the possibility of keeping their arm or leg. This operation remained the standard of care to treat vascular trauma and aneurysms for the next 150 years.

The foundation and rationale behind this surgery proved far more relevant than the technical details and epitomized Hunter's reputation for bringing science to surgical innovation.[12] Whereas other procedures like amputations and cutting for bladder stones evolved empirically, Hunter scientifically developed proximal ligation, identifying and localizing the disease process through vivisecting animals and dissecting human corpses, modes of investigation emerging as increasingly important forms of scientific evidence by the late eighteenth century.[13] He then utilized his experimental knowledge of collateral circulation and arterial anatomy to design an operation to change the natural history of the aneurysm (that is, rupture) and cure the patient.[14] Relying on these results, Hunter reconfigured the old technique by placing his ligature several centimeters above the aneurysm in healthy artery. This seemingly minor alteration avoided the previously common—and lethal— problem where tissue necrosis would cause the suture to fall off, leaving the patient to bleed to death. More generally, this entire process established the fundamental principle of identifying local, anatomic pathology through experimentation and using that knowledge to guide the design of novel operations. This principle, first implemented by Hunter in the 1780s, has shaped the development and practice of surgery since.

The Hunterian operation for aneurysms quickly spread to vessels throughout the human body and to countries all over the Western world, courtesy of Hunter's students. John Abernethy attained fame for the first successful ligation of the external iliac artery for an aneurysm in the pelvis and added the important step of severing the proximal artery to guarantee disruption of blood flow (figure 1.1d).[15] Antonia Scarpa carried Hunter's teaching to Italy, where his 1804 text on aneurysms eventually surpassed his teacher's work in fame and importance.[16] Astley Cooper, perhaps Hunter's best-known pupil, became interested in vascular surgery when he saw his foster brother bleed to death after a wagon wheel ran over his leg and severed the popliteal artery.[17] Simplifying Hunter's technique, Cooper gained recognition by performing the first carotid ligation to cure an aneurysm in the neck as well as a series of nine successful external iliac ligations. Today, Cooper remains famous for the first ligation of the abdominal aorta in 1817, although his patient died forty hours after surgery.[18] His student Valentine Mott brought these principles and techniques to the United States, where he achieved world-wide recognition for ligating the innominate artery in close proximity to the heart in 1818 in addition to 138 other vessels over the course of his career.[19] Mott, Cooper, and Scarpa demonstrate the crucial role of interpersonal relationships in disseminating medical innovations. The active participation of teachers and students in hands-on learning is especially influential in procedural fields like surgery where written communication struggles to convey the tacit knowledge and practical steps vital to its success.[20]

These men and their international professional recognition exemplify how Hunter's operation for aneurysm came to represent surgical excellence in the eighteenth and nineteenth centuries. Surgeons established their reputation by which artery and how many they had successfully ligated.[21] Medical periodicals triumphantly announced these accomplishments, like an article in the inaugural *New England Journal of Medicine and Surgery* (now the *New England Journal of Medicine*) trumpeting the first ligation of the external iliac artery in the United States.[22] Hundreds of books, articles, and pamphlets described and commented on the operation.[23] Samuel Cooper's *A Dictionary for Practical Surgery*, the most popular English-language surgical textbook of the early nineteenth century, dedicated twenty-five pages to aneurysms and their treatment, strongly advocating for Hunter's proximal ligation.[24] The topic frequently headlined conferences and lectures, with the 1843 Hunterian Oration detailing all 389 ligations published in the literature.[25] Contemporary licensing exams tested applicants on the procedure.[26] More than any other operation, arterial ligation for aneurysm defined skilled surgery from John Hunter through the mid-nineteenth century.

The central role of ligation resulted from both its therapeutic potential and its scientific foundation. For much of the eighteenth and nineteenth centuries, arterial ligation for aneurysm was one of the few major operations surgeons could perform to heal patients with a relatively high rate of success, and one of the only elective ones.[27] The union of science and effective surgery enabled its practitioners to proclaim not only their procedural competence but also their academic foundation. This combination provided the potential for improving their stature in the crowded medical marketplace of the nineteenth century.[28] "The history of the operation for the aneurysm would alone show that surgery is capable of making considerable advances to perfection," proclaimed William Hunter, brother of the surgeon and a famous physician in his own right.[29]

Compared to prophylactic, definite amputation, proximal ligation presented obvious benefits to patients, but it inherently cut off blood supply to any tissue beyond the suture, causing patients like Marvin Rynar to suffer. It was still possible for gangrene to develop and require amputation. Even when patients retained their limbs, they often lacked sufficient blood flow to use their arm or leg effectively in work or daily life. Rynar certainly appreciated being alive and keeping his leg, but he also clearly suffered from the sequelae of the procedure; surgeons strove to do better.

New Era of Surgery

The surgical revolution of late nineteenth century has received considerable attention from historians. Anesthesia permitted pain-free operations.[30] As critical but less discussed, ether and chloroform kept patients still throughout a procedure; placing fine, precise stiches into a small artery would be nigh impossible on patients thrashing from the agony of the knife. Joseph Lister described antiseptic surgery in 1866, and although it required decades to gain acceptance, by the 1880s clinicians throughout Europe and the United States routinely practiced anti/aseptic techniques with markedly lower rates of postoperative infection.[31] More importantly, the germ theory contributed to an ontological understanding of disease that led to surgery becoming the cure for many previously untreatable conditions.[32] Differentiating and localizing maladies like appendicitis, tonsillitis, and cancer created targets for operative intervention that could heal patients. Improved outcomes and lack of pain prompted both surgeons and patients to go to the operating room in ever-greater numbers.

These surgeons and patients benefitted from an environment more conducive to successful operations. The rising acceptability of receiving treatment in hospitals over the late nineteenth century led to the relocation of surgery from dining rooms to operating rooms.[33] The controlled space enabled aseptic techniques, and the concentration of patients permitted clinicians to study disease and the impact of their interventions more effectively and efficiently. Electric lighting enabled cases to proceed at any time of day or night with guaranteed illumination that markedly improved visibility.[34] The professionalization of nurses in the late nineteenth century created a skilled assistant who enforced anti/aseptic practice, facilitated the flow of the procedure, and also managed both pre- and postoperative care.[35]

Surgical training improved over the course of the nineteenth century. In Europe, laboratory-based, clinically integrated schools graduated comparatively competent clinicians.[36] Formal medical education lagged in the United States, but individuals interested in surgery frequently enrolled in postgraduate courses or traveled to Europe for further learning.[37] Though idiosyncratic, the preparation of surgical leaders like William Halsted, J. B. Murphy, and Alexis Carrel differed substantially in length, scientific integration, and research emphasis from the informal, stochastic apprenticeships of the Astley Cooper / Valentine Mott generation that prioritized clinical teaching.

Ongoing education relied on both journals and medical conferences, relatively new resources. The industrial revolution catalyzed both, with steam presses churning out thousands of periodicals and steam-powered trains and ships transporting physicians around the world to attend meetings and clinics.[38] The number of medical journals swelled in the nineteenth century: 479 were established in the UK alone between 1800 and 1900, with an exponential increase following 1880.[39] They became the primary transmitter of medical knowledge.[40] Whereas publications on anesthesia in the 1840s circulated in journals, pamphlets, and books, literature discussing asepsis three decades later appeared almost exclusively in periodicals.[41] General titles like the *New England Journal of Medicine* (1812), the *Lancet* (1823), and the *British Medical Journal* (1857) predominated early; specialty titles like *Annals of Surgery* (1885) arrived later and helped nurture professional identity.[42] So too did surgical meetings. Expanding out of general medical congresses from the 1800s, strictly surgical conventions began in the early twentieth century via the Society of Clinical Surgery (1903) for elite practitioners and Franklin Martin's Clinical Congresses (1911) for any interested doctor.[43] Attendees not only heard lectures but also had the unparalleled opportunity to observe operations performed by their inventors. The superiority of this face-to-face teaching over didactics had (and still has) particular value in fields like surgery that involve physical skills and demand procedural competence.[44]

Journals and meetings connected an international web of surgeon-investigators who communicated, collaborated, and competed with one another to advance the field.[45] Citations clearly reveal familiarity with colleagues' work from around the Western world. In place of the individual, isolated efforts of men like John Hunter, a global community of surgeons arose that expedited the creation and the diffusion of technologies and techniques, contributing to the accelerated growth of efforts to repair arteries.

The scientific, educational, and social environments contributed to a dramatic increase in surgery in the late nineteenth and early twentieth centuries. Between 1880 and 1890, the medical literature described more than a hundred new operations.[46] Between 1900 and 1925, the number of surgeries at the University of Pennsylvania Hospital increased from 870 a year to 4,180 a year. At New York Hospital, only 18 percent of inpatients received an operation in 1900, but 69 percent did in 1920.[47] The idea that surgery provided a solution had taken hold. Once rare, elective surgery became the dominant therapy of the era—and, for many conditions, the only effective one.

The manner of surgery changed as well. Operations in the early nineteenth century emphasized speed and flair. With the introduction of anesthesia, surgeons could now take their time; the advent of asepsis prioritized careful dissection, precise tissue handling, and bloodless fields.[48] Operations simultaneously became more precise and more radical, seeking to cure the entire disease with a single procedure.[49] Rynar's surgeon William S. Halsted epitomized and proselytized this new style of surgery.[50] Following medical school and internship in New York, Halsted pursued postgraduate education in Germany, studying with leaders in the field like von Bergmann, Billroth, and Volkmann. He brought their teaching of scientific surgery back to the United States and expanded it by researching broadly applicable subjects such as breast cancer, thyroid disease, intestinal anastomosis, and arterial aneurysms. Meticulous dissection and delicate handling of tissue undergirded his entire practice, enabling Halsted to achieve superior outcomes. Eventually these practice habits came to characterize the best surgery throughout the country.

Vascular surgery both benefitted and differed from the changes of the late nineteenth and early twentieth century. Fragile blood vessels and the tiny, precise sutures used to sew them relied on the new style of Halsted and others. The general increase in the volume of operations led to iatrogenic vascular injuries that inspired clinicians to pursue reparative options. Investigations of other organs like the intestines crossed over to the realm of arterial surgery, sharing similar goals of joining two tubes with no leaks. However, whereas surgeons created many late nineteenth-century operations for nosologically novel diseases like appendicitis or tonsillitis, vascular pathology had not changed.[51] The diseases clinicians confronted—aneurysms and trauma—remained unaltered, as did their proposed etiology. But, over the ensuing decades, the options for treating these conditions diversified considerably.

Plugging Holes While Maintaining Flow:
Operations to Repair Arteries

Early failures attempting to repair blood vessels emphasized the importance of the scientific environment in the late nineteenth century to achieving operative success. While a British surgeon known only as Mr. Hallowell famously repaired a brachial artery with a pin in 1759, this one-off achievement hardly heralded systemic change, and future efforts floundered.[52] Conradus Asman's series of failures in animal experiments during the 1770s proved especially discouraging to subsequent investigators.[53] But, in the late nineteenth century, Alexander Jassinowsky of Dorpat (now Tartu, Estonia) initiated the field of arterial repair by demonstrating its feasibility.[54] He made incisions into the carotid arteries in the necks of dogs then sewed up the lacerations; twenty-two of his twenty-six animals not only lived but also maintained open vessels that permitted blood flow; previous attempts by Asman and others resulted in blood clots clogging the passage. Jassinowsky credited strict asepsis, curved needles, fine silk, and especially proper technique. Like Halsted's work, Jassinowsky prioritized the delicate handling of tissue and avoiding any unnecessary manipulation of the artery itself. Needles sharply penetrated the vessel wall at right angles. Sutures had to exert enough force to seal the hole but not unduly crimp or stricture the vessel. Wound closure could not be so tight as to compress the recently repaired artery yet had to provide secure, waterproof protection to the site. Individually all minor technical points, collectively they determined the difference between success and failure.

Following Jassinowsky's success, other surgeons like John B. Murphy began experimenting with arterial repair. Born to a poor farmer's family, Murphy trained as a doctor in Chicago before traveling to Germany for additional surgical education.[55] Remembered today for the eponymous sign indicating gallbladder inflammation, Murphy rose to national prominence in the late nineteenth century for his work on appendicitis, intestinal anastomosis, and lung-reducing surgery for tuberculosis—and for his treatment of casualties from the 1886 Haymarket Affair, which received widespread media coverage. His interest in vascular surgery stemmed from a colleague who accidentally severed a patient's carotid artery and was unable to repair it; the patient bled to death. Realizing his own inability to overcome such a complication, Murphy resolved to study the subject and began a series of animal trials that resulted in a landmark 1897 paper.[56]

Attempting to mimic his colleague's error, Murphy intentionally lacerated the arteries of animals and sewed them closed. Murphy successfully repaired six of fourteen injuries, a markedly lower percentage than Jassinowsky. Yet, set against the precedent of Asman's failures, even a 43 percent success rate inspired contemporaries. Like his Dorpatian colleague, Murphy also credited asepsis and perfect technique.[57] Following Murphy's article, a number of other surgeons published confirmatory findings.[58] Case reports of surgeons successfully attempting these operations on humans also began to appear.[59] Notably, the literature focused on the practical results obtained in the operating room; expounding theories about which technique might work best without proving it on animals or people was meaningless in the field of surgery. After a brief description of any new technical variations, authors spent the majority of their articles recounting in detail the cases they performed, including the health of the patient/animal, diagnosis (or intentional creation) of vascular pathology, indications for surgery, a step-by-step narration of the procedure, any complications, postoperative course, and autopsy results. Encompassing only the most basic statistical analysis and almost never including control subjects (as was standard for the era), these articles, and thus the profession, relied on descriptive case series to prove the efficacy and utility of surgeries.

Thrombosis—or blood clots at the repair site—caused the majority of failures for Asman, Murphy, and other doctors. Recognition of this problem and understanding its etiology resulted from more than a century of physiology research, as a localist and eventually histological approach overtook humoral and neo-humoral explanations for disease in the nineteenth century. The influence of surgeons like Xavier Bichat and Francois Magendie on early physiological experimentation both enabled and reinforced this local orientation.[60] Bichat's identification of tissue as the fundamental morphological structure held particular value as scientists could extrapolate discoveries on one particular area throughout the human body. At the same time, investigations into the cause and effect of inflammation revealed the centrality of white blood cells.[61] This microscopic orientation synced with increasing attention on histology, driven partly by Rudolf Virchow's foundational work in cellular pathology.[62] Virchow's early studies focused on this problem of thrombosis (blood clots), revealing how inflammation initiated and exacerbated the process.

Subsequent research determined the importance of maintaining the integrity of the intima (the innermost lining of a blood vessel) to obviate intravascular inflammation and thus prevent thrombosis.[63] This finding prompted a debate among surgeons about whether they should penetrate the intima with their sutures. Sewing through the intima was easier to do, particularly on smaller arteries, and enabled more secure connections between vessels, but it did disrupt this inner tissue layer and leave a foreign body (the suture material) in the lumen of the artery as a nidus for clot formation. Therefore, surgeons like Jassinowsky, Murphy, and many early pioneers studiously avoided disrupting the intima while sewing. Other surgeons recognized the technical difficulties inherent in this strategy and developed alternatives. George Dorrance only sewed everted ends while George Brewer eschewed sutures altogether and relied on plaster mini-casts (figures 1.2 and 1.3).[64] The details of their efforts are less meaningful than highlighting how physicians were actively researching this problem and designing creative surgical solutions to a contemporary technical dilemma. While none of these methods saw widespread clinical use, they reflect the ongoing, sputtering efforts of surgeons to repair arteries reliably, efficaciously, and consistently.

The work of Jassinowsky, Murphy, and Brewer focused on arterial trauma and did not address the most common natural arterial pathology of the era: aneurysms. More than a simple hole, aneurysms were expansive dilations of arteries that alternatively threatened to burst and cause a patient to bleed to death or send clots coursing downstream to starve tissue of oxygen and necessary nutrients. Diagnosed by physical exam in the nineteenth century, aneurysms had usually grown quite large by the time they attracted medical attention. Their involved, complex anatomy required the development of sophisticated repair techniques before the field could move beyond Hunterian ligation. Rudolph Matas invented that surgery. A contemporary, friend, and later patient of Halsted, Matas grew up in Louisiana and attended medical school at Tulane, where he had early exposure to vascular ligations.[65] He trained in the United States and Europe, returned to New Orleans, and eventually rose to chair the Department of Surgery at Tulane. His accomplishments spanned the breadth of surgery, including the use of intravenous saline for resuscitation, spinal anesthesia, and positive pressure ventilation. His colleagues elected him to represent America at the 1913 International Medical Congress. He was best known for his treatment of aneurysms through an innovative operation and is regarded as the father of vascular surgery in the United States.[66]

In March 1888, Matas saw Charles Harris, a twenty-six-year-old African American, at Charity Hospital in New Orleans.[67] A hunting buddy had accidentally shot Harris two weeks earlier. He sought medical attention not for the gunshot wound but for a newly developed swelling on his left arm that throbbed and continued to grow; Matas quickly diagnosed a traumatic aneurysm and initially tried to treat it nonoperatively with compression. When

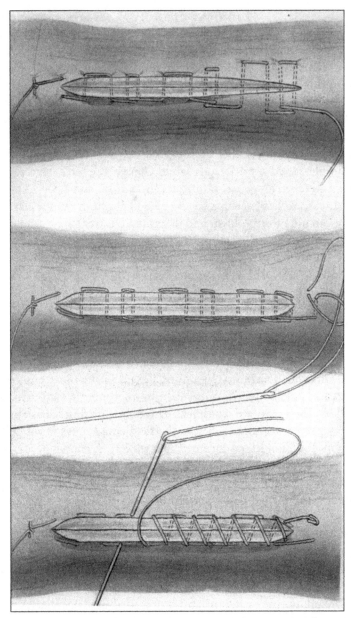

Figure 1.2. Dorrance's everted suture technique. *Top*: The suture pinching up or everting the section of artery to be repaired. Everting the edges meant no foreign bodies or intimal disruption remained in contact with the blood. *Middle*: The completion of the mattress suture line with the knot at the end tied but not tightened. *Bottom*: A line of whip stitches overtop and reinforcing the mattress sutures. Dorrance, "An Experimental Study of Suture of Arteries with a Description of a New Suture."

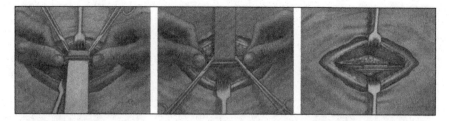

Figure 1.3. Brewer's non-suture method of vessel repair. *Left and center:* The surgeon exposes the artery and uses clamps to place the rectangular plaster bandage underneath it, which is then wrapped around the vessel like toilet paper around its cardboard insert. *Right:* The hole is now covered without any intimal disruption. Brewer, "Some Experiments with a New Method of Closing Wounds of the Larger Arteries."

this attempt failed, Matas performed a standard Hunterian proximal ligation. In the operating room, the aneurysm continued to pulsate and expand; distal ligation also failed. Matas then proceeded to open the aneurysm sac in the style of Antyllus and found a posterior branch vessel feeding the aneurysm, which he sutured closed. "As I look at this open sac," he observed,

> it seems to me there is no great distinction, surgically, between what we have here and the several intestinal orifices Dr. Michinard and I have been suturing all this past winter. . . . In one case we have had to appose serosa to serosa . . . in this instance the inner arterial lining, the intima. . . . [S]o if we bring the lips of these orifices together, we can expect the surfaces to unite in precisely the way as the coats of the bowel unite when sutured. If they unite, there can be no further flow of blood into the tumor.[68]

Relying on his experiences in intestinal surgery, he tacked the edges of the sac down into itself, thus completing the first endoaneurysmorrhaphy (figure 1.4). Matas both cured his patient and developed an entirely new operation for treating arterial aneurysms.

Endoaneurysmorrhaphy—dubbed the Matas operation—spread around the world in the early twentieth century. Matas's 1888 initial publication in the relatively obscure journal *Medical News* received little attention, but his subsequent 1903 article in the leading *Annals of Surgery* brought it to the fore, showing the imperative of both being the first and announcing your discovery in a prominent venue.[69] He carefully delineated the steps of the procedure, including diagrams like those in figure 1.4 to guide other surgeons. The founder of the Cleveland Clinic, George Crile, wrote Matas of his success applying it to a saccular aneurysm, after which the patient kept

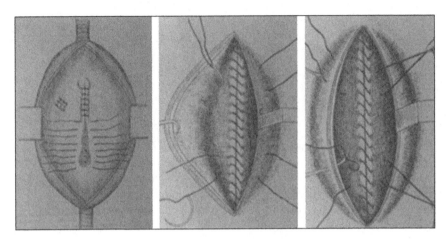

Figure 1.4. Matas operation. *Left*: Normal artery is visible on top and bottom, represented by the short, thin rectangles. The large oval represents the aneurysm sac filleted open. Matas has already sewn closed an opening to a branch artery (see the stitches at 10 o'clock) and is in the process of stitching closed the main connection between the artery and the aneurysm sac (the row of sutures descending down the center of the sac). *Center and right*: Matas is sewing the walls of the aneurysm sac to each other to close the cavity and reinforce the repair. Matas, "An Operation for the Radical Cure of Aneurism Based upon Arteriorrhaphy."

his leg.[70] John Murphy penned, "My method for the management of aneurism . . . is not so good as the endoaneurismorrhaphy of Matas—and that is why I have now abandoned it altogether and use the Matas method as routine. Endoaneurismorrhaphy has come to stay."[71] Shortly after Matas's publication on arterial aneurysms, Warren Stone Bickham expanded its use to arteriovenous fistulae in what became known as the Matas-Bickham operation.[72] That procedure remained the standard of care through World War II.[73] Remarkably, these accolades accrued after Matas had performed exactly two of his eponymous operations, the first of which was an emergent, ad hoc, improvised effort to keep his patient from bleeding to death. Some of these encomia resulted from Matas's existing professional reputation as a leader in the field, but it also reflected a contemporary acceptance of new surgeries after only a few demonstrated successes.

Despite the global fame and distribution of the Matas operation, comparatively few surgeons used it in practice. Between 1903 and 1939, surgeons at the Mayo Clinic performed 14 Matas operations for aneurysms, but they resorted to standard ligation in 123 cases.[74] Rudolph Matas scoured the surgical literature for accounts of its use and by 1916 had identified 354 endoaneurysmorrhaphies.[75] While an impressive and international distribution, 354 over thirteen years hardly represented a commonly practiced procedure. The relative scarcity of aneurysms compared to other surgical diseases, such as appendicitis, provides one explanation for the low number, but the technical inability of most early twentieth-century physicians to perform the procedure successfully had a far greater impact on its infrequency. Why, then, did the profession of surgery value and praise an intervention that benefitted so few patients? The prestige of the commentators offers a partial answer, as men like Crile and Murphy were colleagues of Matas and, as uncommonly well-trained practitioners, had little difficulty replicating his results. More generally, the surgical community championed rare, complex operations such as the endoaneurysmorrhaphy for their potential in curing disease. Often ignoring immediate epidemiological benefit (or lack thereof), surgical praise reflected the faith in the ability of operations to solve medical problems, if not now, then in the future.

Neither the Matas operation nor early versions of arterial repair nor Hunterian ligation could treat the most feared aneurysms: those of the aorta. The aorta is the largest blood vessel in the body, more than an inch in diameter and running from the heart to the navel, where it splits into two arteries that supply each leg. A ruptured aortic aneurysm meant near-instant death for the patient. This lethality attracted medical attention, particularly after the seventeenth century, when physicians like Giovanni Lancisi recognized the condition was a complication of omnipresent syphilis.[76] Surgeons attempted ligation, but it almost always killed the patient.[77] Seeking alternatives, they tried a wide variety of interventions from diet and bed rest to placing compressible metal bands around the artery to filling the aneurysm with metal wire and electrocuting the coils.[78] While none proved successful, their diversity and continued development underscore contemporary confidence in surgery to cure patients. Ultimately, the solution to aortic aneurysms required a new technique: arterial anastomosis.

Arterial Anastomosis

Anastomosis—reconnecting two ends of a divided artery—marked the next major technical development in vascular surgery. It held enormous promise. Arteries severed by knives or bullets could be repaired and aneurysms completely resected with normal blood flow restored. Surgeons dreamed of using anastomosis to reattach amputated limbs and to transplant organs. Yet the technical difficulties of anastomosis tempered these aspirations. Sewing closed a slit in an artery was challenging in its own right and regularly met with failure, but the difficulty of that procedure paled in comparison to anastomosis. Whereas the muscular walls of injured arteries often came together naturally to facilitate suturing, when divided, these same muscles pulled the ends apart, leaving a yawning gap to bridge. For an effective junction of two vessels, surgeons must permanently affix one end of a small, floppy tube to the other end in a manner that did not leak, that kept the passage open for blood to flow, and that did not cause blood clots. (Think of sewing two cooked penne noodles together while keeping the center channel open.) Its execution pushed the limits of surgery in the late nineteenth and early twentieth century.

Much as Jassinowsky had provided proof of concept for suture repair of vessels, Russian army surgeon Nicolai Vladomirovich Eck demonstrated the feasibility of vessel anastomosis. Working with dogs in 1877, Eck performed a side-to-side anastomosis of the vena cava, the largest vein in the body, which returns blood to the heart, and the portal vein, which carries blood from the intestines to the liver. In so doing, he created the world's first portocaval shunt, since dubbed the Eck fistula.[79] The procedure, well known in the contemporary literature, successfully relieved portal hypertension, although it was not used in humans for another sixty-eight years because of challenges in clinical implementation.[80] Most (seven of eight) of the animals died within days from peritonitis or intestinal strangulation (the eighth ran away), but on autopsy their vascular connections were open—the surgery had succeeded. Eck's results, along with the exciting reports of vessel repair discussed above, prompted a flurry of experimental work on anastomosis.

Eck, and Jassinowsky before him, established proof of concept by relying on dogs; neither applied their innovative technique to humans. This dependence on animals as experimental models was a universal method not just for vascular operations but for surgery generally. In contrast, animals had a less prominent role in other fields of medicine. While scientists used them extensively in basic physiology experiments, animals had a more limited role when investigating treatments. Certainly psychoanalysis was nigh impossible to practice on dogs, but even pharmaceutical treatment of medical diseases is difficult to model zoologically, as evident by the millions of mice society continues to cure of cancer without human benefit. In contrast, lacerations in a dog's carotid artery look a lot like lacerations in a person's carotid artery, and doctors assumed what fixed one would work equally well on the other. This homology, combined with the aforementioned emphasis on practically demonstrating new ideas, rendered vivisection crucial to the process of surgical innovation.

The technical difficulties involved in sewing two ends of an artery together—in dogs or humans—led surgeons to consider alternative methods, particularly the use of prosthetic bridges. These prostheses would unite a divided vessel but demanded far less skill and precision since they required only a few stitches to secure them. In 1894, Robert Abbe published his method of using glass tubes to connect two arterial ends (figure 1.5).[81] Recording his success on a cat's aorta, Abbe became the first surgeon to restore continuity to an interrupted artery. However, he pessimistically reflected on the future of the procedure: "I do not expect that this version of surgical possibilities will be realized soon, nor do I think enough has been proved to warrant much hope."[82] Correct in predicting the delayed clinical application of vascular prostheses, Abbe did not anticipate the wave of experimental attempts that followed. Surgeons substituted various materials for Abbe's glass, including ivory, rubber, and, in one case, hollow pigeon bones.[83] Erwin Payr's magnesium rings proved most popular and enduring, though scarcely more successful than previous inventions.[84]

The high rate of failures with prosthetic material prompted other surgeons to try to sew arteries directly to one another. J. B. Murphy, the Chicago surgeon discussed above for his work on repairing arteries, performed the first successful arterial anastomosis in humans.[85] H.V. was a twenty-nine-year-old Italian peddler shot in the thigh in September 1896. When Murphy explored the wound in the operating room, he found the bullet had penetrated through the femoral artery, nearly severing it. Recognizing the impossibility of a simple stitch repair, Murphy removed the damaged segment then restored continuity by inserting one end into the other in what he called the invagination method (figure 1.6). H.V. kept his leg with a fully functioning artery. Murphy's work on this operation reflects the crossover between repairing and anastomosing arteries; many surgeons experimented with both techniques. A major advance in arterial surgery, invagination saw rapid and global application, with Djeineil Pacha in Moscow first repeating it the same year as Murphy's landmark publication.[86] Successful case reports relying on Murphy's invagination technique peppered the medical literature for the next decade.[87]

While Murphy studiously kept his sutures out of the intima, his invagination method violated the newly discovered tenet of intima-to-intima contact. The prioritization of intimal apposition stemmed from contemporaneous work on intestinal anastomosis. Many of the surgeons mentioned, including Halsted, Matas, Murphy, and Abbe, pioneered operations in both fields, as evident from Matas's thought process when devising his endoaneurysmorrhaphy. For intestines, they noted the importance of bringing the serosal

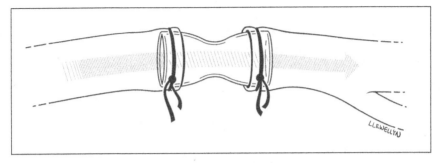

Figure 1.5. Abbe's glass prosthesis bridge. Note the two simple sutures holding the hourglass prosthesis in place. Methods of securing bridging materials varied slightly but remained consistently simpler than suture anastomosis of Eck and others. Figure rendered by Megan Llewellyn, MSMI.

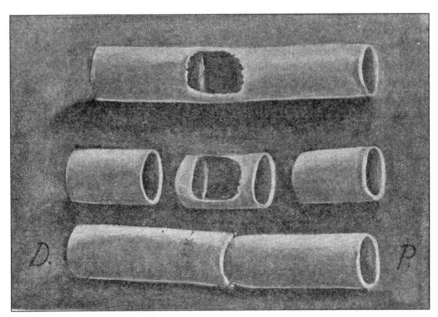

Figure 1.6. Steps of Murphy's operation. *Top*: Artery with a bullet hole in the center, penetrating both the front and back walls of the vessel. *Middle*: Murphy has cut the artery both in front and behind the damaged section to remove it en bloc. *Bottom*: Murphy has inserted one end into the other to recreate continuity. The sutures holding the two segments together did not penetrate the intima of the interior segment. Murphy, "Resection of Arteries and Veins Injured in Continuity."

layer of each end into contact to achieve a watertight seal; surgeons came to understand the intima analogously. Their recognition partly stemmed from gross anatomical observations but also resulted from an increased appreciation of histological homogeneity among tissue types. In his seminal 1906 textbook *Surgery: Its Practices and Principles*, W. W. Keen intoned, "The principle of 'intima to intima' signifies just as much in the plastic surgery of the blood vessels as that of 'serosa to serosa' to the abdominal surgeon."[88] This association highlights the coevolution of intestinal and vascular surgery, with the concurrent and codependent development illustrating the rapid and broad changes to the field in the early twentieth century.

With neither prostheses nor invagination providing the desired intimal connections, surgeons began exploring methods to sew the ends of arteries directly to one another. The concomitant demand to keep suture out of the intima greatly complicated this task and led to creative solutions. Most famously, Mathieu Jaboulay and his intern Eugène Briau at the Hotel-Dieu in Paris invented a U-stitch that everted the anastomosis; dozens of one-off variations appeared in the literature, rarely repeated and even more rarely attempted on humans.[89] Again, these efforts reflect active, international, ongoing experimentation by the surgical profession to solve the problem of arterial disease. In 1899, Julius Dörfler tried puncturing the intima—and to his own surprise, met great success.[90] Using small, curved, cambric needles and silk suture, he successfully anastomosed eleven of twelve dog arteries without any complicating blood clots. As additional investigators pursued vascular research, they slowly accepted and adopted Dörfler's techniques, which reached their apogee through the work of Alexis Carrel and Charles Guthrie.[91]

Alexis Carrel and Charles Guthrie's Triangulation Technique and the Origins of Modern Vessel Repair

Alexis Carrel and Charles Guthrie established the modern method to repair and anastomose arteries. Building off research from the nineteenth century, Carrel and Guthrie perfected, advanced, and disseminated their technique far beyond their predecessors' efforts. More importantly, they demonstrated its practical possibilities, both for vascular surgery per se as well as for blood transfusions and the then-flourishing investigative field of organ transplantation. Never one to shy from publicity, Carrel emerged as a leader in these disciplines, a position both affirmed and promoted by his receipt of the 1912 Nobel Prize in Medicine.

Born on 28 June 1873 in Sainte-Foy-les Lyons, Alexis Carrel was raised by his mother after the 1878 death of his father, a successful textile merchant. He earned both his bachelor's degree in science and his medical doctorate from the University of Lyons, where he worked with the aforementioned surgeon Jaboulay. While he attended medical school, an anarchist stabbed the popular president of France, Marie Francois Sadi Carnot, on 24 June 1894. The wound did not instantly kill President Carnot, but it did sever the portal vein. No doctor caring for the president had the ability to repair a torn blood vessel, and Carnot bled to death. Carrel, shocked by the sense-less death, refused to accept that such a "simple" operation as sewing blood vessels back together proved impossible, inspiring him to pursue a career in vascular surgery.[92]

Carrel initially continued his studies in France, but he immigrated to North America after failing to gain promotion (twice), which he blamed on faculty opposition to his belief in a supernatural cure for a patient with peritoneal tuberculosis at the famous healing shrine of Lourdes.[93] This dis-agreement spawned lifelong animosity between Carrel and the French medi-cal establishment. In 1904, he arrived in Canada where he found no open jobs but did meet Chicago surgeon Carl Beck, who became his academic mentor in the New World.[94] Carrel worked with Beck—even living in his house—for more than a year, developing novel operations like the Beck-Jianu gastrostomy.[95] Beck eventually led Carrel to join the physiology lab of Charles Guthrie. The pair made a powerful research team: in fewer than two years, they published twenty-one papers relating to vascular surgery.[96] Their research changed the field forever.

Charles Claude Guthrie received his MD in 1901 from the University of Missouri School of Medicine, where he subsequently worked as a fellow in pharmacology and physiology. In 1903, he moved to the University of Chi-cago lab of George Stewart, meeting Carrel three years later.[97] Despite the fact that Carrel and Guthrie made their discoveries jointly and coauthored all of their early papers, Carrel received the majority of the credit. His fame came from deliberate self-promotion, and, as an immigrant Frenchman with opinionated views he never hesitated to express, Carrel fit easily into the role of a media darling.[98] Moreover, Carrel was the doer, the surgeon, the person actually connecting vessels. Guthrie's scientific training and physiological background provided the essential foundation for Carrel's success, but think-ers and theorizers, with their intangible contributions, rarely attract adula-tion like the person performing the dramatic action. This tendency further buttressed the authority of surgeons.

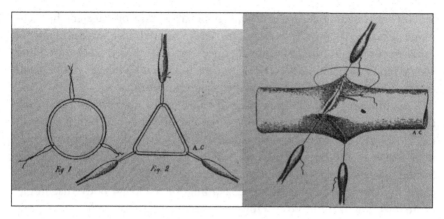

Figure 1.7. Carrel's original triangulation technique. *Left*: Carrel has placed three sutures at equal distance in the wall of the artery. Careful inspection reveals that he specifically avoids puncturing the innermost layer of the vessel wall. An assistant places these sutures on tension, transforming the circle into a triangle. *Right*: Carrel and his assistant have brought the now triangular ends of two arteries together and are anastomosing them with a simple whip stitch, using a manually threaded straight needle. Carrel, "La technique opératoire."

The pair began their investigations by expanding on a French paper Carrel published in 1902 that advocated a novel method of anastomosis via a unique triangulation technique.[99] As seen in figure 1.7, Carrel proposed inserting three equidistant guy sutures into each end of the vessel. With outward traction applied to these sutures, the round vessel becomes a triangle (hence triangulation). The operator would line up the edges of the triangle, suturing them together with a simple over-and-over stitch. The sides of the triangles were straight lines, markedly easier than trying to sew in a circle, particularly with the straight needles common at the time. The guy sutures simultaneously worked to evert the edges of blood vessels, permitting the intima-intima connection deemed essential while keeping suture material outside the lumen.

While innovative, Carrel failed to achieve consistent success before teaming up with Guthrie.[100] Technical failure or blood clots frequently complicated his early efforts. Concern over clotting initially prompted Carrel to avoid the intima, but in 1905 he and Guthrie decided to try puncturing this inner layer. They achieved superior outcomes with surprisingly little thrombosis. While Dörfler had previously demonstrated the efficacy of this maneuver—a priority that Carrel and Guthrie admitted ignorance of but recognized in subsequent articles—it was the Chicago pair who popularized and propagated the technique. Driving the needle through the entire arterial wall was substantially easier than trying to thread it into the media; it also allowed work on smaller vessels and created a more secure connection. Carrel and Guthrie's publications ended the debate over whether to sew through the intima.

They also emphasized the salience of using small, curved needles and silk thread. Straight needles, standard for the era, presented technical difficulties in sewing the connection, particularly for vessels deep in the body or of a smaller diameter; needles shaped like a C ameliorated these challenges. Suture material was widely debated at the time. Many contemporaries advocated for catgut because it dissolves, eliminating a foreign body that might cause infection or thrombosis. However, this dissolvability made connections tenuous and risked the ends coming apart. Carrel and Guthrie (and Dörfler as well) insisted on using silk sutures, which allowed for a thinner thread, greater strength, permanent presence, and more precise stitches to effect the intima-intima connection. Like Jassinowsky and Eck, they conducted their experiments and reached these conclusions through animal vivisection, not performing a single case on humans.

These three major contributions—utilizing silk thread with curved needles, including the intima in the suture, and employing the triangulation technique—revolutionized the potential for vascular surgery. The combination maintained a normal vessel caliber, avoided exposed intima, eliminated foreign bodies like magnesium rings, and greatly simplified the sewing. The fundamentals of the method Carrel and Guthrie established remain in use today. From a technical perspective, vascular surgery had arrived. Actual operations relying on triangulation, however, remained exquisitely rare, with relatively few patients who needed the procedure and even fewer surgeons who could perform it competently.

Despite the total reliance on animals and the infrequency of clinical application, the advance afforded by triangulation attracted the attention of contemporaries. "I told Dr. Halsted of your work yesterday," wrote the famous neurosurgeon Harvey Cushing to Carrel in 1905, "and he was very much excited over your superlatively good results."[101] Letters poured in from surgical greats like J. M. T. Finney at Johns Hopkins, Joseph Bloodgood in New York, Theodor Kocher (who received the first Nobel Prize in surgery) in Switzerland, and many others.[102] Franklin Martin wrote Carrel requesting an article for his increasingly prestigious journal *Surgery, Gynecology, and Obstetrics*.[103] George Crile tried to recruit Carrel to his Cleveland Clinic, and Cushing offered him a place in his lab at Johns Hopkins.[104] It was not just academic surgeons who had an interest: Israel Brown, practicing in

Norfolk, Virginia, asked Carrel for more details on his operation, after begging forgiveness for trespassing on his time.[105] Cushing describes the throng of people pressing to see Carrel operate at the 1905 Society of Clinical Surgery meeting.[106] Clearly, attendees had heard of the triangulation method through articles but either doubted the written word or found that prose and illustrations failed to communicate the new technique effectively. Those who missed the conference demonstration often visited Carrel's lab. Halsted made the trip in February 1907, commenting "how greatly I enjoyed the very beautiful demonstrations. It was not simply the fact that arterial suture can be accomplished in this way that impressed me but the really exquisite manner in which it was accomplished."[107] His letter emphasizes not only the technical details but also the importance of in-person observation for the communication of surgical principles.

In 1912, the Nobel Committee feted Carrel with the highest honor in science, the Nobel Prize in Physiology or Medicine, for "his work on suturing vessels and transplanting organs."[108] At thirty-nine years old, he was the youngest recipient to date. Although Carrel always considered himself a Frenchman, the United States celebrated him as the first American ever to receive this award, and encomia poured in from all corners. The event affirmed the rise of American science for the medical community.[109]

While the rest of the world viewed successful vessel anastomosis as an accomplishment in its own right, both Carrel and Guthrie saw it as a means to greater medical ends, notably organ transplantation. Carrel in particular envisioned banks of spare organs that surgeons could implant into bodies as needed.[110] Though the notion of replacing diseased or disfigured tissue has existed since antiquity, the idea of solid organ transplant emerged under a very specific set of social, medical, and surgical conditions in the late nineteenth century.[111]

Implanted organs require blood to survive. Early attempts to connect them to the host's vasculature relied on Payr's magnesium rings or Murphy's invagination method and repeatedly failed.[112] The anastomosis technique developed by Carrel and Guthrie enabled the transplantation of organs. By October 1905, just a few months into their collaboration, the two published in *Science* their transplantation of a dog's kidney from its usual retroperitoneal location into its neck. They reported that the kidney functioned normally, producing urine and remaining viable.[113] This was the second report of a successful kidney transplant in history; Emerich Ullmann in Austria published the first in 1902.[114]

Carrel and Guthrie expanded their efforts to other organs. They quickly followed their initial article on kidneys with others describing thyroid and ovarian transplants.[115] Operations soon became more elaborate, with Carrel and Guthrie amputating a thigh, then reattaching it in 1906.[116] Head transplants on dogs, while attempted, failed almost immediately.[117] Seizing the inspiration of the Nobel Committee's charge and Carrel's laboratory accomplishments, other investigators carried forward these efforts and even extended them (unsuccessfully) in humans, raising the visibility of arterial repair and its therapeutic potential to the broader public.[118]

Their struggles exposed the challenges of trying to transplant tissue from one animal to another (allografts). Carrel and Guthrie's experiments functioned splendidly in autografts, when they transplanted the same animal's organ from one location to another, but never succeeded when they tried to exchange organs between different animals. Initially concerned that inadequate surgical technique caused their failures, they practiced the operation on autotransplants until consistently achieving success, with organs functioning for years after the operation. They could never duplicate these results in allografts and ultimately concluded some other biological factor (ultimately identified as immune rejection) impeded their efforts.[119] "From a surgical point of view, the problem of grafting is solved," declared Carrel in an interview. "Whether it ever will be viewed from the angle of compatible organs, I cannot tell. Perhaps someday—perhaps never."[120] As Carrel had become the face of organ transplant who had achieved better results than any other surgeon had with autografts, his abandonment of allografts equated to a discipline-wide admission of failure and ultimately shifted surgery away from organ transplantation by 1915.[121] Yet, when it returned after World War II, innovators relied on the very methods and techniques Carrel and Guthrie had pioneered decades earlier.

The notion of transplanting organs intrigued lay society. The popularity of H. G. Wells's contemporary novel *The Island of Dr. Moreau* (1896) and references to Mary Shelley's *Frankenstein* (1818) exposed societal fears of the potential implications of surgically trading body parts.[122] But, whereas these novels portrayed the dark side of science, most of the early twentieth century press lauded surgeons and their accomplishments. Carrel and his organ transplantation in particular were met with public adulation.[123] Dubbed the "Wizard Surgeon" in one newspaper article, accounts abounded on his ability to replace organs and speculated on the possibilities and consequences of these operations when extended to humans, which the press assumed was just a matter of time.[124] Attention exploded after Carrel won the Nobel Prize in 1912.[125]

Ordinary Americans clearly knew all about Carrel and his experiments, as evident from the myriad letters beseeching him to try organ transplantation on their senders.[126] "Can you replace testicles that have been removed for over thirty years[?] You can imagine how anxious a person would be to have it done," implored Zachariah Light, who included a postscript inquiring about the fee.[127] H. R. Polite, an engineer who lost his right hand in an explosion, asked about the possibility of receiving a new one—one of more than two hundred inquiries for an extremity transplant.[128] Indicating magazine articles as her source for information, Courtney C. McIntrick appealed to Carrel to replace the ovaries a surgeon had extirpated years earlier with new ones from a young, refined, educated, white woman. "You have to start your experiments upon humans eventually," McIntrick noted, "so why not me—and now?" she asked, expressing her willingness to die if necessary.[129] But by the time these and other letters arrived, Carrel had already abandoned organ transplant for new pursuits.[130]

Carrel and Guthrie separated in 1906 as they pursued different professional opportunities and each shifted his research away from vascular surgery. Guthrie took a position as chair of the Physiology Department at Washington University for a few years before transferring to the University of Pittsburgh, where he stayed for the remainder of his career.[131] Simon Flexner recruited Carrel to work at the Rockefeller Institute in New York, where he headed the Experimental Surgery Lab until a conflict of egos and scientific agendas with the new director led to his retirement in 1939.[132] While at the Rockefeller, Carrel continued his endeavors on tissue preservation and transplantation, developing some of the very first tissue banks and pioneering the new science of tissue culture.[133]

Carrel continued to glow in the media spotlight for the remainder of his career. Serving in the French army during World War I, he cocreated the Carrel-Dakin system of wound irrigation that dramatically reduced the incidence of infection among Allied wounded. After the war, he returned to New York and paired with aviation legend Charles Lindbergh to develop a perfusion pump to keep organs alive outside the body, a partnership that landed the two of them on the cover of *Time* magazine, again.[134] He also wrote the popular religio-scientific book *Man, the Unknown*, which became the second-best-selling book of 1936.[135] This work exposes some of Carrel's odious, unabashed support of eugenics, anti-Semitism, racism, and sexism.[136] Returning to his homeland of France during World War II, Carrel died there an outcast accused of Nazi collaboration on 5 November 1945, just months after the Allies had liberated Paris.

Effects of Carrel and Guthrie's Work:
Vascular Surgery from 1905 until World War I

In 1913, Bertram Bernheim of Johns Hopkins published the first textbook on vascular surgery. Bernheim, who studied with Carrel, promoted triangulation.[137] Highlighting the preeminence of technique, he recommended that operators remove their (recently invented) gloves to maximize dexterity when performing the anastomosis, even at the cost of sterility. Bernheim's text, along with dozens of articles in journals, proved the superiority of this operation over Murphy's invagination or any of the prosthetic devices, establishing Carrel and Guthrie's method as the definitive mode of vascular surgery.[138] Just two years following Bernheim's textbook, J. Shelton Horsley in Virginia published another, and, in Germany, Ernst Jeger defended his doctoral dissertation on vascular surgery, which he dedicated to Alexis Carrel.[139] The percolation of the subject into Jeger's dissertation as well as American medical student theses reflects its dissemination into medical schools around the world.[140]

Carrel and Guthrie's method for vessel anastomosis also enabled the new practice of blood transfusion. After recognizing the importance of blood, physicians had to figure out how to infuse it.[141] Until the advent of sodium citrate in 1915 permitted the storage of blood without clotting, all transfusions required the donor and recipients to be physically joined by their blood vessels (plastic tubing to facilitate such a connection was also unavailable).[142] Doctors struggled to make this connection. In 1906, renowned Ohio surgeon George Crile adopted Carrel's technique of vessel anastomosis for blood transfusion. Crile had trained in Ohio and New York City and traveled to Germany for experience with modern surgical research. In the late nineteenth century, his pioneering explorations on patients going into shock associated the pathology with low blood pressures, leading him to argue that administering fluid into the patient intravenously could ameliorate the condition. These investigations made shock a relevant, treatable, and surgical condition, with Crile arguing for blood transfusion as the cure. Crile eventually parlayed his success into founding the Cleveland Clinic after World War I.[143]

He described his first clinical experience with blood transfusion in 1906: a twenty-three-year-old patient from whom Crile had surgically removed four kidney stones continued to bleed after the operation, developing life-threatening shock. Paying no attention to recently discovered blood groups, Crile used the triangulation technique and anastomosed the radial artery from the patient's brother to the patient's basilic vein, allowing blood to flow into the dying man and reviving him. "The transformation in these cases," wrote Crile, "has been unequaled in my surgical experience, except in relief from asphyxia by intubation."[144] His extensive experimental and clinical experience led to him writing the seminal textbook in the field, crediting Carrel and his technique of anastomosis in the preface for making modern blood transfusion possible.[145] Other academic surgeons rapidly adopted the practice.[146] "Of all the acquisitions that have come to advance the progress of vascular surgery," intoned Crile's contemporary Rudolph Matas at a meeting for the American Medical Association, "*transfusions* . . . is by far the most valuable and significant in its lifesaving potentialities."[147]

Vein grafts were the apotheosis of vascular surgery at this time. In this procedure, a surgeon repairs a gap in an artery by sewing a piece of vein to each end of the severed vessel to bridge the chasm. Mechanistically, vein grafts paralleled Abbe's glass tubes and other prosthetics previously tried, with several differences. Patient veins were native tissue, thus not subject to rejection. They featured a natural endothelial lining that, like all blood vessels, resisted coagulation. While surgeons previously suggested prostheses for their ease of implantation, venous grafts required two technically demanding anastomoses to function, making it one of the most advanced surgeries of the era. Carrel had performed this operation experimentally on animals. Spanish surgeon José Goyanes recorded the first case in humans in 1906, but the operation achieved worldwide fame in the hands of Erich Lexer in 1907. Having trained in Berlin under Ernst von Bergmann, Lexer was practicing as a professor and surgeon in Königsberg when a sixty-nine-year-old male presented to his clinic suffering from an aneurysm in his axillary artery, under his arm.[148] When Lexer removed the aneurysm, an eight-centimeter divide yawned, too large to allow a primary end-to-end anastomosis. Unaware of Goyanes's earlier work, Lexer harvested the patient's saphenous vein from his leg and used it to repair the defect.[149] The patient died several days later from alcohol withdrawal, but the surgery was such a procedural success and held such great promise that Lexer dubbed it "the ideal operation," a name richly symbolic of the technical prowess required to complete it, the remarkable therapeutic potential it had for patients, and the esteem with which contemporaries regarded the intervention.

Lexer's publication demonstrated the clinical plausibility and efficacy of the operation to surgeons around the world. In 1913, Joseph Pringle, who learned vascular surgery from Carrel in New York before returning home to Glasgow, performed the first venous grafts in the United Kingdom when he repaired a popliteal and a brachial aneurysm (in two different patients)

using saphenous vein grafts and Carrel's technique.[150] Bernheim, the aforementioned textbook author, was the first American to use venous grafting.
Following an unsuccessful attempt in 1909, he tried again in 1915 when
a syphilis patient presented with a popliteal aneurysm.[151] Preoperatively he
noted the absence of collateral circulation, likely leading to amputation if
he ligated. Intraoperatively, he recognized dense adhesions between the popliteal artery and vein, making the Matas operation technically impossible.
Thus, for Bernheim, venous grafts were a method of last resort. Their efficacy in this patient prompted his enthusiasm for more regular utilization.

The method did see more extensive use in the Serbo-Turkish and Serbo-
Bulgarian Wars between 1912 and 1913.[152] Commanding a military hospital, Serbian surgeon Vojislac Soubbotitch prioritized attempts to repair
wounded blood vessels. Importantly, these operations occurred on aneurysms and pseudoaneurysms that developed days to weeks after the initial
injury, not on fresh wounds. Nonetheless, Soubbotitch repaired seventeen
partially torn vessels and recorded fifteen successful Carrel-style anastomoses,
fixing thirty-two out of seventy-seven total vascular wounds.[153] Significantly,
it was not just Soubbotitch performing these operations but rather a cadre of
sixteen different surgeons, indicating the ability to teach and spread the technique. While acknowledging its technical difficulty, Soubbotitch advocated
for the procedure. He recognized the value of this large case series and strove
to publicize it through articles in the medical literature and presentations at
international medical meetings.[154]

The use of Carrel's technique by Soubbotitch, Bernheim, Pringle, Lexer,
and Goyanes represented the global application of advanced vascular surgery,
but the ability to point to specific examples simultaneously demonstrated
the infrequency of these operations. Indeed, Bernheim lamented in his 1916
case report that only seven venous graft operations had been performed in
the world—"a rarity that is most discouraging to those who had hoped for
real practical developments in modern vascular surgery."[155] Despite broad
dissemination of Carrel's techniques and their promise through journals,
textbooks, and the popular media hype surrounding the Nobel Prize, the
vast majority of surgeons, including those in academia, continued to ligate
arteries just as Hunter had done 150 years previous.

Some surgeons outright opposed Carrel-style anastomosis, arguing that
it endangered the patient. In his discussion of Bernheim's paper, William
Halsted called the transplanted venous segment "a menace," arguing the
sutures could foster blood clots that propagated through and destroyed the
vascular system.[156] Rudolph Matas remained firmly convinced that both
end-to-end anastomosis and venous grafts quickly occluded and provided

little long-term benefit. "The alleged success of the 'ideal' operation," Matas noted, "is far more apparent than real."[157] Thus, two of the most famous surgeons of the day, perhaps partially blinded by their allegiance to their own innovative operations, initially rejected what came to form the foundation of modern vascular surgery. Less august surgeons rarely even attempted vascular anastomosis.

This skepticism about Carrel's technique and the more general reluctance to pursue arterial repair expose the crucial difference between the invention of a procedure and its implementation in practice. The conditions of the late nineteenth and early twentieth centuries created a milieu that encouraged dozens of surgeons to explore suturing arteries. Hoping to treat aneurysms and trauma with results superior to ligation, men like Jassinowsky, Murphy, Matas, and Carrel spent thousands of hours (and many hundreds of dogs) in their experimental laboratories pioneering new operations. Carrel in particular invented a successful procedure for which he received global acclaim built on its promise to unite vessels and transplant organs. He deserved these accolades, for his triangulation method was a creative, original, important discovery that endures as the technical foundation of vascular and transplant surgery today, more than a century later. But, at the cusp of World War I, it remained a well-known, lauded technique that hardly anyone actually used on patients. Most surgeons frankly lacked the skills to perform such an intricate operation; others deemed it unnecessary or too risky. Moreover, the relative rarity of vascular pathology denied them occasions to apply the procedure with any regularity. The millions of wounded soldiers in the First World War would soon provide ample opportunities to practice and potentially transform arterial repair from the ideal, textbook operation to one surgeons routinely implemented to preserve the arms and legs of suffering patients.

Chapter Two

An Ideal Rarely Practiced

Arterial Repair and Its Alternatives from World War I to World War II

The carnage of World War I initially provided hope that arterial repair might emerge from the shadows of the ivory tower and enter common practice. Battles resulted in thousands of patients in dire need of vascular surgery. Doctors deployed to the front lines aware of the possibilities of anastomosis. By 1917, military command strongly advocated for repair over ligation. The stalemate of trench warfare enabled the establishment of semipermanent hospitals, which facilitated complex interventions. Still, these operations remained exceptionally rare despite the efforts of a few pioneers. The same conditions that proved promising to the broad application of arterial repair simultaneously undercut its utilization, as millions of casualties overwhelmed meagerly trained medical providers desperately trying to stave off infection and save the lives of their patients, often at the cost of their limbs.

The practice of vascular surgery did not change significantly during World War I, but the results of this conflict stimulated a series of developments. First, recognizing that the practice of surgery had outpaced the competency of general practitioners, leaders of the American profession initiated coordinated efforts to reform, advance, and standardize surgical education into a universal, residency-based system. This process began to create a separate class of physicians who dedicated their professional careers to surgery.[1] Second, exciting new laboratory discoveries such as the blood-thinning drug heparin and the X-ray technique of arteriography promised to facilitate arterial repair and catalyze its postwar adoption. Lastly, a new procedure called sympathectomy came to the fore. Technically simpler than anastomosis, with outcomes reportedly superior to plain ligation, sympathectomy became the face of vascular surgery in the 1930s.

This chapter continues to explore the paradoxical non-adoption of a well-known surgery that almost everyone agreed produced better results for patients. If World War I demonstrated the power of environment to encourage or hinder the practice of surgery, then the years between that war and the next represented concerted social and scientific efforts to change those conditions and make them more amenable to the implementation of advanced operations generally and arterial repair specifically.

World War I: The Persistence of Ligation

The Serbo-Turkish and Serbo-Bulgarian Wars in which Vojislav Soubbotitch fought and repaired arteries foreshadowed World War I, a military and cultural clash that encompassed much of the world. Devastating new killing technologies tormented the battlefield. Aircraft bombed from the sky while submarines stalked the oceans. Great steel tanks rumbled across a no-man's-land crisscrossed by barbed wire and covered by rapid-firing machine guns. In the trenches themselves, soldiers faced fearsome scientific weaponry like flamethrowers and poison gasses.[2] Many new weapons demanded novel medical responses, like special protective gear for chemical warfare.[3] But the vast majority of soldiers were killed and wounded by metallic missiles penetrating their bodies—wounds amenable to standard surgical interventions, including arterial repair.

In an effort to address this epidemic of trauma, warring nations mobilized the intellectual, financial, and human resources of their countries to build a military medical infrastructure for the protection and care of their armies. Recruiting tens of thousands of physicians into uniform, medical departments grew colossally; over 50 percent of British and German doctors and over 22 percent of licensed American physicians joined the military in World War I.[4] Trying to accommodate the aftermath of battle brought thousands of ill-equipped doctors to manage casualties at the front. Most nations established short instructional courses on military medicine. Although helpful, several weeks in a classroom hardly produced experts. Thrown into the crucible, these physicians attempted to address the public health challenges inherent to trench warfare, flu pandemics, and shell shock in addition to caring for the physically maimed.[5]

Surgical care of the wounded advanced considerably throughout the war. Militaries developed evacuation chains to transport casualties to hospitals behind the fighting, although large battles consistently overwhelmed their capacity. Doctors recognized the need for early surgery close to the front lines and organized new units like casualty clearing stations (British), *ambulance chirurgical automobile* (French), and mobile hospitals (American).[6] The nature of combat surgery also changed. Physicians entered World War I relying on precepts learned in the Boer (1899–1902) and Russo-Japanese (1904–5) Wars, where the pristine veldts of South Africa and sterile steppes of Manchuria left wounds uninfected and supported a conservative philosophy of nonintervention.[7] This management strategy failed miserably in the manure-fertilized fields of France where, according to one military medical manual, "the earth teemed with micro-organisms."[8] Infection ran rampant in 1914 and 1915, with tetanus and gas gangrene afflicting 10 to 25 percent of the wounded, half of whom perished.[9]

Recognizing the impossibility of achieving an aseptic field in combat conditions (still a relatively new concept in 1914), surgeons reverted to Listerian antiseptic techniques through a variety of chemical agents.[10] Here again, Alexis Carrel proved central. Having returned to France to serve his home country in its time of peril, Carrel observed that wound infections were killing the majority of his patients. Existing antiseptics like carbolic acid proved too toxic for prolonged use while more mild solutions like hypertonic saline lacked the necessary potency to destroy germs.[11] Carrel worked with Rockefeller Institute chemist Henry Dakin to create a new agent strong enough to cleanse wounds but mild enough to preserve native tissue. Named Dakin's solution, it was essentially dilute bleach balanced to a physiological level of acidity; it remains in use today. Carrel subsequently developed a system of irrigating tubes to perfuse this new solution continuously throughout a soldiers' injuries.[12] Intellectually endorsed by a Nobel laureate, articles describing the treatment quickly proliferated in the medical literatures in France, England, and the United States, where surgical leaders from William Halsted to Basil Hughes strongly endorsed the therapy. Front-line practitioners quickly adopted it as the most effective means of preventing infection.[13] Some doctors came to question the efficacy of the Carrel-Dakin method over surgical management, but Carrel never intended for it to replace an operation.[14] Rather, it was supposed to follow and supplement excision of necrotic tissue and foreign objects. Carrel, and eventually most military physicians, recognized that the definitive answer to wound infection lay in surgery.

Debridement—or the operative extirpation of damaged sinew, necrotic tissue, and foreign bodies—emerged as the most effective treatment for war injuries by surgeons of every nationality. In removing the shell fragments, soiled clothing, and macerated body parts, physicians eliminated sources of contamination and surgically created a clean wound. While some practiced the technique as early as 1914, not until the spring of 1917 did surgeons accept the importance of routine debridement for preventing infections.[15] Refinement of anesthetic techniques and especially improved management of shock permitted surgical intervention on severely injured soldiers, which often involved substantial resections of tissue to ensure efficacy.[16] Soft tissue debridement combined with Carrel-Dakin irrigation significantly lowered infection rates and saved lives; Carrel-style arterial repairs presented a similar opportunity to preserve limbs.

Modern warfare and its advanced armaments increased the incidence of vascular trauma, an observation first noted in the Russo-Japanese War.[17] Rapid-firing machine guns, repeating rifles, and especially the proliferation of high-explosive cannon fire increased the multiplicity of injuries, raising the chances of striking a blood vessel.[18] Artillery, which caused between 5 and 10 percent of wounds in the American Civil and Franco-Prussian Wars, caused approximately 80 percent in World War I.[19] Exploding shells peppered soldiers' bodies with metal fragments.

The majority of survivable injuries struck the arms and legs. Of the 312,457 British casualties who survived to reach medical care in 1914 and 1915, 66 percent were hit in the extremities (34 percent in the upper extremities and 32 percent in the lower).[20] The American Office of the Surgeon General recorded 266,112 wounds among American soldiers in World War I, almost 50 percent of which hit the arms or legs.[21] Yet wounds to the extremities proved relatively nonlethal, killing 4 percent of Americans hit in the arms and 7 percent with leg injuries. This survivability provided surgeons an opportunity to operate and repair the damage.

Given the frequency of extremity injuries, recorded numbers of vascular wounds underrepresent their actual occurrence. No army required physicians to document injuries to blood vessels, nor did the European powers even hazard a guess at overall prevalence. Cumulative American data initially reported 351 arterial injuries in US soldiers, for a preposterously low reported incidence of 0.0002 percent (see table 2.1).[22] A few individual hospitals collected more precise statistics. The 5th Evacuation Hospital recorded 419 wounds in 215 soldiers, seven of which were injuries to the large vessels, or an incidence of 1.67 percent.[23] The 10th Evacuation Hospital reported a 1.1 percent incidence of vascular trauma.[24] A series of 280 general surgical operations at Mobile Hospital #6 revealed six (2.5 percent) vascular injuries.[25] Proportions of 1 to 2 percent, albeit in smaller series of men so grievously injured as to require evacuation, align closely with other armed conflicts and likely represent a more accurate estimate.[26]

Table 2.1. Distribution and mortality of vascular injuries among American soldiers in World War I

	# of cases (% total)[1]		# of deaths (% total)		Case mortality
Femoral	78	22.22%	26	41.94%	33.33%
Popliteal	27	7.69%	1	1.61%	3.70%
Ant. tibial	49	13.96%	10	16.13%	20.40%
Post. tibial	27	7.69%	4	6.45%	15.00%
Carotid	26	7.41%	11	17.74%	42.00%
Axillary	5	1.42%	2	3.23%	40.00%
Brachial	86	24.50%	6	9.68%	6.98%
Radial	41	11.68%	1	1.61%	2.44%
Ulnar	27	7.69%	1	1.61%	3.70%
Total	351		62		17.80%

Source: Table reproduced from *Report of the U.S. Surgeon General's Office, 1920*, 84–85.
Note:
[1] British data revealed a similar distribution: carotid, 1.8%; vertebral, 0.2%; subclavian, 0.7%; axillary 5.4%; brachial, 14.2%; radial 6.4%; ulnar, 2.8%; external iliac, 0.7%; femoral, 18.4%; popliteal, 11.1%; anterior tibial, 5.7%; posterior tibial, 20.9%; various, 10.8%. Bowlby and Wallace, "The Development of British Surgery at the Front," 705–21.

More interesting than the raw numbers of injuries are the categories the American military selected to measure, indicated across the top of table 2.1. In subsequent wars, surgeons gauged their success in treating vascular trauma by the number of limbs saved, but here, and in an analogous table produced by the British, the militaries documented *lives* saved with no data on amputation rates.[27] Such a choice suggests the contemporary irrelevance of attempting to preserve an arm or a leg while facing the daunting task of keeping the wounded alive.

Surgeons and military medical leaders certainly recognized the threat of amputation associated with vascular injuries and strongly recommended Carrel-style reparative operations. Official American military medical doctrine in the war warned, "If there is danger of gangrene resulting from ligation, a primary suture should be performed and the case watched with particular care."[28] George Makins, senior British surgical consultant in France and global authority on vascular surgery; Theodore Tuffier, doyen of French surgery; and Ramuald Weglowski, surgeon general of the Polish army, all fiercely championed vessel repair and venous autografts in their speeches and writings.[29] The Inter-Allied Surgical Conference in 1917 concluded that, for vascular wounds, "the ideal procedure is to restore the integrity of the vessel by suture."[30] Notably, this conclusion differed markedly from the 1915 and 1916 Inter-Allied Conferences, which had advocated for ligation.[31] The shift toward advocating for repair reflected the general 1917 trend toward increasingly radical operative interventions, likely stimulated by the disappointing results following ligation. Emphasizing the repair of damaged arteries, military medical commanders attempted to disseminate the procedure via meetings like the Inter-Allied Surgical Conference, the distribution of circulars, and especially the consultant system, where senior surgeons would tour frontline hospitals, assess their practice, and suggest improvements.

Prewar simplifications of Carrel's original technique facilitated repairing arteries in World War I. In 1914, Paul Moure had devised a method that employed only two guy wires instead of the original three, which permitted a surgeon and a single assistant to complete the operation rather than the two helpers Carrel required.[32] Reducing the number of assistants was especially relevant during the personnel shortage of the Great War. The tiny needles Carrel recommended, while necessary on smaller arteries, were not required for operations on larger vessels in otherwise healthy young men.[33] And although before the war specially schooled operators were considered necessary for delicate vascular surgery, Rudolph Matas argued at a medical meeting that the conflict demonstrated "surgeons of ordinary training" could perform these procedures.[34]

A subset of surgeons did repair arteries and achieved encouraging results, but contrary to Matas's assertion, they were elite, academic practitioners.[35] Just as before the war, the ability to cite the known examples of arterial repair individually demonstrates both its international distribution and its exceptional rarity. American Charles Goodman repaired five popliteal vessels behind the knee (two arteries and three veins) via lateral suture while visiting a casualty clearing station close to the front lines, and all of his patients retained their legs.[36] Germans Herman Kuttner and August Bier (of the Bier block) adopted Moure's two-guy-wire technique and documented at least ninety-three cases of arterial repair.[37] Polish surgeon Ramuald Weglowski recorded fifty-six venous autografts in the war, and fifty of fifty-two surviving patients maintained circulation to the affected extremity.[38] The British reported at least forty-four cases of suture repair, although almost exclusively on delayed presentations of pseudoaneurysms and arteriovenous fistulae rather than fresh combat wounds.[39] Ernst Jeger, a prodigy in vascular surgery who had trained with Carrel and Kuttner, recorded seven successful vascular repairs, including the reattachment of a partially severed arm, on the eastern front. His capture by the Russian army and subsequent death in captivity cut short this promising career.[40]

When suture repair proved challenging to implement, surgeons looked to the technically simpler method of prosthetic bridges. These contraptions involved a short tube that a surgeon could insert into the two ends of a severed artery, forming a tunnel that shunted blood past the site of injury. They functioned identically to the glass tubes of Robert Abbe (see figure 1.5). Subsequent research had since demonstrated the tendency of blood clots to occlude these prostheses after several days, but surgeons did not intend for them to function as permanent bypasses. Rather, they envisioned the tubes providing some blood flow while the body developed collateral circulation. Both therapeutically and technically, they represented an intermediate option between total ligation and permanent suture repair. Surgeons used a variety of devices in World War I, including glass and aluminum models developed by Carrel, but by far the most common prostheses were the paraffin-coated silver Tuffier tubes, named after the renowned French surgeon who invented them. The French and the British utilized them most often, with one British account documenting eleven placements of Tuffier tubes in 218 injured arteries—still an experimental, tiny fraction of vascular wounds.[41] Results by all accounts were equivocal. Interestingly, the intervention never gained acceptance among American surgeons.[42]

Instead of technically demanding suture repairs or technologically advanced prosthetic tubes, surgeons ligated almost every vascular wound they encountered. British corporal George Coppard was struck by a German machine-gun bullet when fighting in the Battle of Cambrai: "I fell as a bullet passed clean through the thickest part of my thigh . . . a spout of blood curved upwards like a scarlet arc, three feet long and thick as a pencil," reflected Coppard in his diary.[43] Fortunately, his mates quickly applied a tourniquet, arrested the bleeding, and rushed him to the nearest casualty clearing station. "The surgeons did their job in a large marquee. When I came to, I saw two half-inch rubber tubes extending through the bandages round my thigh . . . for Lysol to be squirted . . . every two hours." Coppard's doctors had ligated his femoral artery and applied a Carrel-Dakin dressing to stave off gangrene; he kept his leg.

No country collected army-wide data, but statistics from individual units confirm this practice. For example, American surgeons at the 5th Evac Hospital ligated all seven of their vascular cases, as did British captain A. Bourne for the eight patients with vascular trauma he encountered while campaigning in Egypt.[44] Doctors at the hospital center in Langres similarly tied off all twelve cases they reported.[45] Surgical Team #16, at Base Hospital 31, rarely saw the freshly wounded but had a policy that the "treatment of secondary hemorrhage consists of immediate vessel ligation."[46]

Closer to the front lines, Captain Hey's casualty clearing station treated 523 vascular wounds on the first day of the Battle of the Somme; its surgeons ligated all 523 cases.[47] George Dorrance, who in 1906 had published how to repair arteries by way of everted suture (see figure 1.2), ligated every vascular injury that came across his operating table during the war.[48] When surgeons at US Mobile Hospital #6 encountered arterial trauma, they too ligated the vessel—or just prophylactically amputated the limb if blood flow appeared compromised.[49] Notably, Captain Samuel C. Harvey served as chief of surgery at Mobile Hospital #6.[50] Harvey had completed his surgical training at Peter Bent Brigham Hospital under renowned neurosurgeon Harvey Cushing and returned after the war to chair the department of surgery at Yale. An academic well aware of Carrel's technique and its potential to restore blood flow, Harvey nonetheless directed his surgeons to tie off injured arteries, as evident in the following cases.

Private Nicholas Boss of the 165th Infantry Regiment reached Mobile Hospital #6 on 7 November 1918. Captain Wall cared for his injuries, noting "a dirty through and through wound in the right calf." The offending shell fragment had badly fractured the fibula bone and perforated the neighboring blood supply. After thoroughly debriding the wound and extracting the loose bone fragments, "the bleeding posterior tibial [artery was] ligated . . . [and the leg] splinted."[51] Private Peter Griffen, a trooper in the 2nd Cavalry, arrived at Mobile Hospital #6 on 8 November, three days after receiving a missile wound in his left leg. Lieutenant Jackson operated, noting a large collection of blood behind the knee due to wounds of the anterior and posterior tibial arteries. Jackson ligated Griffen's popliteal artery.[52] Unsurprisingly, both Boss and Griffen subsequently required amputation of their lower extremities.[53]

Contemporary military surgeons clearly recognized the risks inherent in tying off arteries. Doctors at the hospital center at Langres noted "ligations of large vessels predisposed enormously to infection with the gas bacillus," and gas gangrene invariably led to amputation (or death).[54] Physicians at Base Hospital #31 similarly listed ligation, along with inadequate debridement, as primary causes of gangrene.[55] Dr. Wall, at Mobile Hospital #6, anticipated at Boss's initial surgery that the case "may come to amputation."[56] That surgeons continued to practice ligation in spite of the acknowledged risks emphasizes how military, logistical, and medical factors constrained the implementation of new techniques and the practice of surgery.

World War I battles involved hundreds of thousands of men, overwhelming military medical units with casualties and forcing triage decisions to prioritize life over limb. In the first three days of the Battle of the Somme, British Hospital #44 received 4,500 wounded.[57] American Mobile Hospital #39, staffed by a half-dozen surgeons, received 201 cases in twenty-four hours, operating on 170 of them.[58] Under such pressure, surgeons adhered to standard triage principles and favored ligation—which required but a few seconds—over time-consuming, technically complex repairs.

A shortage of uniformed doctors further hampered the ability to treat the deluge of wounded men.[59] The French suffered the most, but all countries lacked sufficient surgeons to care for the tens of thousands of casualties created by battle.[60] "It was necessary in some base hospitals," the American surgeon general's report confessed, "for the bacteriologists, ophthalmologists, oto-laryngologists, commanding officers, and adjutants to . . . perform major operations in order to do what they could to prevent loss of life."[61] It remains unclear as to whether having bacteriologists perform major war surgery helped wounded soldiers or just hastened their demise, but it certainly did not lead to the application of highly complex operations to sew arteries back together.

Both the flood of casualties and the logistical considerations of trench warfare led to prolonged delays before operating, which rendered most attempts at vascular repair pointless. At Passchendaele, it took stretcher bearers more than fourteen hours to transport wounded from the battlefield to dressing stations, then several additional hours to reach a hospital with qualified surgeons. Because of the long delay, thousands of British wounded drowned on the battlefield, unable to escape the rainwater rising in newly formed shell holes.[62] Even after arriving at a hospital, the volume of cases meant patients often waited to see a surgeon.[63] It took more than eighteen hours for the majority of American wounded to reach the operating table at Evacuation Hospital #9, and twenty-seven hours at Mobile Hospital #1.[64] Privates Griffen and Boss, the previously mentioned unfortunate American soldier-amputees, underwent surgery *days* after their missile injuries, with gas gangrene already infecting Boss's leg.[65] "Our heaviest work was done during and immediately following the drives at St. Mihiel and Argonne Woods," documented the official report of Base Hospital #35. "At these times men who had been wounded four or five days before and had had only first aid dressings were sometimes received."[66] In such cases, vessel repair proved irrelevant: bleeding had either stopped or had already killed the patient; limbs had either died or demonstrated that they could survive on collateral circulation.

Even when the wounded reached the operating table promptly, the nature of the trauma and the surgery necessary to treat it often precluded arterial repair. As noted, artillery caused over 80 percent of injuries, and "shrapnel makes very bad wounds," wrote British surgeon Arthur Martin. "It rips, tears, and lacerates the tissues, and repair is often impossible in the face of the anatomical devastation."[67] To prevent infection in contaminated injuries, surgeons had to perform radical debridements, excising extensive chunks of tissue including long segments of blood vessels. Even Bertram Bernheim, the skilled surgeon from Johns Hopkins who had undergone specialized training in vascular surgery, had literally written the textbook on the subject, and had brought his own instruments with him to the battlefield in eager anticipation of applying the technique, was stymied by the conditions of the wounds. "Not that the blood vessels were immune from injury or that gaping arteries and veins and vicariously united vessels did not cry out for relief by fine suture or anastomosis. They did, most eloquently, and in great numbers," he wrote before cautioning, "but it would have been a foolhardy man who would have essayed sutures of arterial or venous trunks in the presence of such infection as were the rule in practically all the battle-wounded."[68]

Comparing the successful adoption of abdominal surgery, or laparotomy, against the persistence of vessel ligation reveals the distinctive features of arterial repair. In 1914 and 1915, surgeons treated abdominal wounds conservatively, applying bandages but rarely operating; 80 percent of patients died. Again as part of a general shift to more operative management in 1917, surgeons began opening the abdomen and attempting to repair damaged organs. Mortality, though still high, dropped to 40 percent by the end of the war.[69] Neither vascular nor abdominal wounds were especially common, each afflicting only about 2 percent of soldiers who reached a physician alive. Yet laparotomy had a chance to save lives whereas arterial repair protected limbs. Moreover, debridement, which provided the theoretical rationale for abdominal surgery, often precluded vascular work. Finally, precisely suturing blood vessels demanded a level of technical competence not required in contemporary abdominal trauma operations that eschewed anastomoses in favor of primary repairs.

Surgical management of vascular injuries did evolve over the course of the war in the form of concomitant venous ligation. While military medical leaders championed the superiority of arterial repair, they also realized that the overwhelming majority of surgeons would continue to ligate damaged arteries. This practice resulted in a high rate of amputation as arms and legs died from inadequate blood flow, prompting innovative but technically simple solutions. British consultant George Makins proposed ligating the vein that normally accompanied each artery, even when it was undamaged. He theorized that this therapy would delay blood from leaving the injured extremity, improve oxygenation, and lower the amputation rate.[70] Prior to World War I, surgeons studiously avoided harming an otherwise healthy vein, but the mass casualties and high morbidity led to a reassessment of this practice.[71] Based largely on the statistics Makins provided, the Allies officially adopted concurrent vein ligation as policy at the Inter-Allied Conference of Surgeons in 1917.[72] It became the standard of care for Anglo-American vascular injuries in World War I through World War II.[73]

The adoption of concomitant vein ligation for vascular injuries not only illuminates how combat shapes surgical therapy; it also exemplifies how the medical profession could recognize a problem, identify a solution, and effect change in practice by reeducating doctors to embrace new therapies. Symposia like the Inter-Allied Surgical Conferences functioned as de facto medical meetings where senior leadership from all nations gathered to discuss results from existing practices and propose new management guidelines. They communicated these updates via both courses and publications. The British, for example, would rotate surgeons out of the front line during quiet periods to attend continuing education classes.[74] Benefitting from the lessons of four years of intra-European conflict, the Americans established courses and schools to educate civilian doctors prior to deploying to war. Founded in the fall of 1917, the School of Applied Surgical Mechanics taught care of gunshot wounds and fractures, reportedly improving patient care.[75]

Every country published circulars, textbooks, and memoranda that instructed medical officers how to manage military trauma and updated them with new recommendations throughout the war. The US Army distributed twenty thousand copies of the *Official British Manual of Injuries and Diseases in War*, collated four hundred relevant abstracts into a pamphlet to disperse, and created a manual of surgical anatomy to circulate.[76] The army also printed a series of *Review of War Surgery and Medicine*, journal-size textbooks reviewing military medicine. In the first issue of March 1918, it noted that for vascular wounds, "the ideal procedure is to restore the integrity of the vessel by suture, either lateral or circular as the conditions may demand."[77] Military medical command had clearly identified the problem of excessive amputation from ligation and tried to save limbs by promoting arterial repair through retraining its ranks of physicians. They failed, partly due to the conditions of war but also because the average American military doctor lacked experience and skill, entering the army ill prepared to perform even the most basic operations.

Brigadier General Edward Munson, MC, directed the Army Medical Department training from 1917 through the end of the war. Just to matriculate into his training program, physicians had to have graduated from a reputable medical school, possess a state license to practice medicine, and pass an examination by a board of local doctors. Yet even among these 2,628 selected, pre-screened men who declared themselves surgeons, Munson gave fewer than 1 percent an A, and graded only 20 percent as C or better on an A–F scale. Over two-thirds of the students were incapable of operating independently.[78] Experiences in the aforementioned School of Applied Surgical Mechanics substantiated Munson's conclusions: intended to focus on complicated war surgery, the class spent most of its time instructing students how to remove an appendix and repair an inguinal hernia, among the most basic operations a surgeon performs.[79] For every Bernheim, Dorrance, or Cushing who deployed to Europe, thousands of poorly trained practitioners accompanied them. Recognizing these deficiencies, the leaders of American surgery returned home and in the interwar period worked to reform surgical education.

The Development of American Surgical Education between the World Wars

Following World War I, the American surgical profession entered a time of transition. The war keenly demonstrated the "topography" of surgeons that existed in this country.[80] The vast majority of general practitioners, who frequently performed minor operations, had attended some lectures on surgery in medical school; younger ones may have spent a few months as a student on a surgical service in a hospital and possibly dedicated a further three months to the discipline during a rotating internship, during which he may or may not have actually performed any procedures. Some general practitioners obtained additional training through attending postgraduate courses or just through years of experience. An older elite composed of men like J. M. T. Finney, appointed chief surgical consultant for the American Expeditionary Force, and Cleveland Clinic founder George Crile, who commanded the first US hospital deployed in the war, held leadership positions in the profession.[81] The doyens of this generation encompassed both academics like William Halsted as well as clinicians like the Mayo brothers who had cobbled together their surgical training. Lacking formal opportunities, they variously traveled to Europe (especially Germany), served as house officers in an inchoate system, attended postgraduate courses, apprenticed themselves to older clinicians, and to a great extent were self-taught.[82] This ad hoc, highly individualized manner of education served well enough for Halsted, Finney, Crile, the Mayos, and a few others, but it could not systematically train a majority of American surgeons.

William Halsted sought to formalize the academic educational process by creating a residency program at Johns Hopkins University. Halsted had completed medical school and a house officership in New York prior to spending two years in Germany and Austria.[83] In addition to learning the science and practice of surgery, he also came to appreciate their educational system. When Halsted became chief of surgery at Johns Hopkins in 1889, he worked with William Osler, chief of medicine, to "adopt as closely as feasible the German plan."[84] Halsted created a pyramidal program that brought residents through a multiyear training regimen focusing on both patient care and research. He deliberately aimed to "produce not only surgeons but surgeons of the highest type, men who will stimulate the first youths of our country to study surgery and to devote their energies and their lives to raising the standard of surgical science."[85] He succeeded, as his trainees chaired departments around the country.[86]

The Hopkins model extended across the United States, with its graduates the most ardent missionaries. Of Halsted's seventeen chief residents, eleven went on to establish similar residency programs.[87] Other surgeons, like longtime friends and fellow chairs of surgery Allen O. Whipple (Columbia) and Evarts Graham (Washington University), never trained directly under Halsted but nonetheless consciously created consonant programs.[88] Graham in particular standardized Halsted's amorphous system into a set-length, graded curriculum where residents earned increased responsibility as they advanced. This stepwise permutation, widely adopted by the 1920s, was critical in surgery to ensure graduates received appropriate operative exposure.[89] By the 1920s, residency, either at Hopkins or an analogous program, became required for appointments at academic hospitals and research institutions. Yet it remained exquisitely rare for the vast majority of practicing US doctors.

Most American doctors in the early twentieth century—including the thirty thousand in the US Army during World War I—lacked access to either the idiosyncratic model of the Finney/Crile generation or the nascent Halstedian residencies. Many of the older physicians had no formal clinical training at all, given the inferior state of American medical schools in the late nineteenth and early twentieth centuries.[90] The 1910 Flexner report catalyzed improvements in medical schools, but it simultaneously distracted attention from graduate medical education.[91] In 1900, fewer than 50 percent of physicians pursued any additional schooling after graduation; until 1914, no state required any postdoctorate education for licensure.[92]

While limited training proved adequate for most practitioners in the late nineteenth and early twentieth centuries, changes in surgery rendered it unsafe and outmoded by the 1930s. Until the twentieth century, surgeons' practice typically involved draining abscesses, setting fractures, and maybe appendectomies, a spectrum sufficiently addressed through informal apprenticeships.[93] But the surgical revolution described in chapter 1 created an array of new operations like vascular anastomosis and concordantly demanded improved graduate education. In 1933 and 1935, the leaders of the American Surgical Association, the oldest and most prestigious organization in the field, dedicated their presidential addresses to the problem "where fingers replace brains and handicraft outruns science."[94] Tellingly, their concerns centered on the ability of doctors to navigate physiology and pathology, not just technical prowess, as the theory and practice of surgery shifted from speedy, dramatic performances to slow, meticulous, yet radical operations that exceeded the abilities of internship-trained generalists.[95] At the same time, leaders of the American Surgical Association recognized the scarce opportunities for further training.[96] In 1935, fewer than thirty-five Halsted-style residencies existed in the country, with each graduating a single chief resident: "not a drop in the bucket towards supplying the need for surgeons through the country," according to Eugene Pool, professor of surgery at Columbia.[97]

Aware of the problem, the American surgical profession tried to redress it in the 1930s. Hospitals were creating residencies in all fields, not only to educate young clinicians but also to provide the medical institutions with cheap, skilled labor.[98] Partly in response to these weaker programs, organizations like the American Medical Association and particularly the American College of Surgeons enumerated criteria for acceptable residencies and established national inspection systems to evaluate them. Notably, the stimulus to improve surgical education came from within medicine; neither government regulation nor popular dissatisfaction drove this campaign. While some general practitioners accused surgical leaders of acting out of economic self-interest, reformers insisted they prioritized patient care as they sought to eliminate medically unnecessary procedures performed by untrained physicians. This internal effort to regulate training and thus entry into field exemplifies the salience of self-improvement, quality control, and autoregulation in the profession.[99]

This same idea of self-regulation also inspired the creation of the American Board of Surgery. In the 1930s, a group of young academic surgeons led by Evarts Graham grew dissatisfied with the current state of the profession.[100] Specifically, these so-called Young Turks believed that the existing system of educating and certifying surgeons was inadequate given rapid advances in the field. At the same time, other disciplines were already establishing boards, including surgical subspecialties.[101] Fearing for both the quality of surgery and its splintering into dozens of fiefdoms, in 1937 the Young Turks founded the American Board of Surgery.[102] To become board certified, one had to complete an approved three-year residency and pass rigorous exams. Initially limited to a select few academic surgeons, board status nonetheless influenced the overall trajectory of training by raising expectations and, more importantly, ultimately compelling other organizations to match its standards.[103]

The American College of Surgeons (ACS) was a leader in evaluating residency programs. It viewed this mission as fundamental to its core purpose of improving American surgery and analogous to its existing efforts investigating and grading hospitals.[104] The college also feared irrelevancy following the formation of the board, prompting it to raise its own requirements and insist on residency for fellowship. Now that it demanded residency, the ACS shouldered the responsibility of inspecting and approving programs.[105] The ACS Committee on Graduate Training in Surgery first met in November 1937, with four charges: (1) establish minimum standards, (2) ascertain which hospitals were capable of meeting those standards, (3) help create residencies, and (4) provide means of periodic inspection.[106] "There are really two problems that confronted us," noted an internal report from a subsequent meeting. "One was the ideal training for the surgeon and the other was the graduate training which is necessary for every man to have before he can become a member of the American College of Surgeons."[107] Despite having two problems, the committee sought a single system of training. This decision created tension between elites, who thought the standards too low, and community practitioners who considered them too stringent, but the organization repeatedly rebuffed suggestions to adopt a two-tier system in its effort to preserve professional unity.

Building off the American Medical Association's (AMA) extant inspections, the ACS committee outlined a model that included three postgraduate years in an ACS-approved hospital, competent and engaged faculty, broad clinical experiences, instruction in basic science, and exposure to research.[108] However, the committee deliberately avoided imposing strict, specific criteria.[109] Recognizing that conditions and opportunities differed considerably around the country, it insisted "the emphasis should be on standards, not on standardization."[110] Following a survey to elucidate basic factual information, the college deployed a trained surgeon-inspector to evaluate each program. The system mirrored its existing hospital inspection initiative and relied on much of the same infrastructure. Given that the ACS did not publish which residencies failed and paid for the entire process, programs had few costs and numerous potential benefits to requesting approval.[111] Determined to advance surgical education and not just judge that which already existed, the college worked with substandard programs, often provisionally approving them as an incentive while helping improve their curricula.

The inaugural inspection in 1937 evaluated 270 hospitals, approved 89 (33 percent) fully, 46 (17 percent) provisionally, and rejected 135 (50 percent).[112] The results limned the current state of surgical education. Variability characterized the findings: "One of the most striking impressions as a result of this study is the complete lack of a basic standard or uniformity in the methods of graduate training," noted the final report.[113] Both structure and educational content differed among hospitals, with residencies ranging from one to five years in length.[114] Programs varied tremendously, with some eliding entire disciplines like urology, orthopedics, or thoracic surgery, raising the question of what "general surgery" included.[115] The surveyors repeatedly lambasted the lack of basic science, postmortem examinations, and formal didactic teaching conferences, particularly in community hospitals.[116]

The college published its findings in the 1939 *Bulletin of the American College of Surgeons* that it freely distributed throughout the country.[117] The printing and distribution cost the college $9,000 in 1938 ($155,000 in 2017 USD)—a significant expenditure for a nonprofit organization during the Great Depression. Such spending highlights the priority the college placed on disseminating both its requirements and a list of the programs that satisfied them.[118] Letters from deans of academic institutions like Yale, smaller schools like the College of Medical Evangelists in Loma Linda, California, and the Women's Medical College of Pennsylvania praised the report and pledged to raise their institutions to its standards.[119] J. Curran, dean of the Long Island College of Medicine, "believe[d] it to be one of the finest things of the kind I have seen," a sentiment Dean C. Poynter of the University of Nebraska echoed while adding somewhat wistfully, "I wish it were as easy to get this program started as it is to talk about it. Certainly the movement is in the right direction and out of it should come a generation of very much better trained men than the last generation furnished."[120]

The next generation of students and teachers appeared eager for this opportunity. Interns commenced writing the college, querying which hospitals had or would receive approval to make their residency decisions. Inspectors conducting the surveys "found great interest in the subject manifested on the part of hospital superintendents, attending staffs and particularly resident staffs who are desirous of seeing facilities improved."[121] After the release of the report, more than one hundred hospitals contacted the college asking to be inspected in 1940.[122] Programs wanted the ACS's imprimatur to attract better-qualified students, and residents sought out ACS-approved programs to ensure entrance into the college and boards, with all the advantages membership entailed.[123] Less cynically, there remained a real commitment to improving the quality of education and a desire among house staff to receive the best training possible. While this era lacks confirmatory data, the benefits of having someone with three years of structured training operate instead of a general practitioner seemed self-evident to contemporaries.

As organizations like the American Board of Surgery came to depend on college inspection and approval, and, as more hospitals sought certification, the rather generic provisions applied in 1938 gave way to increasingly detailed criteria in 1941, when the college published eleven full pages of specifications.[124] This shift signified a notable departure in surgical education, transitioning from highly variable experiences around the country to a more rigid national standard that, ideally, ensured every graduate from an approved program would possess a common set of intellectual and technical abilities, irrespective of whether they came from an academic or community hospital.[125] Requirements emphasized an educated faculty to teach not just surgery but also pathology, radiology, and anatomy, buttressed by new attention to physiology, then viewed as the vanguard of surgical research.[126] The committee focused on both the quantity and variety of cases residents performed. It also continued to mandate research, which particularly challenged community programs. These 1941 standards expose the extent that surgical residency had changed since its inception at Johns Hopkins. Fundamentally, its underlying purpose had metamorphized from producing "surgeons of the highest type" who populated the ranks of research institutions to training both academicians and especially practicing community surgeons. This transition paralleled developments in graduate medical education for other specialties, sacrificing elements of rigor and original investigation for broad applicability.[127]

Form followed function. Surgery residencies began shifting away from Halsted's pyramidal construction, which intentionally produced a limited number of surgical professors. While castoffs in the 1910s had adequate training to perform standard operations and sufficient credentials to land work as surgeons, by the 1930s they lacked both. In 1940, Edward Churchill, chair at the prestigious Massachusetts General Hospital, publicly broke with Halsted's pyramid, commenting that "half a surgical training is about as useful as half a billiard ball."[128] He established a rectangular program that expected everyone accepted as a resident to complete all four years of training, arguing this arrangement would produce desperately needed surgeons in a more collegial environment.[129] This was not the first rectangular program, but it set a prestigious precedent that others could follow.[130] Churchill and others similarly shifted the focus of even academically affiliated programs to producing more community practitioners.[131]

The symbiotic efforts between the college and residencies led to a significant increase in approved programs in the late 1930s. By 1938, the ACS had approved 135 hospitals producing 380 surgeons a year; the 1939 report approved 179 hospitals producing 580 surgeons—an impressive surge but still not close to reaching the stated goal of having a residency-trained surgeon complete each of the estimated 2.5 million operations performed every year.[132] Nor did the average American practitioner yet appreciate the need for prolonged, poorly compensated training, with most doctors continuing to enter practice immediately after internship. Residency, though steadily growing, remained an exceptional experience. With the onset of World War II, reform efforts paused.

Technological Change in the Interwar Wars: Preventing Clots and Visualizing Vessels

While the surgical profession worked to transform its educational foundation for community practitioners in the interwar years, academic physicians continued research efforts in laboratories and clinics around the country. Over the course of these decades, investigations produced a number of exciting medical developments. Electroencephalograms (EEGs) measured brain waves while pacemakers kept hearts beating.[133] New drugs like sulfas fought bacteria, insulin cured diabetes, and vitamins promised better health.[134] In tropical medicine, atabrine helped prevent malaria while Max Theiler's yellow fever vaccine raised hopes of eradicating that infection.[135] Surgically, Graham performed the first one-stage pneumonectomy, and Whipple created his eponymous operation for treating pancreatic cancer, procedures that also remained limited in application for decades.[136]

For vascular surgery, these years lacked the explosion of technical innovation that characterized the late nineteenth and early twentieth centuries; Carrel's method remained predominant. Instead, as part of this wave of science, surgeons established technologies surrounding the repair of arteries that enabled, facilitated, and supported its implementation. In particular, two major discoveries reshaped the field: heparin, a drug that prevents blood clots and increases the success rate of arterial repair; and arteriography, or the ability to visualize arteries with X-rays. Understanding the invention and application of these ancillary technologies provides critical insight into the practice of arterial repair in subsequent years.

Heparin

By preventing blood from clotting, the drug heparin had the potential to eliminate the most common complication of arterial suturing. While the precise origins of heparin remain shrouded in controversy, the process began in the physiology lab of William Henry Howell at Johns Hopkins.[137] In 1916, second-year medical student Jay McClean isolated an anticoagulant substance he dubbed heparphosphatid.[138] Howell and his laboratory then spent the next several years refining the substance, identifying its function, evaluating its clinical utility, and ultimately naming it heparin because of its apparent concentration in dog livers (*hepar* is the Greek root word for "liver").[139] By the early 1920s, Howell and others had initiated human trials, but the side effects proved too toxic for clinical use, causing fevers, nausea, vomiting, and severe headaches in the majority of patients.[140] These adverse effects resulted from impurities remaining in the drug samples, reflecting the intricate biochemical challenges of extracting pure heparin from animal organs.

A research group in Toronto established a new isolation methodology that led to purer yields of heparin, allowing for increased use in the laboratories and the clinic.[141] Charles Best, already famous for his role in the development of insulin, led the Canadian effort. The work on insulin in Toronto had established a collaborative scientific environment comfortable with complex chemical extraction of biological substances; previous partnerships with industry provided both finances and industrial capacity to mass-produce the new drug.[142] Best leveraged this infrastructure to great success with heparin. In 1933, the Toronto team published three key papers that established a new and improved method of isolating and purifying heparin from organs other than dog liver.[143] By 1936, they were routinely producing enough pure heparin to begin clinical trials.[144] Physicians, searching for an anticoagulation drug for years, hoped heparin could either prevent or help the body dissolve unnecessary blood clots. Chemicals identified earlier like hirudin (derived from leech saliva) proved impossible to isolate in clinically significant, economically viable quantities. Citrate helped doctors store blood for later transfusion but did not prove safe for injecting into patients. With the research of Best's group, heparin promised both availability and nontoxicity.

Gordon Murray, a surgeon in Toronto, conducted most of the early research proving the clinical utility of heparin.[145] Long interested in vascular surgery, he experimented with various treatments of blood clots but found that, despite his interventions, most patients died.[146] After learning of Swedish surgeon Clarence Crafoord's success administering heparin, Murray approached Best's group.[147] In a series of collaborative efforts, Best and Murray demonstrated the ability of heparin to prevent and treat blood clots in arteries and veins.[148] Murray specifically explored the benefits of heparin in vascular surgery. Well acquainted with Carrel's technique of anastomosis, he also recognized its limitations: the manipulation and sewing of arteries initiated an inflammatory response that frequently resulted in thromboses, particularly in small vessels. Relying again on a series of more than fifty dog experiments, Murray conclusively proved the ability of heparin to prevent clots and keep arterial anastomoses (including venous grafts) patent.[149] This evidence, echoed quickly in the literature, held the potential to change vascular surgery by making arterial repair more reliable and less technically demanding. Publishing the results in 1940, Murray hoped heparin would help save limbs in the now-raging Second World War.

Arteriography

While heparin facilitated the implementation of arterial repair, the new imaging methodology of arteriography—or X-rays of arteries—enabled surgeons to view the entire length of blood vessels, determine which intervention would most benefit the patient, and evaluate how effectively a procedure treated the vascular disease. Arteriography quickly followed the birth of radiology in concept but required decades to achieve meaningful, broad use in practice. Just a year after William Roentgen announced his discovery of X-rays in 1895, two German scientists published a report of the first arteriogram.[150] It featured the amputated limb of a corpse and served no clinical benefit, but it did provide a proof-of-concept upon which future investigators could expand. Unlike bone, arteries and veins do not normally appear on standard X-rays.[151] To view them, doctors have to inject a dye, or contrast, into the vessel. Scientists grasped this underlying concept almost immediately but spent the next half century experimenting to identify a dye that was metallic enough to provide suitably high-quality images without being so toxic as to kill or sicken the patient.

The effort to image blood vessels occurred simultaneously with—and benefitted from—contemporaneous efforts to visualize the brain, gastrointestinal tract, and genitourinary system. X-rays provided an exciting opportunity to see inside living bodies for the first time, and doctors in all specialties began exploring its potential. Extensive investigations in the 1910s–20s established the efficacy of iodine-based compounds to image the bladder.[152] Lipiodol, a fat-emulsion containing iodine, subsequently became the standard contrast agent for neurological, urological, and reproductive systems through the 1950s. But the dye failed when injected systemically, precipitating blood clots that caused stroke and death when two Frenchman tried using Lipiodol in the first arteriogram on a living patient in 1923.[153] Two German scientists and the American surgeon Barney Brooks followed with clinical arteriograms employing strontium bromide (1923) and sodium iodide dye (1924), respectively, but such cases remained rare.[154]

These early contrast agents had severe side effects, causing nausea, vomiting, excruciating pain, and allergic reactions. Worse, their noxious insult to the artery itself could result in spasming of the blood vessel or the propagation of blood clots, compromising distal circulation. Despite these side effects, the dyes were not strong enough to provide clear images, especially of the smaller arteries. Vascular leader Rudolph Matas considered arteriograms in the 1930s "hazardous and contraindicated in all cases of preexisting or threatened ischemia from arterial disease," and surgeons rarely used the technology before the development of safe, effective contrast mediums.[155]

Portuguese physician and future Nobel laureate Egas Moniz transformed arteriography into a viable clinical technology by identifying a more tolerable dye.[156] As a neurologist familiar with studies on Lipiodol, he sought to apply the technique to visualize the cerebral arteries. Initially, he would surgically expose the carotid arteries on both sides of the neck in order to see the entire brain.[157] But the sodium iodide he used at first continued to cause the same severe side effects in patients, notably pain, nausea, and vomiting; moreover, the images produced, while serviceable, poorly differentiated finer anatomy.[158] In 1927, Moniz tried a new agent, thorium dioxide (Thorotrast), which provided exquisite detail with fewer side effects. Thorium-based dyes, championed by Moniz, would remain the standard of care into the 1950s, when subsequent research revealed that they caused cancer.[159]

It was not just the dye but also the entire process of performing an arteriogram, which in itself was a major surgical procedure in the 1920s and 1930s, that limited its application. The physician prepared the patient's arm or leg sterilely and used a scalpel to cut down and dissect out the artery. With a syringe, the doctor then injected contrast and had to coordinate timing of the X-ray exposure to obtain the clearest image of the entire vessel. The operation required general anesthesia both for the cutdown portion and to prevent the patient from flinching from the pain caused by the injected sodium-based dye; movement would obscure the radiograph.[160] Technological limitations often separated the surgical suite and the X-ray equipment in different parts of the hospital. Pioneering vascular surgeon W. Andrew Dale recalled exposing his patients' femoral artery in the operating room, covering the leg with a sterile towel, wheeling the patient to the radiology suite for an X-ray, then taking them back to the OR to close the wound—a process that both increased the risk of infection and likely reduced application of the procedure.[161]

Despite these difficulties, the medical literature touted the benefits of arteriograms. Surgeons could identify where vessels constricted, the location of aneurysms, and the extent of collateral circulation. Postoperative films assessed the quality of any repair.[162] Yet, similar to plain X-rays, arteriograms remained rare in clinical practice for decades.[163] While the Mayo Clinic completed its first arteriography in 1932 with Moniz's Thorotrast (imported from Germany), the procedure did not become common until the opening of the cardiovascular lab at St. Mary's Hospital in Rochester, Minnesota, in 1960.[164]

Technological limitations like the side effects of dyes and the requirement for arterial cutdowns partially explain surgeons' reluctance to employ arteriograms, but equally important was its (f)utility. Given the infrequency of arterial repair and the few surgeons who could perform the operation competently, most doctors had little use for images of the artery.[165] In these early decades, such films might provide some diagnostic insight, but, without an available therapy, arteriography served more academic than practical value.

Sympathectomy: A Replacement for Repair?

"Sympathectomy" does not mean the surgical removal of sympathy. Quite the opposite, the advent and promotion of this operation reflected professional concerns that the challenging technique of anastomosis exceeded the capability of most surgeons, leaving them unable to help their patients. Sympathectomy refers to the interruption of specific nerve impulses that control the muscle layer around arteries. Lacking nervous stimulation, the muscle relaxes, causing arteries to dilate; the larger diameter tube thus increases blood flow to a region. This new operation represented a possible therapeutic solution to a number of different vascular diseases, including aneurysms, and it was a procedure simple enough for most surgeons to execute successfully. This ease of application combined with perceived efficacy drove case numbers into the thousands, making sympathectomy the face of vascular surgery in the interwar era.

Sympathetic nerves, first identified in 1752 by Jacques Winslow (of foramen of Winslow fame), are part of the autonomic system, meaning they function involuntarily.[166] In 1851, French physiologist Claude Bernard first reported that severing a sympathetic nerve resulted in the dilation of blood vessels.[167] His countryman Mathieu Jaboulay performed the first known sympathectomy when he extirpated nerve bundles in the pelvis to relieve pain in a patient's lower urinary system.[168] Jaboulay's student René Leriche completed the first sympathectomy for peripheral vascular disease in 1913.[169] The support of Leriche, an internationally renowned vascular surgeon who presented his work at medical meetings around the world, helped promote the procedure even as other researchers repeatedly demonstrated the inefficacy of his periarterial technique.[170]

Instead, a translumbar approach invented by two previously obscure Australians proved both more effective and more popular, particularly after surgeons at the respected Mayo Clinic adopted, verified, and heralded this method. Norman D. Royale, an Australian scientist, reasoned that the increased blood flow sympathectomy caused could improve muscle function in cases of spastic paralysis. With his surgical colleague John I. Hunter, the pair published a series of articles in 1924 demonstrating the efficacy of their technique, which involved severing the chain of sympathetic nerves running next to the spine.[171] News of their success spread rapidly around the world, with William Mayo writing to Royale how "my colleagues in the Clinic have been deeply interested in your researches."[172] Reports of the apparent miracle cure appeared in newspapers across the country, including a front-page article in the *New York Times*.[173] Reading these articles, patients subsequently wrote to their doctors, "hoping against hope [sympathectomy] is not the common newspaper dud."[174] This popular and medical fame prompted the American College of Surgeons to invite Royale to deliver its prestigious John B. Murphy Oration at the 1924 Clinical Congress.[175]

A series of personal connections facilitated bringing sympathectomy to the United States and establishing its utility for vascular disease. Following Royale's Murphy Oration, Franklin Martin (founder of the American College of Surgeons) and William Mayo traveled to the University of Sydney to watch Hunter operate and learn his technique of paraspinal interruption, again emphasizing the importance of in-person communication for the transfer of surgical knowledge.[176] They brought this procedure home to Chicago and Rochester, respectively. In Chicago, Loyal Davis and Allen Kanavel quickly proved the superiority of the Australian technique over Leriche's periarterial method while simultaneously demonstrating its inefficacy in treating spastic paralysis, the condition for which Royale had invented the intervention.[177] In Rochester, neurosurgeon Alfred Adson (of Adson forceps fame) similarly showed sympathectomies did not cure spastic paralysis in his patient. But his colleague George Brown in internal medicine, who was also following the case, did notice that the patient's leg on the side Adson operated was markedly warmer than the other. Working with Charles Sheard in the department of biophysics, Brown utilized an advanced temperature control room and vascular laboratory to transform this incidental, subjective observation into a carefully measured analysis of the temperature differential that he quickly associated with increased blood flow. This conclusion led Brown, already interested in vascular conditions, to hypothesize that sympathectomies might treat peripheral vascular disease, which is fundamentally a problem of blood flow. Brown and Adson performed their first surgery for presumed Raynaud's disease in March 1925.[178] "I assisted at this operation," recalled W. McKay Craig, then a neurosurgery trainee; "the patient was completely relieved of his circulatory difficulty."[179]

As indications for the procedure expanded, the surgical approach changed. Initially, Adson made a long incision from the breastbone to the pubic bone, pushed the intestines to the side, and accessed the spinal cord from the front of the body. The invasiveness of this operation limited it to otherwise healthy individuals and still caused four of the first hundred patients to die. Adson's trainee and later successor at Mayo, W. McKay Craig, subsequently developed a translumbar approach in the 1930s, coming from the back with far less disruption of tissue. This new method allowed patients to recover faster and helped avoid complications.[180] Others developed even less-invasive modalities. Trying to design a test to determine which patients would benefit from the surgery, James White injected Novocain into the sympathetic ganglion, which blocked transmissions as effectively as surgery.[181] Like a dentist's shot, though, the nerve block wore off in a few hours. Building on this research, Paul Flothow, another surgical resident at Mayo, proved that ethanol injections permanently interrupted nervous signals.[182] Craig's translumbar approach and Flothow's ethanol injections defined sympathectomies through the 1950s.

By the 1930s, doctors around the world were practicing sympathectomies. The operation featured as the topic for both the presidential address to the American Surgical Association in 1932 and the Hunterian Lecture at the Royal College of Surgeons in 1933 in London.[183] The number of surgeries increased substantially, with the Mayo Clinic performing 18 sympathectomies in 1925 (0.18 percent of total operations) and peaking at 266 (2.8 percent) by 1937.[184] The usage rose so dramatically because the indications for the procedure broadened exponentially. Whereas Royale and Hunter proposed three treatable diseases, by the 1930s, Mayo surgeons had performed sympathectomies on patients for diagnoses ranging from menstrual cramps to epilepsy to arthritis to migraines to constipation.[185] Ultimately, the literature documented at least sixty different indications. This expansion resulted from early enthusiasm for a novel operation that physicians hoped might alleviate otherwise intractable maladies.[186] Subsequent research soon disproved the efficacy of sympathectomy for the majority of these conditions. However, repeated studies, including those using the new technology of arteriograms to show increased blood flow, did demonstrate the success of the operation in treating vascular diseases like Raynaud's, Buerger's, and atherosclerosis, for which it became a popular therapy through the 1950s.[187] In 1949, King George VI of England asked British surgeon James Learmonth (who had worked for five years at the Mayo Clinic with Adson) to treat his Buerger's disease, a pathology of the small arteries typically associated with smoking. Learmonth performed a lumbar sympathectomy and saved the king from amputation.[188]

Sympathectomy soon became an adjunct to other operations, particularly aneurysm repair. For vascular diseases like Raynaud's and Buerger's, removing the sympathetic nerves prompted dilation of the main arterial channel. When Mims Gage, a surgeon at Tulane University who had apprenticed with Rudolph Matas, proposed applying the technique for aneurysms, he anticipated ligating the main artery and counted on sympathectomy to improve the collateral circulation. When attempting this combination sympathectomy-ligation operation for an iliac artery aneurysm in 1934, Gage cured the patient without requiring an amputation.[189] A year later, confronting a popliteal aneurysm, Clarence Bird recalled Gage's experience. "If others share my feelings," Bird wrote, "they approach the obliteration of a popliteal aneurism with misgivings and will be grateful for any aid which may provide further assurance that the collateral circulation will be adequate."[190] Applying a sympathectomy, he successfully ligated the popliteal artery while avoiding amputation. Other surgeons soon followed suit.[191] This modality quickly expanded into trauma surgery as well where the sympathectomy not only relieved the presumed vasospasm that doctors believed resulted from injury but also similarly dilated the collateral circulation in anticipation of ligating an injured main arterial trunk.[192]

Sympathectomy was a far cry from the "ideal operation" that Goyanes and Lexer pioneered in 1906/7. Comparatively easier to perform, it provided a viable, practical, simpler, and seemingly equally effective alternative to technically demanding Carrel-style repairs. From the 1930s, sympathectomies dominated the practice of vascular surgery and were applied to an extraordinarily wide range of conditions in ever-increasing numbers. Surgeons came to rely on it, usually in conjunction with arterial ligation, to treat vascular trauma for the next twenty years, including when they deployed to fight in World War II.

Conclusion: Arteries Left Unrepaired

Arriving with general advances in surgical technique and therapy in the early twentieth century, the arterial repair methods of Alexis Carrel excited surgeons with its possibilities. The First World War doused that enthusiasm as the conditions of that conflict—namely triage, long delays to care, grossly infected wounds, and ill-prepared surgeons—combined to eliminate opportunities to sew wounded blood vessels back together successfully. In the 1920s and 1930s, the efforts of the medical community to mandate and establish surgical residencies would end up addressing one of these important limitations. Other developments in the lab like the drug heparin and the new imaging modality of arteriograms promised to facilitate vascular surgery.

Yet arterial repairs between the world wars remained exceptionally uncommon, even among the elite institutions in the country. Barnes Hospital in St. Louis, Missouri, associated with Washington University School of Medicine, did not note a single arterial suture in its operating room schedules between 1934 and 1937.[193] Between 1893 and 1939, surgeons at the Mayo Clinic performed 1,832 sympathectomies. They ligated 148 arteries to treat aneurysms. In all those years, they repaired only two vessels.[194] When Americans deployed to fight the next World War, arterial repair remained an ideal rarely practiced.

Chapter Three

Opportunities Realized and Discarded

The Management of Vascular Trauma in World War II

In World War II, only 1 percent of all wounds among American soldiers directly afflicted the vascular system, but these injuries caused a disproportionate 20 percent of amputations. Given these severe consequences, trauma to major arteries attracted extensive medical attention before, during, and after the conflict. Even more than the First World War, the Second World War offered surgeons opportunities to repair vessels and not just ligate them, providing them the chance to preserve arms and legs. Better-trained surgeons worked in conditions markedly improved from the trenches of World War I while retaining extraordinary autonomy of practice and freedom from regulatory oversight. Major battles continued to create thousands of bleeding patients in desperate need of vascular surgery. Medical advances like heparin, arteriograms, and sulfa antibiotics in the interbellum years as well as penicillin and blood transfusion early in the war promised greater success and started to alter both physician and patient expectations: whereas before saving lives was the priority, the conditions of the Second World War made it possible for doctors to focus on life *and* limb.

Despite these developments, the American military medical leadership entered World War II strongly recommending ligation and sympathectomy for vascular trauma. They believed the speed, simplicity, and effectiveness of this combination therapy superseded any potential benefits of anastomosis. Once again, high rates of amputation proved this prescription wrong. By the end of the war, the prodigious loss of limbs prompted a previously undescribed shift from ligating to repairing arterial injuries on both the front lines and in army hospitals in the United States. Surgeons who had transformed their practice saved the arms and legs of hundreds of Americans, foreshadowing future care. However, when leaders in American surgery wrote several seminal articles downplaying the transition to repairing arteries and its role in military medicine, the therapy faded from use. Only after hundreds of additional amputations during the Korean War did doctors return to arterial repair as the preferred practice, poignantly demonstrating the power of memory and history in shaping the care of patients.

Creating Opportunities for Arterial Repair: Military Medicine in World War II

Military medicine in World War II built on the experiences of the Great War as well as developments in the interwar period to minister to the millions of soldiers, sailors, airmen, marines, and civilians affected by the conflict.[1] The integration of medical officers into battle planning—perhaps the most important lesson learned from World War I—engendered cooperation between the two professions and obviated many complications of casualty evacuation. Patients also benefitted from new technologies. Sulfa drugs emerged in the 1930s, dramatically reducing infections. The US Army alone used more than four million pounds of this pharmaceutical.[2] The new tetanus and yellow fever vaccines effectively eliminated those diseases from the American military.[3] The insecticide DDT helped control typhus, trench fever, and other louse-borne diseases.[4] Together with the novel synthetic drug Atabrine and improved individual discipline, DDT contributed to the precipitous decline in malaria rates, especially in the Pacific theaters.[5]

The nature of the war altered both the types of wounds and therapies for them. Its mechanization—with exponentially greater numbers of battling airplanes, trucks, tanks, and ships than ever before—significantly increased the frequency of burns, prompting new modes of management that focused on fluid resuscitation and preventing infection with tannic acid and other medicaments.[6] Unlike the static trench combat that characterized World War I, mobility dominated the Second World War. Units hopscotched around the islands of the Pacific, motored across the deserts of North Africa, slogged over Italian mountain ranges, and bulldozed through the plains of northern Europe. This movement constantly shifted the front lines, challenging the evacuation system established in World War I. Yet the commitment to forward surgery remained, with field and evacuation hospitals replacing the old casualty clearing stations. As in World War I, artillery continued to cause the vast majority of casualties.[7] Those wounded benefitted from two major medical developments: blood transfusion and penicillin.

Transfusing blood facilitated the practice of arterial repair by keeping injured soldiers alive long enough to reach a surgeon and replenishing blood lost while operating on the vessels. The practice began in World War I, but its application was haphazard, irregular, and, as judged by all retrospective studies, insufficient.[8] In the years after the 1918 armistice, substantial data revealed the importance of fluid resuscitation in wounded soldiers.[9] Based on their experience during and after the First World War, the British Army Medical Service established the Army Blood Transfusion Service in April 1939 to coordinate transfusions.[10] Whereas the British utilized whole blood almost exclusively, the Americans originally depended on albumin and plasma.[11] Blood, which requires strict temperature control, timely transport, and precise crossmatching of donor to recipient, initially appeared impractical: "it is," the future chief of the American army blood services in World War II, Douglass Kendrick, wrote in 1941, "considered out of the question to supply preserved blood to the combat zone."[12]

Plasma had several major advantages: freeze dried, it was light and easily shipped to forward units; it did not require refrigeration; it could be stored for up to three years; it did not have to be matched to soldiers' blood type; and interwar studies seemed to indicate efficacy on par with whole blood.[13] "We now have a very excellent blood substitute," remarked Kendrick. "For our purposes in warfare, plasma is infinitely superior to blood."[14] The Red Cross collected voluminous amounts, shipping ten million units overseas.[15] Albumin initially appeared even more efficient than plasma, being one-fifth the weight, one-sixth the bulk, and, heat sterilized, eliminating the risks of hepatitis that plasma carried.[16] Developed for the navy specifically to avoid having to coordinate the unwieldy logistics of whole blood on ships navigating the oceans, albumin relied on the novel process of fractionating blood into its constituent parts and infusing the protein-rich portion into the veins to maintain circulation. Its development relied on research funded by the federal government but carried out in academia, an innovative arrangement that came to characterize scientific innovation in World War II.[17]

While touted as efficient replacements, plasma and albumin could not transport oxygen and as such failed to resuscitate the wounded effectively.[18] "Whole blood was found to be an absolute necessity," remarked the commanding officer of the 33rd Field Hospital.[19] Edward D. Churchill, chair of surgery at Massachusetts General Hospital and theater consultant (whose implementation of rectangular residencies was discussed in the previous chapter), led the effort to switch from plasma to whole blood.[20] When the military proved recalcitrant to change, Churchill went public with his protests to the *New York Times*.[21] Shortly thereafter, the US Army affirmed its commitment to whole blood transfusion and began procuring the necessary equipment.

Hospitals in North Africa, lacking established blood banks, began collecting the life-sustaining liquid from anyone available. "We bled our [own] personnel and the lightly wounded," recalled the chief of the 3rd Auxiliary Surgery Group.[22] In acquiring donations, one physician attached to the 8th Evac insisted, "whiskey of the American variety played a most important part" as medical officers resorted to bribing reluctant soldiers for a pint.[23] By spring of 1944, the American army created specific units to collect blood from soldiers to supply the field and evacuation hospitals.[24] These units drew blood from whomever they could, leading the chief surgeon to issue an official order forbidding front-line combatants from donating.[25] Similar efforts transpired in the European and Pacific campaigns.[26]

The volume of casualties in both the Pacific and Europe required more blood than local units could provide. A tremendous national effort ensued that relied upon Charles Drew's concept of banking. The American Red Cross collected blood in the United States, designed refrigerated transportation systems, and delivered it abroad.[27] By the end of the war, roughly 388,000 units of blood were shipped overseas, enabling the successful resuscitation of wounded soldiers and providing opportunities for surgeons to attempt elaborate and complex procedures, including those on blood vessels.[28] Furthermore, the regular use of local blood banks provided a safety net during cases that risked substantial blood loss, like vascular operations. Arterial anastomosis, which had permitted some of the earliest trials of blood transfusion by George Crile, now relied on this same technology to facilitate its regular integration into military medicine.

If blood aided patients through the surgery, then antibiotics helped keep them alive postoperatively by preventing infections. Initially, military doctors turned to sulfas.[29] Gerhard Domagk discovered the basic mechanism behind the pharmaceutical in 1932, published his results in 1935, and received a Nobel Prize in 1939. Physician scientists in France, England, and the United States quickly began experimenting with and using various formulations of the drug, which effectively treated pneumonia, gonorrhea, meningitis, bacillary dysentery, and hemolytic streptococcal infections, all diseases that had previously devastated armies but had comparatively little effect on American troops in World War II because of sulfanilamide and sulfadiazine. From Pearl Harbor onward, the US military advocated for both the topical and oral administration of sulfas to combat casualties, although by 1943 studies began to question their efficacy in treating war wounds.

The success of sulfas created a chemotherapeutic culture of practice that encouraged the use of the even more effective drug, penicillin. Discovered fortuitously by Alexander Fleming in 1928, the penicillin mold languished in laboratories around the world for much of the next decade.[30] Chemists Ernst Chain and Norman Heatley, working with pathologist Howard Florey, determined how to isolate the active ingredient in the late 1930s, and the drug cured laboratory mice for the first time just as Hitler conquered France. Florey and Heatley turned to the United States to mass-produce the drug; the surface fermentation methods employed in England required more bedpans than the country could spare. Twenty American pharmaceutical companies collaborated, sharing information and ideas in unprecedented (and unrepeated) cooperation that epitomized the federal-private-academic research enterprise characteristic of World War II. They eventually established a process of deep fermentation that allowed for mass production. Penicillin, which in 1943 cost $9,000 per ounce (250 times the price of gold), became widely available by 1944.[31] The US Army recognized the need to educate its medical corps officers about this novel pharmaceutical and initiated courses to familiarize them with the new drug.[32] By February 1944, the abundance of penicillin allowed authorities to recommend its liberal use in the wounded, and medical officers rapidly took advantage of the perceived panacea for their patients, many of whom had suffered wounds to the vascular system.[33]

Penicillin benefited these patients in multiple ways. Certainly, it treated postoperative infections, curing otherwise moribund soldiers. This application proved particularly valuable in vascular cases where infected blood clots—which existing sulfa drugs could not address—threatened limbs. But by 1945 doctors also used penicillin prophylactically, administering it to the wounded whom they thought were likely to develop an infection. This strategy had the greatest potential to facilitate arterial repair because it allowed surgeons to debride less tissue, confident that penicillin would eradicate the bacteria their scalpels missed. Vessels that World War I surgeons would have extirpated to eliminate the risk of infection now remained in situ for surgeons to repair.

Prewar Plans for Vascular Surgery in World War II

The delayed entrance of the United States into World War II enabled the Army Medical Department's planners to coordinate and execute an educational program to teach inexperienced physicians how to care for the combat wounded, including those with vascular injuries. The National Research Council published a series of military surgical manuals to instruct civilian physicians about topics specific to military medicine, with the fifth volume covering the vascular system.[34] Authors included Arthur Allen, Gezá de Takats, and Daniel C. Elkin, three nationally known academic surgeons who had dedicated their careers to studying vascular disease. Other prominent surgeons including Emile Holman, Halsted's last resident and chair of the surgery department at Stanford, published articles in the medical literature such as "War Injuries to Arteries and Their Treatment" to serve as primers for medical officers perhaps unaccustomed to managing vascular trauma.[35] Some personnel had the opportunity to participate in refresher courses with sessions dedicated to this subject, such as the one at Tulane University taught by Rudolph Matas, although most classes were discontinued by the fall of 1943, when the majority of surgeons had already deployed.[36] Importantly, even though these fora carried the imprimatur of the military, the content and instruction came from civilian academicians, not career military physicians. While this arrangement had the benefit of providing young surgeons with the latest recommendations from true experts in the field, it also came with the limitation of a civilian perspective on wartime pathology.

These publications and classes continually emphasized ligation, often providing detailed, step-by-step instructions and anatomical illustrations to teach neophyte doctors.[37] The military officially ordered its practitioners to tie off damaged arteries in Surgeon General's Office Circular Letter 178 of 1943, later reinforced by War Department Technical Bulletin Medical 147 of 1945.[38] In keeping with doctrine established in the First World War, most sources advised ligating the corresponding vein, too, followed by a sympathectomy.[39] If publications mentioned arterial repair at all, they cautioned against its perceived perils and recommended surgeons rarely perform the procedure.[40] Instructional material stressed the importance of using the drug heparin to prevent blood clots from forming in the vessels.[41] Prescriptions for postoperative care focused on maximizing blood flow to an extremity post-ligation by prohibiting smoking, ensuring appropriate temperature control, and, in some cases, advocating alcohol consumption (alcohol dilates blood vessels). Specific protocols varied greatly. This education continued throughout the war in the form of official circulars and medical conferences reminding uniformed doctors of appropriate treatment and instructing them in new guidelines.[42] Less officially, senior academic surgeons served as consultants who, while outside the formal chain of command, would tour military hospitals teaching the young physicians.[43] These circulars and consultants continued to recommend ligation.

The sources deemphasized arterial repair for several reasons. Eminent surgeons questioned whether an average operator on the battlefield could perform a Carrel-style anastomosis. Publications noted the likely long delay between wounding and the operating table, potentially precluding any benefit to restoring circulation. Authors feared presumed complications of arterial repair, like the stitches falling apart and resulting in severe bleeding, aneurysms forming at a weakened suture line, or clots propagating up the vessel. But, most importantly, they genuinely believed that ligation combined with sympathectomy was not only sufficient but actually the preferred choice given its simplicity, speed, efficacy at staunching bleeding, and acceptably low risk of limb loss, as documented in the surgical literature of the 1920s and 1930s. Based on these civilian-generated data, prewar predictions of amputation rates following ligation and sympathectomy appeared acceptably—and later embarrassingly—low (see table 3.1).

The Practice of Vascular Surgery in World War II

Injuries to the vascular system constituted approximately 1 percent of total wounds—a figure that assuredly underestimated the true incidence.[44] This 1 percent reflected only trauma to arteries in the extremities, where they were responsible for at least one out of every five amputations. When reported, trauma to intra-abdominal arteries had extremely high mortality rates.[45] A 1946 article documented almost 2,500 vascular injuries. Vessels most commonly wounded included the brachial (24 percent of all arterial injuries), femoral (21 percent), popliteal (20 percent), and tibial (20 percent) arteries.[46]

Combat medics served as first responders and had received specific training that focused on controlling bleeding.[47] Manuals stressed applying direct pressure, recommending tourniquets only as a last resort. Stretcher bearers carried the wounded men to the nearest battalion aid station that, while normally staffed by a physician, stabilized casualties but rarely provided definitive treatment. Patients were evacuated to the rear, with 10 to 20 percent of the most severely wounded proceeding immediately to surgery at a field hospital, usually located five to ten miles behind the front lines. The remainder continued farther back to a larger evacuation hospital where they either recovered and returned to their units or required transport back to the United States.[48] Most vascular surgery occurred at field and evacuation hospitals. Because of the island-hopping nature of fighting in the Pacific, this echeloning of care proved impossible and led to specific constraints on the practice of vascular surgery.[49]

Surgeons in World War II largely followed the directions of the military medical manuals and ligated vascular wounds. For example, the 3rd Army suffered 362 cases of arterial injuries fighting in Europe from August through November of 1944; surgeons tied off 346 (96 percent) of them.[50] Data from the Surgeon General's Office revealed 1,639 ligations in 1,774 vascular injuries (92 percent) in Europe and North Africa.[51] Data from the Pacific theaters, while more scattered, report an even greater reliance on ligation.[52] Sources across the war confirm these trends.[53] With the more limited debridement penicillin permitted, surgeons could ligate vessels closer to the site of trauma, preserving not only more of the main artery but also the collateral branches deliquescing from it.[54] Limbs, or at least longer stumps, thus had a greater chance of survival. However, compared to civilian cases, the gross trauma inherent in war wounds frequently destroyed collateral circulation as well as the main arterial channel, dooming chances for recovery.[55] This pathology proved especially true for landmine injuries, which, largely absent from the World War I battlefields, now notoriously mangled lower extremities and their blood supply.[56]

Surgeons continued to ligate the concomitant vein in an effort to preserve limbs. Although most manuals and directives issued to military surgeons recommended this procedure, the frequency of its application remains difficult to determine. Some surgeons reported taking the vein in almost every operation.[57] Others never did.[58] Over the course of the war, evidence mounted against its efficacy.[59] "Surgeons who have had experience with this procedure," noted the surgeon general's annual report in 1945, "have observed no beneficial effects from its performance."[60] An Inter-Allied Medical Conference in the European theater in December 1944 concluded that simultaneous venous ligation did not prove beneficial and ought not to be done.[61] Conferences like this one mirrored similar symposia in World War I and brought together military medical leaders from multiple nations to discuss current modes of treatment along with means to improve them.[62] They represented professional and institutional commitment to real-time reforms in patient care and, in this case, the ongoing, high-level interest in vascular surgery. However, front-line surgeons continued doing what they believed best treated their patients, highlighting their practical autonomy from command interference.

The use of sympathectomy similarly reflected the individualized practice of a procedure that came under increasing clinical suspicion during the war. The therapy received strong recommendations in the prewar literature as well as publications issued during the conflict, and doctors applied it to most of their vascular patients.[63] The 95th Evacuation Hospital reported performing sympathetic blocks in "nearly most every" case.[64] In their 487 vascular cases, the 3rd Auxiliary Surgical Group applied sympathetic blocks in 340 (70 percent), and in 94 percent of their ligations.[65] The Inter-Allied Surgery Conference continued to call for "more general use . . . of sympathetic blocks in an attempt to improve collateral circulation," demonstrating its perceived effectiveness.[66] Surgeons predominantly relied on chemical injections (Novocain) rather than an operation to interrupt the sympathetic ganglions, minimizing the risks to the patient through an easier, less invasive intervention.

Not every surgeon remained convinced of the ability of sympathectomy to stave off amputation. "We used Novocain sympathetic block only a few times," recalled the chief of surgery at the 4th General Hospital in Melbourne; "the results were equivocal."[67] On the other side of the world, the 9th Evacuation Hospital used Novocain regularly in the eighty-eight vascular injuries it reported in Africa and Europe, but its "observations and experiences cannot prove that this treatment has in any way influenced the outcome."[68] Several large, retrospective case series also did not show significant benefit or harm from the practice.[69] Sympathectomy worked by dilating collateral arteries; when enemy munitions, particularly landmines and other explosive ordnance, shredded those vessels, the intervention failed. Despite the statistical ambivalence, most American surgeons remained convinced of the importance of the technique and regularly credited sympathectomy for saving limbs.[70]

Physicians in World War II relied on other interwar inventions like arteriograms and heparin far less frequently. While front-line hospitals had X-ray equipment readily available, physicians did not perform arteriography. It is not clear whether they lacked access to contrast agents, worried about possible side effects, had no time to utilize them in the rush of casualties following a battle, or doubted its utility. Given the standard treatment of ligation, the few clinicians who tried arteriography found it was not helpful in guiding therapy or predicting outcomes.[71]

Heparin similarly went unused, despite it being widely known and strongly recommended in articles and instructions issued to military medical officers before the war.[72] Some units complained about the unavailability of the drug.[73] Others felt uncomfortable prescribing it in forward areas where it proved challenging to check labs regularly or observe patients continuously.[74] Serving as director of the Surgical Consultants Division of the Office of the Surgeon General, Michael E. DeBakey came to oppose the wartime use of heparin.[75] He maintained that it was too risky to prescribe anticoagulant medication in war wounded whose greatest peril was bleeding to death. As a result of DeBakey's opposition, surgical consultants restricted the delivery of heparin only to those hospitals with personnel familiar with its use, significantly limiting its distribution and utilization.[76]

Not yet a household name or even a senior figure in the surgery world, DeBakey relied on his position in the Office of the Surgeon General to influence American military practice. Born in 1908, DeBakey grew up in Louisiana as the son of Lebanese immigrants and completed both undergraduate and medical school at Tulane in New Orleans, Louisiana. Despite lacking a formal residency, he was unusually well trained for his era, particularly in the management of vascular disease, studying under Rudolf Matas and Alton Ochsner in the United States as well as René Leriche, Martin Kirschner, João Cid dos Santos, and Jean Kunlin in Europe. DeBakey would assume a towering position in American surgery over the second half of the twentieth century, leading Baylor College of Medicine to become an international center for cardiovascular research and care, appearing on the cover of *Time* magazine, and receiving an abundance of encomia including the Lasker Award, the Presidential Medal of Freedom, and, in recognition of his global reputation, the USSR's Academy of Science Jubilee Medal.[77] But during the Second World War, he as yet lacked this stature.

Instead, without issuing direct orders, DeBakey leveraged the authority of the Surgeon General's Office to convince officers more senior than he of the dangers of heparin. Many front-line practitioners lacked access to journals and colleagues, much less their own laboratories, cutting them off from traditional sources of information and verification. The Surgeon General's Office became the official conduit, digesting periodical literature and scientific investigations to produce reports and issue opinions about new discoveries and their proper use. This process undeniably added an additional filter of expert interpretation, but the advantage of a standardized approach to casualty care appealed to military medical leaders like DeBakey. Second, his role required him to travel extensively around Europe, where he developed personal relationships with many American surgeons. These connections not only helped DeBakey promulgate his ideas about heparin and sympathectomy but also centered him in a professional network that took on increased importance in later years.

Despite prewar optimism for ligation, sympathectomy, and (the rarely used) heparin, this triple therapy resulted in an unexpectedly high percentage of amputations. Prior to the war, vascular leaders like Danial Elkin

Table 3.1. Table comparing the predicted with actual amputation rates by artery, demonstrating markedly more amputations than had been anticipated and exposing the failure of ligation + sympathectomy to manage vascular trauma in World War II.

Artery	Expected Amputation Rate[1]	Actual Amputation Rate[2]
Internal Carotid[3]	30%	30%
Subclavian	9%	29%
Axillary	9%	43%
Brachial	3%	27%
Common Iliac	50%	53%
External Iliac	13%	47%
Common Femoral	21%	81%
Superficial Femoral	10%	55%
Popliteal	0%[4]	73%
Anterior Tibial	3%	9%
Posterior Tibial	3%	14%

Notes:

[1] *Burns, Shock, Wound Healing, and Vascular Injuries*, 211.

[2] DeBakey and Simeone, "Acute Battle-Incurred Arterial Injuries," 69. These data also include results from the eighty-one repaired arteries, so the actual percentages for amputation following ligation would be slightly higher.

[3] "Amputation" following ligation of the carotid artery refers to severe and irreversible neurologic damage.

[4] This is so far-fetched that presumably it was a typo or oversight, although the manual spelled out "none" rather than using arabic numerals so the mistake was larger than just dropping a digit.

and Gezá de Takats had anticipated relatively little limb loss following this therapy, based on their civilian experience.[78] They were wrong. Table 3.1 shows that the actual rate of amputation far exceeded the prediction for every single artery, sometimes by as much as fivefold. In the 2,471 vascular wounds DeBakey and his junior colleague Fiorindo Simeone cataloged, fully 40 percent—or 995 arms and legs—required amputation; other studies suggested similar or higher percentages.[79] That the military tracked amputations following vascular injury distinguished the Second World War from the First, when only life or death was recorded. This difference between the wars reflected the increasing expectation of saving both life and limb by the 1940s. The dissonance between expectations and what actually transpired partly resulted from the attempt to apply civilian experience to a military environment. Ligations in civilian practice often treated vascular disease like aneurysms, which allowed the body years to develop a robust collateral circulation to supply vital oxygen and nutrients to the extremities. Instantaneous wartime trauma provided no such luxury, and healthy young males had minimal preexisting collaterals. Vascular trauma certainly afflicted civilians' arteries as well, but the knives or low velocity gunshots typical in urban violence rarely interrupted more than a single artery, leaving extant collateral circulation in place. Military trauma—high explosives, blast injuries, shell fragments—often annihilated all arteries such that ligation frequently led to limb loss. The excessively high amputation rate following ligation led to the deployment of a novel technology to restore the continuity of severed vessels.

The Office of the Surgeon General introduced a new tool in World War II designed to facilitate the repair of arteries and enable average operators to practice advanced vascular surgery. Arthur H. Blakemore and Jere W. Lord devised a prosthetic device to anastomose arteries without technically demanding suturing. Blakemore, a Johns Hopkins medical graduate who assembled his surgery training at Hopkins, Henry Ford Hospital in Detroit, and Roosevelt Hospital in New York, focused his research on vascular operations as a professor at Columbia Presbyterian Medical Center.[80] In reading the literature from the First World War, Blakemore noted the high amputation rate and recognized the effect losing limbs had not only on the individual but also to the society responsible for supporting the disabled.[81] He conceded the inevitability of many of these amputations in World War I but believed that modern medicine combined with careful surgical debridement would alter the calculus. "We are now compelled to recognize them [amputations] for what they actually are, namely, a problem in vascular surgery," wrote Blakemore in 1942.[82] His collaborator, Lord, earned his MD from Johns Hopkins before completing a surgical residency at Cornell in the 1930s and securing a faculty position at New York University Hospital.[83] Together in New York City, the pair developed the Lord-Blakemore tube to solve the problem of amputation resulting from vascular insufficiency.

They worked to devise a method that linked severed arteries via tension-free vein grafts but did not require time-consuming, intricate suturing.[84] The invention involved taking a segment of a wounded soldier's vein, inserting it through a Vitallium alloy tube, and using that construction to bridge gaps in damaged arteries (figure 3.1). Although this technique clearly derived from early prosthetic anastomosis devices like Abbe's glass, Payr's magnesium, and Tuffier's silver tubes, it had the significant advantage of creating a span totally lined by intima, theoretically lessening the incidence of thrombosis.[85]

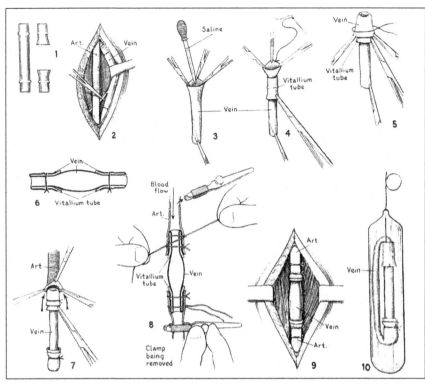

Figure 3.1. 1945 depiction of application Lord-Blakemore tubes. The precise method underwent several minor variations among their publications. (1) Two variants of the tubes for a short or long graft. (2–3) Harvesting and preparing the vein. (4) Pulling the harvested vein through the tube. (5) Wrapping the end of the vein around the tube to ensure intima-intima connections; surgeons complained this step was the most time consuming and frustrating. (6) The Vitallium vein prosthetic graft ready to implant. (7) Inserting the cuffed end of the prosthesis into the end of an artery. (8) Securing the prosthesis in place with a simple loop tie around its end. (9) The completed procedure. (10) Pre-prepared prostheses preserved in vacuum tube to distribute to forward surgeons (no evidence of their actual distribution exists). Blakemore and Lord, "A Nonsuture Method of Blood Vessel Anastomosis," *JAMA*, see 686 for diagram. Copyright © American Medical Association. All rights reserved. Reproduced with permission.

A variety of experiments in laboratory animals proved its efficacy, and later trials successfully demonstrated its use in civilian patients.[86]

Blakemore and Lord emphasized the expediency and ease of the technique when advocating for its use in war. Instead of lengthy, intricate suturing, surgeons just inserted the vein-covered Vitallium tube into the end of the torn artery and looped a single thread around the overlap to secure it in place. "The method is so simple," Blakemore and Lord wrote, "that it has proven within the realm of successful accomplishment by third-year medical students."[87] They believed even "the average operator" could complete the procedure in fifteen minutes by relying on prefabricated, freeze-dried prostheses stored in vessel banks.[88] They made these claims, however, before the technology ever went to war.

Blakemore-Lord tubes failed in combat. Surgeons generally acknowledged knowing about the technique, and the 3rd Army even distributed Blakemore and Lord's publications to all hospitals, but the tubes themselves remained quite rare.[89] There is limited evidence of their use in the Pacific theaters and only about forty documented implantations in the North African, Mediterranean, and European theaters combined.[90] Their two advantages—simplicity and speed—proved overoptimistic. In a 1944 conference between British and American military medical leaders, every single participant criticized the technical difficulty of the method.[91] Simeone, who amassed prodigious experience sewing arteries in the war, averaged 2.9 hours per case over a series of thirteen operations with the Blakemore-Lord tube, longer than a suture anastomosis would require.[92]

When surgeons did use the new technology, it failed to prevent amputation. The residency-trained Simeone tried applying Lord-Blakemore tubes thirteen times in Italy; eight (61 percent) of those soldiers lost their legs. Doctors in Europe using the tubes at the 9th Evacuation Hospital (50 percent amputation rate) and in the 3rd Army (63 percent) met similar results.[93] The likelihood of limb loss in these series exceeded the risks of ligation while requiring significantly more time and resources. Other vascular prostheses made from glass and plastic fared similarly.[94] While the Lord-Blakemore Vitallium tubes featured prominently in the medical literature and conferences of World War II, its rare use, technical challenges, and poor outcomes rendered it irrelevant to military medicine. Tellingly, despite its limited distribution, no American military hospitals requested additional tubes.[95] Publications on the technology ceased after World War II, and it never gained traction in the civilian surgery community. Its failure demonstrated the broader inadequacy of shortcuts for vascular anastomosis.

The Shift to Arterial Repair, 1945

While most surgeons deploying to Europe or the Mediterranean were aware of the possibility of repairing arteries, few doctors attempted the procedure before 1945. Of the 362 vascular injuries in the 3rd Army marching across France in 1944, surgeons attempted only sixteen repairs (4.4 percent), ten of which failed and required amputation.[96] DeBakey and Simeone's report, which largely reflects casualties in North Africa and the Mediterranean, identified only eighty-one instances of arterial suture in 2,471 cases, or a 3.3 percent repair rate; all but three were simple arteriorrhaphy; none involved venous autografts.[97] Individual experiences confirmed these trends.

By 1945, practice began to change, and surgeons repaired arteries more often. Three main reasons explain the shift. First, by 1945, the military environment in the European and Mediterranean theaters of operations improved as the Allies fought a different style of war. The Battle of the Bulge was the last offensive gasp from the Wehrmacht, and Germany's defeat meant final victory in Europe became a question no longer of if but of when.[98] Huge battles with thousands of simultaneous casualties ceased: the rate of wounded soldiers per day fell threefold from 1944 to 1945 in both the 1st and 3rd Armies.[99] As such, triage became less relevant, and surgeons had most time to focus on individual patients. A surfeit of supplies accumulated as lines stabilized. Hospitals became fixed facilities that featured more advanced technology. With control of the skies enabling free daytime movement behind the lines via both truck and airplane ambulances, hospitals could support each other, transferring patients or personnel to accommodate local needs. The entire military evacuation network developed into a robust, efficient infrastructure that rapidly transported wounded soldiers to appropriate facilities. Feelings of confidence and security among troops—medical and otherwise—grew with victory in sight, an attitude that encouraged bold innovation. This scenario contrasted sharply with the Pacific theaters where the archipelagic nature of the campaigns and the vast distances involved led to tenuous supply chains, prolonged evacuation times, delayed care, and obstacles to networking among medical units. The lack of a contemporaneous transition to repairing arteries in the Pacific despite nearly identical patients, pathologies, practitioners, and technology reinforces the importance of the particular environment of war in determining patient care.[100]

Second, by 1945 surgeons had more experience. In a few months of combat, they had treated more vascular trauma than they would manage over decades in their civilian practices. Surgery, a manual skill, improves with repetition.[101] Months of operating on wounded soldiers made practitioners more adroit, evident not just in the increased proportion of arterial repair but also in improvement in other areas, like thoracic surgery.[102]

Third, surgeons grew disgusted with consistently abysmal rates of amputation following ligation. "In spite of the well-known poor results reported following vascular suture and anastomosis," reported one team in 1945, "we elected to try it in preference to the seemingly invariably disastrous ligation."[103] The same volume that empowered surgeons with greater skills and knowledge simultaneously demonstrated the repeated consequences of ligation. In a report to the theater surgeon, Simeone found "the poor results when lacerated major arteries were ligated led surgeons in forward areas to suture lacerations of the vessels whenever possible."[104] Granted tremendous practical autonomy and freedom from regulatory oversight, surgeons began attempting this new procedure. One evacuation hospital in Europe, for example, "distressed" over the high amputation rates following ligation, transitioned from tying off 100 percent of its damaged arteries in 1944 to repairing 23 percent in 1945.[105] Surgeons in the 3rd Army "were thoroughly indoctrinated with the importance of attempting repair of major vascular injuries" by 1945.[106] Not every unit met with success, but most hospitals at least tried suturing arteries before the end of war.[107]

The auxiliary surgical groups exhibited the most pronounced shift towards arterial repair due to the quality of their personnel and their extensive experience. The army formed the aux groups to push advanced surgery forward on the battlefield, effectively creating medical "fire brigades" of unusually well-trained surgeons that traveled to wherever casualties were heaviest.[108] Five aux groups operated in roughly fifty teams each, consisting of a surgeon, assistant surgeon, anesthetist, and a few enlisted men. Leaders of the groups handpicked team members, who often came from university departments, had completed some form of graduate surgical education, and were generally more skilled than the average military medical officer in World War II. Designed to function at the level of field hospitals, teams moved from unit to unit, operating on the recently wounded but leaving postoperative and nursing care to regular field hospital staff. In this peripatetic existence, they amassed voluminous experience; teams belonging to the 3rd Aux logged an average of 814 cases in the ten-month European campaign alone (for comparison, modern surgery residents must complete 850 cases over five years to graduate).[109]

In 1945, they put that skill and experience to use repairing arteries. Out of 220 documented vascular injuries seen by 2nd Aux teams, surgeons repaired twenty, or 9 percent.[110] The 3rd Aux was even more ambitious. From D-Day to December 1944, their groups repaired a trifling fifteen arteries, but, disgusted with the high rate of amputation that followed ligation, 3rd Aux surgeons repaired 107 out of 487 (22 percent) of their vascular cases between December 1944 and VE Day.[111] These 107 repairs the 3rd Aux alone performed exceeded the total number (81) of repairs DeBakey cites for the entire war, demonstrating both the shift to arterial repair in 1945 and the failure of DeBakey and Simeone's study to capture the transition.

Sewing arteries together demonstrably saved limbs. The 50 percent amputation rate following ligation dropped to 35 percent when surgeons repaired arteries, according to DeBakey and Simeone's data.[112] The 2nd Aux doctors demonstrated even greater success, nearly halving their amputation rate (44 to 25 percent) when they anastomosed or sutured vessels.[113] The difference allowed hundreds of men to return home with arms and legs intact and thus avoid the challenges associated with disability in mid-twentieth-century America.[114] Certainly, these numbers reflect a selection bias, with surgeons choosing ligation in more complicated cases.[115] Furthermore, while the record clearly demonstrates a turn toward fixing arteries in the latter months of the war, ligation remained predominate. Even the 3rd Aux, which had the highest repair rate in the records (22 percent), still tied off the majority of damaged arteries. Nonetheless, a clear change of practice transpired as surgeons in Europe and Italy came to recognize the inadequacy of ligation as well as the superiority of repair, and began suturing torn vessels in ever-increasing numbers.

Shift to Arterial Repair II:
Military Vascular Surgery in the Continental United States

The shift to arterial repair also occurred in stateside military hospitals. While front-line medical units cared for actively bleeding patients, trauma to blood vessels could also cause more chronic problems, specifically pseudoaneurysms and arteriovenous fistulae (abnormal connections between arteries and veins). Neither condition was imminently fatal, but both required surgical correction. The military ordered physicians to send these patients back to the United States where experts in vascular surgery could evaluate and ultimately treat them.[116] Most deployed surgeons welcomed the opportunity to transfer such cases, particularly the fistulae.[117] Over the course of the war, stateside military vascular centers treated 221 pseudoaneurysms and 593 arteriovenous fistulae—numbers that far exceeded any previous collection of these pathologies.[118]

Vascular centers were part of a larger hospital system designed to provide wounded soldiers with specialized care. The surgeon general established this network in 1943 to concentrate both matériel and especially personnel resources for specific injuries, like brain, spine, eye, and vascular pathologies. By 1945, fifty-eight specialty centers existed, comprising thirty-three thousand beds.[119] The hospitals not only delivered expert care to complicated patients but also provided an unprecedented concentration of case material that enabled research into otherwise uncommon diseases. Surgeons recognized the research potential of these centers. "The importance of being able to study a large series of vascular cases, heretofore never assembled at one place, even over life times of experience, was judged to be a rare opportunity," asserted a 1945 report, "not only in the care of wounded and injured soldiers but for the overall scientific knowledge of these conditions."[120]

The recently invented American C-54 four-engine transport plane permitted transoceanic carriage, a capability new to World War II that made these centers possible. Like blood transfusion, medical evacuation by airplane began in World War I on a small scale, but limited aeronautical technology bridled the ability of aircraft to serve as effective ambulances in the Great War. As more powerful aerial platforms emerged in the 1930s, long-distance transport by airplane became more feasible, as demonstrated by Nazi forces in the Spanish Civil War. Importantly, all patients received definitive surgical care in Europe or the Pacific; only then did they fly to America for specialized attention, usually just a few weeks after sustaining their injury. Technology permitting expeditious transport empowered surgeons in the United States to access patients at a speed unimaginable to First World War doctors, enabling prompt intervention by subject matter experts. By the end of the war, almost 1.2 million wounded Americans benefitted from aerial medical evacuation.[121]

Several vascular surgery centers existed during World War II, although no more than three at a given time. In the spring of 1943, War Department Memorandum 40–14–43 established the first two, at Letterman Army Hospital in San Francisco and Ashford General Hospital in White Sulphur Springs, West Virginia. Ashford Hospital, so named for the famous army sanitarian Bailey K. Ashford, took over the grounds of the luxurious Greenbrier Hotel and established a two-thousand-bed hospital, six hundred of which were reserved for vascular patients evacuated from the European and Mediterranean theaters. With three vascular surgery specialists, Ashford served as the prototype for the other centers.[122] The hospital at Letterman existed for only a few months before eventually moving to DeWitt General Hospital in Auburn, California, accepting casualties from the Pacific.[123] The third major vascular center was founded in May 1944 at Mayo General Hospital in Galesburg, Illinois, which at its peak incorporated more than seven hundred beds.[124]

The concentration of both esoteric physical tools and skilled personnel created facilities able to provide vascular care that exceeded the capability of most academic medical centers of the era. The hospitals accumulated highly specific equipment to aid diagnosis of vascular diseases, like oscillometers, plethysmographs, and precisely controlled temperature rooms that were unavailable to other medical units.[125] The leadership at these centers represented the elite of American vascular surgery in the 1940s. Daniel C. Elkin, at Ashford, earned his MD at Emory before completing a surgery residency at Brigham Hospital in Boston, where he trained under the pioneering cardiovascular surgeon Elliot Cutler. Before the war, Elkin chaired the Department of Surgery at Emory, where he became a national authority on vascular disease; after the war he served as the fourth president of the Society for Vascular Surgery.[126] Harris B. Shumacker Jr. completed medical school and internship at Johns Hopkins before finishing his residency at Yale. He returned to Hopkins to lead its nascent vascular division in the 1930s. After being medically evacuated from the Southwest Pacific theater, Shumacker took charge of the center at Mayo; he later became the thirteenth president of the Society for Vascular Surgery.[127] DeWitt Hospital had two chief surgeons over the course of the war. Ambrose H. Storck, who had trained under Rudolph Matas and Alton Ochsner in New Orleans, initially held the position. He was succeeded by Norman Freeman in 1944, who had completed residency with Isidor Ravdin in Philadelphia at the University of Pennsylvania Hospital before becoming one of the first surgeons in the United States to limit his practice to cardiovascular patients in the 1930s.[128]

Initially, physicians at these centers followed standard practice and ligated damaged blood vessels. Because surgeons like Elkin did not consider pseudoaneurysms or arteriovenous fistulae "emergency operations," they often waited three to four months for collateral circulation to develop before taking the patient to the operating room, hoping this delay would minimize the risk of subsequent amputation.[129] In 585 operations on arteriovenous fistulae in 1943 and 1944, surgeons ligated 551 (94 percent), repairing only thirty-four lesions of the femoral or popliteal arteries.[130] They similarly occluded the main artery of 99 percent of pseudoaneurysms, through either simple ligation or obliterative Matas operations.[131] Results proved unexpectedly disappointing.

While the delay-and-ligate strategy effectively treated pseudoaneurysms and fistulae and largely prevented amputation, it led to severe symptoms of vascular insufficiency. Patients complained of leg pain, temperature sensitivity, and an inability to walk such that, though retaining their physical extremities, they became de facto disabled—just like Marvin Rynar from 1909. Objective laboratory tests substantiated the significantly diminished blood flow to arms and legs.[132] These outcomes surprised the surgeons. General medical consensus before the war held that collateral circulation enabled most patients to regain normal function following ligation. It was only with the concentration of hundreds of cases, made possible by war trauma and the specialized centers, that physicians both recognized and amassed convincing evidence to prove that vascular insufficiency following delayed ligation was not an exception but rather the rule. This observation represented a major shift in the understanding of vascular disease and its treatment. It also highlighted the perils of relying on personal experience and a small sample size to draw general conclusions.

The realization prompted surgeons to revolutionize their practice. For centuries—ever since John Hunter—surgeons had been ecstatic to save a patient's limb. Now, in 1945, this result was no longer good enough. Developments in medicine and surgery advanced the goal of vascular intervention from saving an arm or a leg to preserving a healthy, functioning extremity. Accomplishing that goal necessitated arterial repair. Shumacker and Freeman both believed their facilities could accomplish this restorative objective and began suturing arteries in 1945. At Mayo General Hospital repairs consisted of only 3 percent (4/138) of operations in the last few months of 1944, but, after recognizing their potential, Shumacker "decided that repair would be carried out in every instance in which it could possibly be performed" and sutured 53 percent (30/57) thereafter; at DeWitt, 34 percent (23/67) patients received reparative surgeries between June and November 1945.[133] Freeman had 18 successes in these 23 attempts, relying chiefly on primary arteriorrhaphy (including one remarkable case on the aorta) and a single end-to-end anastomosis. Shumaker's group was more aggressive, employing ten end-to-end anastomoses (one failure) and six venous autografts (one failure).[134]

Like their brethren closer to combat, surgeons at these centers relied on penicillin to prevent and control infection. Mayo and especially DeWitt Hospital utilized arteriograms often to identify the specific pathology and to confirm the success of their operations (figure 3.2).[135] Heparin proved even more important for patent repairs at Mayo and Dewitt.[136] "The success with which restoration of arteries and veins can be accomplished with the use of anti-coagulants has been striking," as Storck observed heparin keeping anastomoses open and free from clot without evidence of massive bleeding, the feared side effect of the drug.[137] Again much discussed, the effects of sympathectomy remained equivocal.[138]

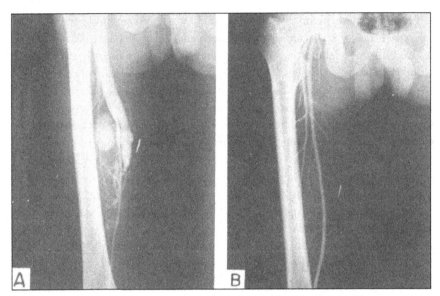

Figure 3.2. The successful repair of an arteriovenous fistula portrayed by an arteriogram. Films show a patient's thigh, with the long, thick white line on the left
being the femur bone. (A) Film taken before the operation shows thickening of the
femoral vein (the shorter, thick white vertical line to the right of the femur) under
the high pressure of arterial flow and a false aneurysm (the egg-shaped structure
between the white lines). Note how the blood flow stops mid-thigh. (B) Film taken
after a reparative operation has a much thinner white line on the right, which
depicts blood and contrast flowing through the now mended femoral artery. On
both images, the small, short white line farthest right is a piece of shell fragment
remaining in the patient's thigh muscle. Storck, "Evaluation of the Vascular Status
in Traumatic and Nontraumatic Lesions of the Blood Vessels," 53.

Elkin at Ashford generally eschewed the new technologies of heparin and
arteriography while continuing to ligate patients' vessels because of his fear
of the possible complications of arterial suturing. "On theoretic grounds it
would seem best to repair the opening in both artery and vein," acknowledged Elkin, "but this is technically difficult and may result in secondary
hemorrhage, thrombosis, or recurrence."[139] These concerns from the chief
surgeon prevented any arteriorrhaphies at Ashford, despite its demograph-
ics, pathologies, and resources being identical to the two other facilities. The
absence of repairs highlights the inherent power of the military hierarchy
to shape clinical decisions. It stresses the importance of local context to the
diffusion of innovations, including surgical technique.[140] The persistence
of ligation also demonstrates the differences in practical autonomy between

the front lines, where individual surgeons could largely determine their own practice, and the home front, where they had to follow orders. Finally, the legitimate divergence of the hospitals leaders' choice of therapy exposes the contemporary uncertainty over the proper treatment for these patients.

Freeman and Shumacker ultimately proved Elkin's worries unfounded. The incidence of hemorrhage and infections approached zero, and the feared propagation of thrombus throughout an artery never materialized. New aneurysms did not form at the allegedly weakened suture lines. Surgeons could reach these definitive conclusions only because the war had concentrated scores of patients with repaired arteries at a few locations, providing a heretofore unique opportunity to study the consequences and implications of the operation. Importantly, patients experienced dramatic clinical improvement: those who underwent successful arterial repair consistently reported fewer symptoms of vascular insufficiency than did those patients who endured traditional ligation. Freeman and Shumacker came to favor reparative operations and emphatically urged their application whenever and wherever possible.[141]

The experiences at these stateside military vascular centers thus demonstrated the potential of vascular surgery when appropriately trained, adequately equipped surgeons managed patients under particular conditions. Specifically, under the leadership of young, residency-educated surgeons, arterial repair was demonstrably effective. And, importantly, it succeeded in large enough numbers of "average" cases to prove not just its feasibility but its superiority when compared to arterial ligation. This success echoed the accomplishments of the auxiliary surgery groups in Europe. The impact of these conclusions, however, was fleeting.

The Failure of Success

Janus-faced about their performance in World War II, surgeons at once complimented their management of vascular wounds while simultaneously regretting their inability to demonstrate significantly better outcomes than the British had achieved in the First World War. In a 1946 article, Charles Odom, who had served as command surgeon for General Patton's 3rd Army, defended his results against criticism of poor or inadequate operations while at the same time concluding that "continued emphasis should be placed on vascular surgery, in order to bring this field abreast of other surgical specialties."[142] Odom and others clearly recognized the potential of arterial repair to save limbs and at least partially lamented their inability to effect it more widely.

Several factors prevented anastomosis from becoming more common in the Second World War. Again, the constant mobility of hospital units presented obstacles to the performance of advanced surgery; the synchronous success at US-based vascular centers highlights the importance of stability and resource concentration. As in World War I, military circumstances led to protracted delays between injury and definitive treatment. The longer the wait, the higher the risk of amputation, and even arterial repair could not save limbs following intervals of more than eight to ten hours.[143] No single source documents the average time between wounding and surgery. Individual units cited widely varying statistics, though most reported operating on the majority of patients within twelve hours of injury.[144] While undoubtedly shorter than the waits in the First World War, the delays certainly limited opportunities to repair arteries.

Furthermore, frontline military units had to triage their wounded, which presented challenges to the practice of time-consuming arterial repair. Large battles swamped medical units with casualties. For example, one evacuation hospital performed four thousand operations in the thirty-one days after D-Day.[145] Arterial repair inarguably took longer than simple ligation; one unit clocked repair operations requiring nearly four hours compared to sixty-two minutes for ligation.[146] Luther Wolff commanded a general surgical team in the 2nd Aux, which, toward the end of the war, received an assistant professor of surgery from a prestigious American university as a replacement for a departing surgeon. This professor began operating on a patient with an injury to the femoral artery, attempting to repair the injury via a saphenous vein graft. "Finally, after about three hours of this professor of surgery fooling around with the vein transplant, I had to order him to go ahead and ligate the artery, since it was so imperative that we get to the abdominal cases in the shortest possible time," wrote Wolff in his diary. "Theoretically, he was doing the proper thing, but from a practical standpoint . . . it was obviously not the time or place for this type of surgery."[147] Wolff went on to acknowledge the risk of amputation, but you could not sacrifice one soldier's life to save another's limb.

Moreover, unlike this professor in the aux group, most surgeons lacked any prewar experience suturing arteries together. While approved surgery residencies had begun to proliferate before World War II, they remained rare in the 1930s. The military recognized the paucity of well-trained surgeons, but it insisted on a ratio of 6.5 physicians (and 0.5 surgeons) for every 1,000 troops, citing the importance of having ample resources to treat casualties after a battle.[148] This proportion required almost 40 percent of practicing doctors in the United States to don a uniform, and it dramatically influenced medical education. Medical schools, traditionally four years long, shortened their curriculum to three years to graduate physicians more rapidly for the war effort.[149] Many of the faculty deployed overseas, depleting the teaching ranks and leaving those doctors who remained home overwhelmed with clinical responsibilities.

Postgraduate education also deteriorated.[150] It suffered from the same shortage of faculty, except unlike students, interns and residents had to help care for patients, sacrificing learning for service. For the first time since Halsted started his program at Johns Hopkins, the number of surgical residents in America decreased—by 45 percent.[151] Additionally, residencies shortened considerably as the military forced the acceptance of the 9–9–9 paradigm: All medical school graduates served a nine-month rotating internship, which included two months of surgery. Thereafter two-thirds deployed overseas, and one-third remained for another nine months of specialty training. After eighteen months, half of the remaining residents shipped overseas and half continued their graduate medical education. Of the roughly sixty thousand medical officers in World War II, approximately eighteen thousand came through this system, meaning twelve thousand doctors in World War II had only nine months of graduate training with two months of surgery.[152]

This arrangement did not create competent surgeons. While initially accepting the 9–9–9 plan as a military necessity, the American College of Surgeons came to believe it "seriously retarded education in the medical and surgical specialties."[153] Evarts Graham, who chaired the National Research Council's Committee on Surgery during the war, railed against the plan in both professional journals and lay publications like the *Saturday Evening Post*: "Shall we send our men into battle with Civil War muskets if the supply of modern firearms is deficient? Of course not. Anybody can see how ridiculous and murderous that would be," inveighed Graham. "But perhaps only doctors themselves can appreciate how murderous a half-baked medical officer can be."[154] This dissatisfaction extended to the front lines, where senior officers commented on the ineptness of young doctors. The chief of surgery at the 18th General Hospital begged his superiors to "try to supply more experienced surgeons at the front," complaining that the newly minted practitioners simply could not operate.[155] Other sources flat out criticized the recent graduates' lack of basic proficiency in such core disciplines as anatomy. "It was nothing unusual," remarked one senior physician, "to see an officer operating with an open textbook alongside the patient."[156] Ben Eisemen, who after the war introduced Goretex grafts into vascular surgery and chaired departments at Kentucky and Colorado, had participated in this expedited educational track: "When we went to war, hell, I hadn't done any operations at all!"[157] His first laparotomy was on a dog in medical school; his second, on a wounded soldier at Normandy.[158] Expecting surgeons with no training to perform technically advanced arterial repair was unrealistic.

Despite these challenges and limitations, both the aux groups on the frontlines and the vascular centers stateside had clearly and unequivocally proven that well-trained surgeons could repair arteries under combat conditions and achieve results superior to ligation, but these lessons were ignored in the postwar years because of the inaccurate conclusions of DeBakey and Simeone. Their landmark 1946 *Annals of Surgery* paper came to define vascular surgery in World War II; the literature cites it more than a thousand times as both doctors and historians have relied upon the data.[159] Initially, the publication established its authority partly from the personal relationships DeBakey cultivated during the war but mostly by its thorough, scientific portrayal of events. Featuring almost 2,500 cases, the article easily represents the broadest overview of the topic, with other accounts rarely eclipsing one hundred cases. With access to statistics from the Office of the Surgeon General, DeBakey and Simeone provide a detailed literature review before analyzing nearly every aspect of vascular trauma in the Second World War, including incidence, anatomic variability, and assessment of all known interventions. DeBakey's growing international reputation in the postwar years only further solidified the authority of this seemingly comprehensive article.

DeBakey and Simeone reached several important conclusions. First, surgeons repaired only a tiny fraction (3 percent) of vascular injuries. Furthermore, they noted that while 40 percent of patients lost their limbs, 60 percent kept their extremities, and these outcomes, while not ideal, were acceptable in wartime. Finally, they denied complex arterial repair a role in future military surgery. "It is clear," they wrote, "that no procedure other than ligation is applicable to the majority of vascular injuries which come under the military surgeon's observation."[160] They cited triage concerns, suboptimal operating conditions, and especially long lag times between wounding and surgery to justify this verdict. These findings became accepted as the true experience of vascular surgery in the Second World War.

While DeBakey and Simeone inarguably presented the largest collection of vascular cases in World War II, their article suffered some methodological flaws that influenced its conclusions and, ultimately, the future practice of vascular surgery. The text asserted that they analyzed 2,471 cases compiled piecemeal from various military units, but a close reading of the article and follow-up publication reveals that almost all statistics, graphs, and tables rely on a subset of 1,500 cases. These 1,500 derive directly from a report

Simeone authored during the war.[161] However, Simeone's report drew on the records of only four hospitals, all of which predominantly served in the North African and Mediterranean theaters, and he largely stopped collecting data in December 1944.[162] Thus, critically, the article completely missed the shift to repairing arteries in 1945.

The failure of the article to capture this transition hurt the future practice of vascular surgery. It inaccurately presented arterial repair as an experimental, unproven, and, in some cases, unjustifiable procedure while continuing to advocate for ligation. How a society or group remembers and understands the past often differs from actual events, and this divergence can have lasting effects.[163] In this unfortunate, archetypal case, DeBakey's authoritative article led to surgeons ligating vascular wounds for years to come, damning hundreds of patients to unnecessary amputations as a result of inaccurate history. It ultimately required the war in Korea to make adoption of arterial repair permanent.

Chapter Four

Reshaping Surgical Infrastructure between World War II and the Korean War

The end of World War II had proven arterial repair both feasible and, in most cases, a superior operation to ligation, but in the postwar years surgeons again returned to tying off blood vessels. With Carrel's technique well established, it required a series of scientific and professional developments to make the practice of vascular anastomosis widespread. In the short time between World War II and the Korean War, there were no technical advances, no neoteric diagnostic technology invented, and no novel instrumentation introduced. Rather, the supporting infrastructure around the practice of vascular surgery changed in four interrelated ways. First, rapid progress in heart surgery sparked additional research on related topics, particularly the preservation and use of blood vessels for grafts. Second, anesthesiology transitioned from a nurse-centric service to a physician-driven specialty that facilitated surgeons safely performing increasingly invasive operations, like those on large blood vessels. Third, the Society for Vascular Surgery, founded in 1947, created the space for the presentation and appreciation of research while fostering a sense of professional community. Finally and most importantly, residencies, which had educated only a select few doctors before the war, graduated into a standardized and ubiquitous route of surgical education, producing a cadre of well-trained operators. These four contextual changes all occurred outside the operating room but nonetheless proved crucial to the eventual adoption of arterial repair by creating a fertile milieu that enabled its rapid, broad use in the Korean War and the years thereafter.

Vascular Surgery Research between World War II and Korea: Cardiac Surgery and Vessel Banks

The paucity of arterial repair in World War II and the resulting high amputation rate following ligation disappointed many young surgeons who returned to the United States determined to establish reparative procedures. Allan Callow, who served as a battalion surgeon in the Pacific and landed on Tarawa with the third assault wave, recalled in a later interview, "Since I saw so many arms, legs, and lives lost in the war [from vascular trauma], I th[ought] I'd like to do something with arterial surgery."[1] Callow and fellow academic surgeons re-demonstrated the efficacy of arterial repair and further refined operative techniques.[2] Some researchers focused their attention on innovative material for grafts, looking to new synthetics like plastic and Lucite.[3] Most physicians investigating grafts, chastened by the failure of the Lord-Blakemore Vitallium tubes in World War II, retreated from artificial components and concentrated their efforts on biological products, taking tissue from humans. Surgeons fiercely debated between using patients' extra veins, which were readily available and remained alive but risked dilating under arterial pressure, and using preserved arteries from deceased donors, which were dead tissue, albeit physiologically homologous to the vessel being repaired.[4] Neither veins that came from the patient's own body nor cadaveric arteries posed risks of rejection that had doomed Carrel's earlier transplants.

Research in arterial repair expanded as a result of the war, but its clinical practice remained limited. Several small series of repairs appeared in the literature.[5] Michael DeBakey, a future leader of vascular surgery, performed 110 surgical operations from November 1948 through 1949; only two involved anastomosing blood vessels.[6] In all of 1946, surgeons at the prominent Massachusetts General Hospital repaired only a single artery: Claude Welch, another World War II surgeon distressed over the high amputation rates he witnessed in Italy, sutured the severed popliteal artery of a local football player, saving his leg.[7] DeBakey at Baylor and Welch at Massachusetts General represented the elite of American surgery; the infrequency of this operation by these surgeons signified its relative scarcity in hospital around the country where most doctors continued to resort to ligation.[8]

The sputtering practice of peripheral arterial repair contrasted with an explosive growth in heart surgery that stimulated research beneficial to both fields. In 1944 in Sweden, Clarence Crafoord bypassed an aortic coarctation (narrowing) with the subclavian artery, attracting international attention.[9] That same year, Alfred Blalock at Johns Hopkins performed the first "blue baby" operation to relieve the symptoms of tetralogy of Fallot, a complex congenital heart defect that his cardiologist colleague Helen Taussig was diagnosing in her pediatric patients. Unable to offer anything but palliative management for dying babies, Taussig discussed the possibility of a surgical treatment with Blalock. Again perfecting the procedure first on dogs, he ultimately anastomosed the subclavian artery to the pulmonary artery with the critical assistance of his African American laboratory technician, Vivian Thomas. This anatomical rearrangement bypassed the right heart and better oxygenated the blood. It is difficult to overstate the medical or social impact of this surgery. It certainly was the most famous operation of the decade and received widespread coverage both in the lay and medical press.[10] The success rapidly drew patients desperately needing the operation to Johns Hopkins (the alternative was death) as well as visiting surgeons hoping to learn the technique. It also spurred the innovation of new procedures for other heart conditions, many of which similarly relied on the fundamental technique of arterial repair.[11]

These new cardiovascular surgeries and the excitement surrounding them prompted further research on blood vessel grafts. While Crafoord's and Blalock's original procedures depended on end-to-end anastomosis, surgeons soon found that the ends of an artery were sometimes too far apart to pull into apposition. In these situations, the operations required a graft to bridge the gap. Veins, traditionally used in this role since Goyanes's and Lexer's ideal operation in 1906/7, provided an early answer, but the size mismatch between smaller veins and large arteries complicated the technique.[12] Heart surgeons turned their attention to arterial grafts.[13] Problematically, while veins can be harvested from the patient during the same operation, appropriately sized arteries had to come from cadavers—humans do not have large, lengthy arteries to spare. Thus, arterial grafts required hospitals to exert significant, systemic efforts to collect, catalog, and store them to ensure an adequate inventory for patients.

The increasing prevalence of cardiovascular surgery generated an escalating need for arterial graft material, which led to the establishment of vessel banks. The idea of storing blood vessels (and other body parts) for later use originated long before the 1940s: Alexis Carrel suggested the idea near the turn of the century, remarking that "it would be very convenient for the surgeon . . . to keep in store pieces of skin, periosteum, bone, cartilage, blood-vessels, omentum and fat, ready to be used."[14] Carrel and his former collaborator Charles Guthrie worked independently on preserving blood vessels and demonstrating the suitability of these stored grafts in vascular surgery.[15] They examined tissue culture and cryopreservation as two technologies to preserve organs.

Tissue culture involves the growth and replication of cells outside of the body, a field inaugurated in 1907 by Ross Harrison at Yale and made clinically practical by Carrel the following decade.[16] This modality had the advantage of keeping the tissue alive throughout the storage process but required exceedingly precise technique to execute successfully. The other option, cryopreservation, froze cells in a state of arrested animation, as recently detailed in Joanna Radin's book *Life on Ice*.[17] Carrel, again involved from the beginning, used his previous experience with tissue culture to assess the vitality of the tissue post-thawing and conducted a variety of experiments demonstrating that arteries did survive the freezing process and could be used as grafts.[18]

Although vessel preservation techniques were available by the 1910s, they had little clinical utility until the surgical advances of Blalock and Crafoord required the use of arterial grafts to repair heart defects. Leading pediatric surgeon Robert E. Gross particularly advocated for the use of preserved arteries over venous conduits. He specifically came to favor tissue-culture preserved vessels, believing the process of freezing destroyed the functionality of grafts.[19] Gross established his reputation in the 1930s by pioneering a new operation to ligate the ductus arteriosus, another congenital heart defect. Following Blalock's demonstration of the successful blue baby operation, Gross adopted it in Boston and rapidly accumulated nine successful tetralogy repairs using preserved arteries.[20] His prior reputation as a leader in pediatric cardiac surgery and his extensive, successful experience—more than most of his contemporaries—combined to create a voice of authority that shaped national practice in favor of tissue culture in the late 1940s.[21] However, this method presented severe logistical challenges: arteries lasted only six weeks, and, given the difficulties of obtaining consent from next of kin and harvesting fresh grafts sterilely within the necessary few hours postmortem, tissue banks never contained enough specimens. The expense of equipment and personnel also limited its applicability to only the best-funded institutions. More importantly, and partly in response to these limitations, a bevy of new studies countermanded Gross's original findings and proved the suitability of freeze-dried grafts.[22] As a result of these findings, artery banks based on cryopreservation began proliferating around the country.[23] These repositories facilitated vascular and cardiovascular surgery, not only helping patients through the provision of grafts but also exposing young trainees to both more operations and the opportunity to gain experience by harvesting the vessels.[24] Initially limited to academic institutions, citywide collectives formed in the early 1950s, allowing broader access to local hospitals. When surgeons returned from the Korean War technically prepared to start repairing arteries, the infrastructure for providing necessary grafts was ready and waiting for them.

The Development of Anesthesia

These new, complex cardiac surgeries, particularly on children, required advanced anesthesia care to keep patients alive throughout the operation. In the years following World War II, anesthesia moved from a nurse-driven aux-iliary service to a new medical specialty better prepared to support patients during invasive procedures. After its discovery in the mid-nineteenth cen-tury, the application of anesthesia diffused relatively rapidly throughout the United States; by the Civil War, surgeons used anesthesia in essentially all their cases.[25] The comparatively simple and relatively safe administration of ether, the drug of choice in America, enabled nonphysician practitioners to function as anesthetists. In the United States, nurses, medical students, and other ancillary personnel typically put patients to sleep.[26] Waking them up proved more challenging. Mayo Clinic anesthesiologist John S. Lundy, an early leader in the profession, recalled that, prior to World War II, "there was a tendency for only those physicians who were incompetent in general prac-tice or in other branches to limit themselves to the practice of anesthesia."[27] The quality of anesthesia care had direct and obvious influences on surgeons' ability to perform complicated operations safely.

Like surgery, the discipline of anesthesia had started to professionalize in the late 1930s.[28] The field was becoming more complex with the introduc-tion of new anesthetic drugs, advanced delivery devices, and more compli-cated modalities for controlling the airway.[29] Leaders in the field formed professional organizations such as the American Society of Anesthetists, rec-ognizing both the structural benefits of these societies as well as the need to produce highly trained clinicians.[30] By 1938, students sat for the first board exams in anesthesiology, paralleling the establishment of surgical boards (1937). In 1940, the discipline became an official section of the American Medical Association.[31]

These reforms occurred too late and involved too few doctors to affect care in World War II, where the almost amateur application of anesthesia hindered combat surgery.[32] While a few wartime practitioners had com-pleted formal postgraduate education in anesthesia, the majority had no background prior to donning a uniform. The army established six-week instructional programs (later twelve weeks) in an effort to teach general med-ical officers the basics of the practice.[33] Subsequently deemed some of the most effective medical trainings conducted by the military, the courses used didactic and hands-on lessons to explain the fundamentals of general and regional anesthesia.[34] Even with these classes, a severe shortage of personnel existed, and enlisted men often functioned as anesthetists.[35] In North Africa, 20 percent of so-called anesthetic specialists had no coursework in the discipline at all; a further 15 percent had fewer than three months of schooling.[36] Endotracheal intubation, the use of a flexible plastic tube to protect the airway while the patient is asleep, exposed the challenges of relying on minimally trained anesthetists: while intubation allows for definitive airway control, enabling deeper anesthesia and facilitating operations in the chest, only 3 percent of cases in the European theater were intubated due, in part, to amateur providers.[37]

World War II catalyzed the maturation of anesthesia from a craft into a profession.[38] The short training programs during the war imbued enthusiasm for the specialty, and almost 80 percent of their graduates sought formal education upon returning home, becoming full-fledged anesthesiologists.[39] The membership of the American Society of Anesthesiology expanded over 600 percent from 1940 to 1960; the number of residency spots increased tenfold during that time. Board certification more than tripled between 1945 and 1955. The field grew much faster than the rest of medicine: whereas there were fewer than five anesthesiologists per 1,000 physicians in 1940, by 1955 that proportion reached twenty-two per 1,000.[40] These numerous, better-educated anesthesia practitioners would provide superior care in the Korean War and beyond, again creating a clinical infrastructure to support more complex operations, like arterial repair.

Professional Home:
The Creation of the Society for Vascular Surgery

The network of vessel banks and the professionalization of anesthesia would assist surgeons repairing arteries in the operating room; the Society for Vascular Surgery provided them a forum to present, explore, discuss, and transmit research on these operations. In the nineteenth and early twentieth centuries, a variety of organizations like the American Surgical Association and American College of Surgeons formed to fill both professional and intellectual needs.[41] As general surgery research increasingly splintered into various subdisciplines—at least at the highest levels of the profession—practitioners sought spaces to discuss topics of special concern.[42] Functioning as communities of individuals sharing similar interests, societies served as vehicles to communicate new discoveries and enabled groups of surgeons to establish organizational identities that proved crucial to the professionalization of both surgical and medical specialties.[43]

The Society for Vascular Surgery (SVS) was formed in the years surrounding World War II.[44] By the late 1930s, pioneers like J. Ross Veal in Louisiana and George D. Lilly in Miami, Florida, recognized the potential advantages of an organization dedicated to the field. They sought a gathering of like-minded physicians with whom they could exchange ideas on how to advance the scientific understanding of vascular disease and its treatment; later, they sought to use this group to advocate for their professional interests as well. Veal started campaigning for an association in 1938, but the Second World War interrupted planning. After the war, Veal and other academic leaders moved quickly to establish the society, which held its first formal meeting on 8 June 1947. Thirty-one academic surgeons composed the charter membership; notably, only one dedicated his practice exclusively to vascular surgery.[45] The others worked as general surgeons with an interest in blood vessels, a practice model common for the era.

With an exclusively elite, academic membership, the organization worked hard to cater to general practitioners. The SVS intentionally scheduled its meetings to coincide with the annual AMA conference, the biggest medical event of the year. The AMA regularly drew tens of thousands of physicians and surgeons in the 1940s and 1950s. With weekend and evening presentations to encourage attendance around AMA sessions, the SVS wanted to educate nonspecialists about vascular surgery; it even hosted expert panels to which doctors could submit questions on vascular diseases and their treatment. More than five hundred general practitioners came to the initial SVS meeting, demonstrating a high level of interest in the nascent SVS and the field it represented.[46]

Over the next decade, the SVS formalized and expanded while simultaneously becoming more exclusive. At its initial meeting, the entire annual budget was the cost of lunch for the members, which treasurer Harris B. Shumacker collected by actually passing his hat around the table for contributions.[47] During the 1940s, members wrote and adopted bylaws and a constitution that articulated their mission statement. The society prioritized researching the science behind arterial and venous diseases, developing surgical therapies for these conditions, and providing continuing education in vascular surgery to specialists and nonspecialists alike. By 1952, SVS meetings separated from the AMA as the society turned increasingly internalist.

The programs of annual meeting clearly reflected these developments. Early papers focused on veins and often featured nonoperative management.

Varicose veins were a favorite topic, with an array of suggested treatments for specialists and generalists alike. There was not a single talk on peripheral arterial repair until 1949, and no presidential address touched on the subject until the ninth annual meeting in 1955.[48] These more advanced presentations also signaled a shift in intended audience, being clearly aimed at those dedicating their careers to the management of vascular disease. Still, arterial repair remained a rare subject until after the Korean War. When it did appear, the SVS had been meeting for a half dozen years and readily provided the professional infrastructure to share, discuss, and advocate for the operation.

The Making of the Modern Surgeon: The Proliferation and Standardization of the Residency Education System

Vessel banks, improved anesthesia, and new societies would matter little without surgeons capable of suturing arteries together. World War II catalyzed the rapid expansion of postgraduate training in the United States, transforming the profession and practice of surgery into a true specialty.[49] The war years themselves undermined residencies, shortening their length and compromising their quality through the 9–9–9 system. But the war experience simultaneously highlighted both the professional and clinical benefits of postgraduate education. The military recognized the superiority of board-certified practitioners, granting them higher rank, better pay, and more appealing assignments than generalists self-identifying as surgeons.[50] After the war, the federal government continued to demonstrate preference for board-certified physicians by awarding them salaries 25 percent greater than their nonboarded colleagues at federal facilities like Public Health and Veterans Administration (VA) hospitals.[51] These perquisites led to a rush of military medical veterans pursuing board certification—and the residency experience required therefore. A survey conducted by the American Medical Association revealed that 80 percent of uniformed doctors in World War II intended to pursue additional schooling after the war, with 63 percent planning on board certification. Using those survey results, the American College of Surgeons predicted ten thousand men would apply for a spot in a surgical residency; before the war, the college had approved only approximately six hundred positions per year.[52]

The critical role of the GI Bill for funding residency education in the 1950s reveals the importance of the US government in expanding these opportunities. Prior to federal support in the post–World War II era, hospitals provided surgical residents with room, board, and perhaps a pittance of a stipend.[53] When residency training became eligible for GI Bill funds—a freighted decision that officially declared it education, not on-the-job training—it provided the young housestaff with a reasonable salary and relieved hospitals of their financial responsibility to trainees.[54] These actions both created more positions as well as increased the number of recent medical school graduates able and willing to spend a further three to four years in a residency. This early, vital participation of the government came two decades prior to the Medicare and Medicaid legislation that is traditionally associated with federal support of graduate medical education.[55]

The federal government also physically created thousands of additional residency positions as military and especially veterans' hospitals expanded. A legacy of World War I, the VA hospital system grew in size to accommodate those returning from the Second World War.[56] In 1946, the VA planned to increase by sixty thousand beds, offering a wealth of clinical material.[57] Given the patient population, doctors working in these institutions cared for the sequelae of war trauma, including the same pseudoaneurysms and arteriovenous fistulae that Elkin and Shumacker had treated at their military centers during the war. These pathologies, uncommon in civilian facilities, further exposed young trainees to vascular surgery.

VA hospitals also provided an increasingly rare opportunity for residents to treat patients while minimally supervised. Senior surgeons prized the decision making that independence required. Yet, after World War II, they grew increasingly concerned that the rise of health insurance would eliminate the charity patients whom the residents had traditionally treated without much oversight. VA facilities guaranteed housestaff that autonomy, a perceived critical component of surgical training, and helped make the hospitals appealing partners to university-based programs filled with paying, private patients who were off limits to the residents.[58]

Postwar leaders also worked to transform the veterans' system from isolated outposts to ones closely integrated with academic medical centers. In 1944, only five VA hospitals had any association with an academic medical center. By 1946, more than thirty affiliations existed (out of 109 facilities), with additional attachments forming through the 1940s and 1950s.[59] This partnering uplifted veterans' facilities, brought elite faculty into the institutions, and produced a real incentive to develop qualified residency programs. Many of the professors had served in World War II, where they encountered profligate vascular trauma; some had since joined the SVS. These experiences allowed them to bring arterial repair into residency programs' curricula via the operating room, through lectures, on rounds, and in journal clubs, introducing trainees to the subject. More broadly, the academic affiliation provided residents at VA hospitals access to female and pediatric patients as well as the research resources and didactic lessons that remained crucial components of graduate medical education; simultaneously doctors at university-based institutions were exposed to the veteran patient population.[60]

The number of approved surgical residencies at VA facilities increased exponentially after the war. In the initial American College of Surgeons (ACS) survey of twenty VA hospitals in 1944, only seven had general surgery departments certified to educate residents, and these had received only provisional approval.[61] By August 1947, the college had accredited fifty-one VA hospitals for 750 surgical residency slots per year—more than all sanctioned civilian positions created between Halsted's program and the end of World War II.[62] By 1949, VA hospitals had established themselves as official, accredited, and acclaimed sites of graduate medical education, training 2,500 surgical residents a year in seventy-four locales.[63]

Approved residencies also expanded into military hospitals in the postwar years. Prior to World War II, the ACS refused to certify any military training program, with inspections revealing none satisfied their requirements.[64] During the Second World War, the army declined any external inspections, instead focusing on producing as many medical officers as possible to accommodate war needs.[65] The Public Health Service and the navy, however, faced fewer personnel demands. The navy in particular had officers serving in the college and placed early value on specialists in their base hospitals.[66] The navy began to reorganize its programs during the war, and by VJ Day, the ACS had conditionally approved thirty-two general surgery residencies in naval hospitals as well as ten programs in Public Health Service institutions.[67]

After the war ended, the military had the time and resources to dedicate to reorganizing surgical training along ACS guidelines. More importantly, a dearth of uniformed doctors made it urgent that the army and navy establish approved residencies as a recruitment incentive. When conscription ended in 1945, doctors fled uniformed service, with fewer than one thousand drafted physicians (out of a pool of more than fifty thousand) electing to remain in the army.[68] By late 1946, all branches, but especially the army, suffered from a severe shortage of medical officers.[69] The services believed that providing sanctioned residency positions, both in military hospitals and through federally sponsored programs in civilian facilities, would attract young physicians to the armed forces.[70] The navy and Public Health Service continued to expand their offerings, and the army now became amenable to restructuring its residencies to meet ACS standards.[71] Like VA facilities, military hospitals struggled to provide trainees access to female and pediatric patients. Smaller posts lacked research opportunities and didactic instruction. Unlike the VA system, military hospitals rarely partnered with neighboring academic medical centers. Moreover, faculty (and sometimes residents) rotated among different duty stations, complicating any ability to build a stable training environment.[72]

The ACS faced a dilemma: it wanted to maintain high standards but also felt a patriotic duty to cooperate with the army and navy, in which many college officers had served during the world wars.[73] The ACS ultimately compromised on some of its standards, like basic science classes and minimal faculty turnover, to accommodate the specific circumstances of the armed services. By July 1950 when the United States entered the Korean War, all major military hospitals (eight army, eight navy, and five Public Health) had ACS approved surgical residencies; 215 army doctors had completed their graduate medical education, and the number of board-certified physicians in the army had more than doubled since 1946.[74]

The decision of the VA and military hospitals to pursue ACS certification illustrates how broadly ACS standards were accepted among surgeons, trainees, and residency directors. Government hospitals had no obligation to seek accreditation, being able to establish their own licensing policies. The armed forces using approved residencies as a recruitment tool demonstrated both the popularity of the programs among postwar doctors and their relative scarcity in the civilian world. The strategy proved effective, resolving the physician shortage of 1946 and creating a surplus of uniformed doctors such that the secretary of defense ordered the downsizing of military residency programs in the fall of 1950.[75]

Meanwhile, surgical training positions at civilian hospitals were increasing rapidly. This rise partly reflected the growing number of civilian health-care facilities: the 1946 Hill-Burton Act funded the construction of thousands of hospitals around the country, adding tens of thousands of new beds for patients requiring medical and surgical care.[76] Before the 1940s, most hospitals did not need housestaff to function, but, by the 1950s and 1960s, medicine became ever more complicated. Technologies like hemodialysis, new lab tests, and other interventions required physician oversight, and hospitals came to depend on residents to provide the necessary around-the-clock labor.[77] Realizing both their own needs and those of the thousands of young military medical veterans looking for places to train, hospitals applied to the ACS and AMA in droves for accreditation of their residency programs.[78]

Both organizations hurried to approve residencies in the postwar years. Adjusting their criteria in 1945 to match those of the American Board of Surgery, the college now required residents participate in at least three years of post-internship training while maintaining their insistence on broad clinical exposure, basic science instruction, and original research.[79] The growing length reflected the changing practice of surgery as more advanced operations like the blue baby repairs and the complex perioperative management around them demanded additional education. The AMA did not change its standards, still catering to a membership composed mostly of general practitioners who occasionally operated; it had minimal interest in fostering a class of full-time surgeons. Both groups saw the rapid approval of programs—even if provisional—as having two main advantages. First, they believed they owed veterans for their wartime sacrifice, and, as one set of ACS minutes reflected, establishing education opportunities was "the most useful and patriotic activity in which the College could engage."[80] Second, they realized hospitals would institute residencies with or without official sanction and concluded that having some oversight had the potential to strengthen programs, or at the very least monitor them.[81]

Both the AMA and ACS expedited their inspection process in an effort to evaluate as many hospitals as possible. Before World War II, the AMA had approved 610 hospitals for 5,256 residency slots, numbers that nearly doubled to 1,017 programs and more than 12,000 spots by early 1948.[82] From 1941 to 1945, the number of ACS-sanctioned residencies barely budged (514 to 578), but, from 1945 to 1950, it jumped nearly twofold (578 to 1,129); programs in general surgery specifically exhibited a similar trend, more than doubling from 188 in 1945 to 454 in 1950 (figure 4.1).

The rush to certify hospitals successfully established educational opportunities for veterans, but the expediency also admitted subpar residencies. An ACS report from 1947 demonstrates the loosening of its requirements, compromising on criteria like basic science and breadth of clinical exposure.[83] The AMA freely admitted to lower standards than the college or the board, again reflecting its primary membership of general practitioners rather than full-time surgeons. Yet the postwar speed of accreditation caused programs to be included that could not even reach the AMA's minimal standards. By 1948, the AMA acknowledged a backlog of 550 residencies that it had approved without ever inspecting; another 350 on its list were long overdue for mandatory reinspection.[84] Collectively, these represented almost half of all AMA-sanctioned residencies. By 1946, the American Board of Surgery, the organization with the highest standards, recognized the comparatively poor quality of residency programs being ratified.[85] "It was clear to the American Board," remarked its president, Warfield Firor, that "too many candidates were coming up to take the examination and failing, obviously not having had adequate training."[86] The board briefly tried to start its own

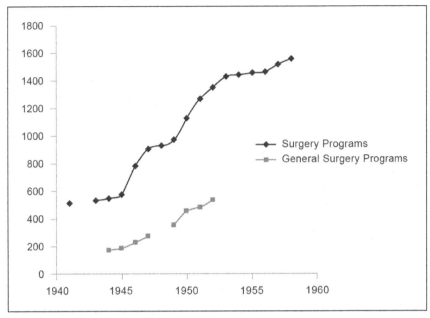

Figure 4.1. Increase in ACS approved surgical residency programs, 1940–60. Note the relatively flat line during the war years followed by a rapid, sustained spike in approved programs after World War II. Data do not reflect AMA approvals. Surgery programs included general surgery, otolaryngology, obstetrics and gynecology, neurosurgery, urology, thoracic surgery, and ophthalmology. Data compiled from numerous documents in ACS archives.

evaluation system but found the task too big to accomplish alone.[87] Indeed, the rapid expansion of hospitals and programs around the country made it financially and logistically impossible for any single organization to inspect, assess, and appropriately credential all surgery residency programs throughout the United States and Canada. Over the next several years, the board, the college, and the AMA hammered out a tripartite agreement confirming mutually agreeable standards and a unified inspection service in what became known as the Residency Review Committee.[88]

The emergence and work of this committee confirmed the importance of surgical residencies to both the profession and practice of the discipline. Through the 1960s, board certification remained rare and mostly limited to the academic elite.[89] Instead, completion of an approved residency increasingly determined who was operating in 1950s America.[90] Practically, local hospitals controlled who could operate by extending or denying surgical privileges to individual doctors. By the late 1950s, some were reserving this permission to physicians who had completed ACS-approved residencies, as evident by the lawsuits several general practitioners filed to protest this delineation.[91] General practitioners still performed a significant number of operations—especially in more rural parts of the country—but the number was shrinking and becoming concentrated on the relatively less-complex cases like hemorrhoids and appendectomies. In a study relying on Blue Cross / Blue Shield data (an admittedly nonrandom sample), the American Surgical Association found that, by 1957, residency-trained surgeons were performing greater than 60 percent of gastrectomies, radical mastectomies, and thyroidectomies (vascular operations were not studied).[92]

For residency to function as a de facto metric of qualification, everyone had to agree on what satisfactory surgical training entailed—a contentious process that lasted many years and ultimately resulted in the Residency Review Committee. Residencies also had to break out of their sequestered academic confines and become a universally available pathway. In this transformation, they sacrificed some of the exclusivity, science, and rigor characteristic of university programs in the 1920s for a more democratic, clinically oriented experience at community and government hospitals in the 1950s.

The proliferation of residencies and the expectation of completing one to become a surgeon led to a new generation of surgical housestaff, many of whom were gaining exposure to vascular surgery for the first time. Some attended meetings of the Society for Vascular Surgery or read the resulting journal articles in the literature. Others worked with faculty who had experimented with arterial repair in World War II and were testing novel techniques in their laboratories. Those at academic institutions witnessed the excitement and curative potential of vascular anastomosis in heart surgery and often participated in the harvest of arteries for institutional vessel banks. All residents were working with more competent, better-trained anesthesiologists, a specialty that underwent a similar, concurrent professionalization. When these surgeons later deployed to Korea, they went to war with far greater training, significantly more experience, and a much stronger background than did their predecessors in World War II. These infrastructural seeds combined to prepare the Korean War surgeon to sew damaged arteries together.

Chapter Five

An Ideal Implemented

Arterial Repair in the Korean War

The Korean War transformed vascular surgery from a practice based primarily on ligation to one of arterial repair. Bookended by the global cataclysm of World War II and the society-wrenching quagmire in Vietnam, Korea has suffered from inattention in lay and academic sources alike. This disregard extends to the medical and scientific aspects of the conflict. Yet the war proved crucial for establishing arterial repair as the standard of care for traumatic injuries to blood vessels. This sea change in vascular surgery over the course of three years of fighting demonstrates the importance of the particular milieu of the Korean War. The nature of combat, with relatively stable lines by 1951, total control of the air, and a robust supply chain created conditions amenable to surgical innovation while still resulting in the thousands of casualties needed to improve vascular management. Uniformed clinicians retained the freedom to experiment. Medical advances such as more powerful antibiotics, massive blood transfusions, artificial kidneys, and more advanced anesthesia care helped keep the wounded alive to and through prolonged operations. A cadre of young, bold, residency-trained surgeons capitalized on these circumstances to repair arteries in ever increasing numbers.

Seesawing to Stability:
Brief Military History of the Korean War

Dramatically different from the totality of World Wars I and II, the comparatively limited engagement in Korea against technologically inferior foes fostered an environment conducive to medical innovation. After largely escaping the destruction of World War II, Korea fell prey to international politics that artificially divided the peninsula into a Communist north under Soviet influence and an anti-Communist south backed by the United States. Leaders of both North and South Korea wanted to unify the country under their rule.[1] On 25 June 1950, the North Korean army launched a surprise attack across the 38th parallel. With South Korean forces reeling in retreat and Western fears of a domino effect in full bloom, the United Nations voted to dispatch an international force to defend the South.[2]

The war proceeded in four distinct stages (figure 5.1). First, North Korean armies drove UN forces south into a desperately defended position, the Pusan Perimeter.[3] The peninsula of Korea both hemmed in UN forces while also limiting fighting to a discrete geographic area. Despite the tenuous situation on the ground, the US Air Force quickly established control over the skies that it maintained for the duration, and the US Navy rapidly dominated the seas.[4] These achievements limited North Korean forces to a land war while providing safe aerial and nautical evacuation routes for US casualties. After General Douglas MacArthur's audacious amphibious landing at Inchon on 15 September 1950, the tide turned. The second phase (September–November 1950) featured an aggressive UN offensive up the peninsula, nearly reaching the border of China. During the third period (November 1950–spring 1951), China entered the war and pushed the UN armies back to roughly the 38th parallel.[5] Finally, the conflict entered its ultimate and longest stage (spring 1951–July 1953), of World War I–style positional warfare.[6]

The suddenness of the fighting exposed the unpreparedness of American forces, both militarily and medically.[7] Demobilization following VJ Day eviscerated not only the infantry and armor branches but also the Army Medical Department.[8] The 1948 Selective Service Act helped fill the ranks of fighting units, but, unlike its World War II predecessor, it did not conscript physicians. The military implemented various incentives, including significantly increasing residency opportunities, in attempts to recruit more doctors. Despite these efforts, when the North Koreans invaded there were only 185 American doctors assigned to the Far East Command, with a grand total of five board-certified surgeons.[9] Desperate to provide sufficient medical care to GIs fighting in Korea, the Eighty-First Congress passed Public Law 779, better known as the Doctor Draft, in September 1950.[10] Significantly, the draft prioritized clinicians in residency, who deployed with minimal military training to care for the one hundred thousand Americans wounded in the war.[11]

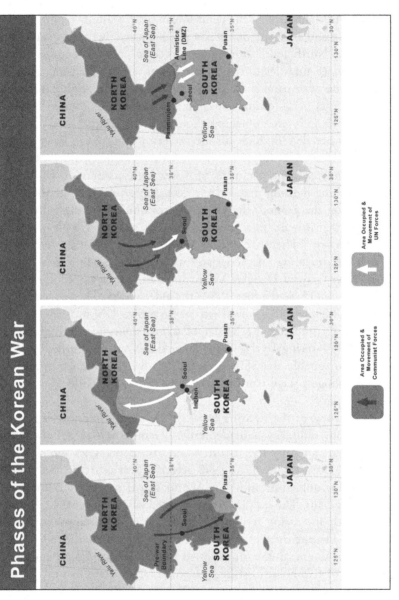

Figure 5.1. Four strategic stages of the Korean War. Note how these first three stages involved large movements up and down the peninsula but that stable front lines characterized the final and longest stage, from the spring of 1951 until the end of the war in the summer of 1953. This stability would prove crucial to the uptake of arterial repair. Map created by Scott Behm.

Blood and Snow:
Creating a Supportive Medical Infrastructure in the Korean War

Soldiers and marines injured in Korea accessed a military medical network modeled after the European Theater of Operations in World War II. After receiving basic first aid from a medic, injured soldiers arrived at battalion aid stations for initial care.[12] Here, general medical officers without any residency training provided lifesaving but limited interventions: stopping bleeding, applying dressings, administering antibiotics, and, if indicated, evacuating the patient to the next echelon, division clearing stations, which stabilized the casualties until they could reach a surgical hospital.[13] By the end of the war, doctors at the division level were performing minor operations, but regulations explicitly forbade vascular surgery. The general medical officers there lacked residency training, and high command feared their interventions might worsen arterial injuries, especially after repair became common in 1952.[14] Wounded marines followed a similar chain of evacuation, though one that emphasized earlier surgery; notably, injured marines were more likely to survive than their army counterparts.[15]

Mobile army surgical hospitals provided most of the definitive surgical care for soldiers and marines, including the majority of the vascular surgery. While the 1970s TV show *M*A*S*H* cemented the fame of these units, they emerged from World War I–era US Army efforts to offer forward surgical care.[16] The auxiliary surgical teams that functioned so efficiently in World War II in this capacity failed to establish themselves in Korea. The army lacked the necessary hospital beds, surgeons, and nursing staff in any one location to deliver postoperative care for the additional cases the aux teams would perform.[17] In their stead, the army developed a mobile, self-sufficient sixty-bed hospital designed to support an infantry division.[18] On paper, MASHs included fourteen physicians (of whom five were surgeons), twelve nurses, two medical service corps officers to manage administration, and ninety-seven enlisted men, although they rarely deployed with their full complement of physicians, much less surgeons. Among the fourteen medical doctors were residency-trained radiologists, and while no evidence of front-line arteriograms has surfaced, forward hospitals acquired increasingly advanced X-ray machines throughout the war to aid diagnosis.[19] The fourteen doctors also included at least one residency-trained anesthesiologist, and nitrous oxide eventually replaced the simpler methods of drip ether and chloroform as their anesthetic agent of choice.[20]

Three MASHs left for Korea at the start of hostilities; three additional American hospitals and one Norwegian MASH followed. Intended as pure surgical support for the severely wounded, MASHs shunted medical or otherwise stable patients to other units and grew into mini–evacuation hospitals. Sheer volume dictated their expansion in both bed capacity (sixty to two hundred) and the range of services they provided.[21] Later in the war, as the front stabilized, some MASHs specialized, with the 8209th incorporating a neurosurgery team and the 8228th ministering to all hemorrhagic fever and cold injury (e.g., frostbite, trench foot, and hypothermia) patients.[22]

The MASH was not the only novel feature of military medicine in Korea. The army developed and prescribed the anti-malaria medication primaquine in response to the epidemic of vivax malaria; the new and frightening disease dubbed Korean hemorrhagic fever spawned extensive research efforts.[23] Hemodialysis, invented after World War II, deployed to war for the first time in Korea, helping save the lives of wounded soldiers suffering from acute renal failure.[24] The mortality of soldiers with severe acute kidney injury dropped from 90 percent in World War II to 55 percent in Korea for those who reached the dialysis unit.[25] Surgically, however, the expansion of blood transfusions and antibiotics most dramatically improved outcomes and fostered conditions for arterial repair to flourish.

Blood transfusions grew from the World War II experience, which had previously demonstrated its life-saving properties over plasma. Whereas in World War II military units supplied much of their own blood, in Korea it almost exclusively came from Japan or the United States.[26] (It is interesting that, despite being an implacable foe five years earlier, the Japanese so willingly donated to American soldiers.) The international collection and transportation of perishable blood products represented one of the most challenging and successful logistical endeavors of the war. Doctors in Korea transfused enormous quantities: in World War II, the average American casualty received 0.45 units; by the end of the Korean War, this number had quadrupled to 1.9 units.[27] "The quantity of blood given in the forward hospitals was truly staggering," remarked Paul W. Sanger, who commanded the 38th Evac Hospital in World War II before serving in Korea as a consultant.[28] Despite the increased volume of transfusions, no report, interview, or memoir cited a shortage of blood products.

If blood kept patients alive before and during surgery, then an expanded antibiotic armamentarium benefitted them postoperatively. As sulfa drugs fell into disuse, new medications like streptomycin and the tetracycline family (the first so-called broad-spectrum antibiotics) joined penicillin to aid in the control of infections.[29] Given the Korean custom of using human excrement to fertilize fields, these novel agents took on particular importance and were used extensively. "Every patient in the chain of evacuation received intramuscular injections of penicillin and streptomycin at noon and midnight," recalled navy surgeon Howard Browne.[30] The rate of gas gangrene, which had been a major problem in World War I and remained troublesome in World War II, dropped to an all-time low of 0.8 percent in Korea; no soldier died from it.[31] Infections certainly existed—one study revealed 3.9 percent of wounds at an evacuation hospital had "serious infections"—and vascular patients, with diminished blood flow, were at greater risk than others.[32] But, to an extent not previously possible, physicians and surgeons were able to control infection and focus their attention on other problems.

Developments in large-scale blood transfusion, new malaria drugs, the artificial kidney, and arterial repair represented just a few aspects of medical innovation that occurred during the conflict. Whereas research in World War II stemmed mostly from individual initiative, in Korea, the army sought to centralize that effort. "Just as the staff of a tuberculosis hospital studies tuberculosis, or a cancer hospital studies cancer, the Army Medical Corps should study trauma," asserted one report justifying official, team-based military medical investigation in Korea.[33] In 1951, the army sent Fiorindo Simeone, DeBakey's coauthor on the World War II vascular surgery study, to Korea with a team to identify military medical problems that could benefit from further experimentation. "Shortly after arriving in Korea in December 1951," a team member recalled, "it became apparent that one of the major problems confronting the surgeons was the management of casualties with arterial wounds."[34] Conducting high-level clinical research in the third world, much less the third world at war, challenged the investigators who mostly published case series.[35] Nonetheless, the team, composed of young, eager, resourceful doctors, established the importance of certain medical and surgical interventions—like repairing rent arteries.[36]

Vascular Surgery in the Korean War

Vascular surgery in the Korean War developed in four overlapping waves. In 1950, the administration of Walter Reed Army Hospital in Washington, DC, allocated a ward dedicated to treating chronic vascular patients, which quickly and decisively (re)demonstrated the superiority of arterial repair over ligation. Simultaneously in Korea, various surgeons in both the army and the navy bucked regulations and explored front-line arterial repair. The proofs of concept set forth by both the Walter Reed team and these individual surgeons allowed the army to send vascular surgery research teams to Korea, which definitively proved the suitability and superiority of the technique. Finally, members of these teams transitioned into the role of specialized surgeons who not only treated hundreds of cases themselves but also taught MASH surgeons how to perform the intricate operations. While chronologically overlapping, each phase provided the evidence and the motivation to proceed to the next, until arterial repair became standard of care.

Walter Reed

The success of the vascular surgery hospitals in World War II led to the 1950 establishment of a similar center during the Korean War at Walter Reed, the army's flagship hospital.[37] Career army officer Brigadier General Sam Seeley, MC, chaired its Surgery Department.[38] Despite having no formal background in vascular surgery, he recognized the value of specialized care for these patients and created a semi-independent vascular section, with Lieutenant Colonel Carl W. Hughes, MC, and Major Edward J. Jahnke Jr., MC, in charge of clinical and investigative work. All army vascular patients from the Korean War who required further management came to Walter Reed.[39] This category excluded acute vascular trauma, which surgeons treated in-theater with arterial ligation. Most patients arriving at Walter Reed suffered from traumatic pseudoaneurysms and arteriovenous fistulae, analogous to the majority of cases at the World War II vascular centers.[40]

Doctors at Walter Reed initially tied off damaged vessels until results from isolated arterial repairs clearly proved superior, prompting the hospital to change its management of vascular casualties by the end of 1950. The early reliance on ligation largely resulted from the recommendations of Daniel C. Elkin, who had directed the vascular center at Ashford Hospital in West Virginia during World War II. Elkin conservatively eschewed arterial repair, believing its risks outweighed potential benefits.[41] Although data from the other hospitals contradicted his argument, this information remained largely unpublished and thus unknown. In contrast, as chairman of surgery at Emory with an international reputation, Elkin commanded authority. Following Elkin's advice, the Walter Reed team began ligating all damaged arteries, reserving anastomoses for a select few cases when limb loss appeared imminent.[42]

In following their patients, the team found the results of repair "were so gratifying that we now attempt to restore the continuity of all major arteries."[43] They used a modified Carrel technique to perform the anastomoses.[44] Arterial repair staved off amputation and almost entirely eliminated the debilitating symptoms of arterial insufficiency such as pain, cold intolerance, and nonhealing ulcers.[45] Whereas 24 percent of patients who underwent ligation developed serious signs of arterial insufficiency, only 2.8 percent of patients who received arterial repairs did, and this difference improved to 44 percent versus 5 percent when specific to lower extremity pathology.[46] Based on these data, Seeley and his team made it "policy to re-establish the continuity of all major vessels by suture anastomosis, homologous artery graft, or autogenous vein graft."[47] As a result, while doctors repaired only 55 percent of the first sixty-four cases in 1950, in 1951 they sutured or anastomosed 87 percent of all torn vessels.[48] A navy team, working independently on the West Coast with wounded marines, simultaneously came to the same conclusions and modified their protocol to favor reparative operations as well.[49]

The success of arterial repair at Walter Reed spurred efforts to change practice in Korea. Largely due to the conclusions of DeBakey and Simeone's famous article, the military insisted combat surgeons ligate vascular injuries in Korea. But physicians like Seeley, Hughes, and Jahnke had (re)proven the superiority of routine arterial repair. They recognized that the concentration of cases at both Walter Reed and Korean MASHs created an unparalleled opportunity to test, implement, and establish these interventions.[50] They convinced the army to form a mobile research team to travel to Korea where they could not only try repairing arteries in combat but also, and more importantly, transfer their knowledge to surgeons on the battlefield and spread the technique throughout the peninsula.[51] A team was ready to ship out in the summer of 1951, but the stalemate that resulted from promised peace talks following a successful UN offensive delayed deployment of the research units.[52] The war in Korea, however, raged on.

Rogue Surgeons

While Seeley, Jahnke, and Hughes were re-recognizing the suitability of arterial repair in Washington, DC, surgeons on the front lines in Korea regularly faced vascular trauma in the combat casualties admitted to their aid stations, MASHs, and other hospitals. Official medical doctrine, carried over from World War II, insisted on ligating injured vessels in all but the most extraordinary cases. Most doctors complied, and amputation rates unsurprisingly paralleled those from World War II. Some surgeons, however, defied regulations and insisted on repairing vascular damage, as evident in these three case studies, presented in chronological order. Notably, the episodes happened independently, with no communication among the parties. The spontaneous occurrences of three entirely separate, concurrent incidences of arterial repair exposes how the confluence of military, medical, and social conditions in Korea created a propitious environment that shaped surgical practice.

Hermes C. Grillo performed one of the first venous grafts in Korea in a dirt-floored tent a few miles behind the main line of resistance.[53] Grillo grew up in Providence, Rhode Island, and graduated with a degree in chemistry from Brown University in 1943. He matriculated into Harvard Medical School during World War II as part of the V-12 program, which aimed to produce officers for the US Navy/Marines by selecting individuals to graduate from college or professional school rather than serve as enlisted men. Receiving his MD in 1947 (at age twenty-three), he missed active duty in that war. Following medical school, Grillo earned a position as a surgical resident at Massachusetts General Hospital, then under the direction of Edward Churchill, who had served as an influential surgical consultant in World War II. When Congress passed the Doctor Draft that prioritized conscription of previous V-12 members, Grillo volunteered to join the military, allowing him to choose the navy, which he envisioned involving a relaxing Mediterranean cruise. Assigned instead to the 1st Marine Division, he arrived in Korea in February 1951.

With three and a half years of formal residency, Grillo had as much surgical training as anyone else in the entire division. Assigned to Dog Medical Company (functionally a mini-MASH that supported a single regiment close to the front lines), he operated on hundreds of freshly wounded American, Korean, and Chinese soldiers. Conditions were austere. The unit lacked any X-ray equipment and had a bare 80-watt bulb as its operating light. Without tissue retractors, Grillo improvised: he asked his engineering department to fashion some out of spent 155mm artillery shell casings. The hospital had no suction, forcing him to mop out any blood and detritus that accumulated in body cavities. Cleanliness was less than ideal: "It was aesthetically troublesome to me to be sewing up someone's intestine and have a fly sit on it," recalled Grillo in a later interview. "This didn't seem to do anyone any harm; the patients did all right, but it was very upsetting to me."[54] Despite these limitations, Grillo and his team handled general, neurological, urological, orthopedic, thoracic, and vascular trauma.

In April 1951, a young wounded marine arrived at Dog Company with multiple wounds from shell fragments and bullets, including one in his upper thigh. After debriding and controlling the trunk wounds, Grillo turned his attention to the leg, where it became apparent that the patient had a damaged femoral artery. "I couldn't bear just tying off the artery" and risking amputation, remembered Grillo. He recalled an episode during residency when he had seen one of the senior surgeons, Robert Linton, perform a vein graft to save a patient's leg. This operation was so rare at the time that subsequently "[I] ran to the library and I read all of Carrel and Guthrie's stuff and I thought, 'God this is exciting.'" Now in Korea, Grillo marshaled this education and "decided that the only thing I could do [for the wounded marine] was to take a piece of saphenous vein and put it in."[55] After the surgery, Grillo evacuated the patient to the nearest hospital ship, where he subsequently died of renal failure; an autopsy demonstrated a patent graft. Grillo performed several other primary suture repairs while in Korea, including one on the pulmonary artery.

Otto Apel and his colleagues at the 8076th MASH created a veritable vascular center during their tours in Korea.[56] Like Grillo, Apel participated in the V-12 program as a medical student at Columbia University but graduated after World War II ended. He pursued a surgical residency at St. Luke's Hospital in Cleveland. When the Korean War started and the Doctor Draft passed, Apel found himself in army green, deployed to the 8076th MASH in the spring of 1951 after only two years of residency training. Also facing thousands of casualties, Apel and the chief surgeon of the 8076th, John Coleman, refused to accept ligation as the definitive treatment for arterial wounds given the high rate of amputation that followed. They too turned toward arterial repair.

Coleman made his initial forays with this procedure on wounded Chinese and North Korean prisoners. After several attempts, he confided in Apel, and the two worked together to practice suturing vessels. Neither surgeon had performed this operation—nor even seen it performed—during their years in residency; it was just not common. However, both had read extensively about vascular surgery in the literature, and, with an abundance of patients, they began perfecting their technique. They suffered from a dearth of appropriate equipment: without vascular clamps, they used Penrose drains to occlude arteries; only thick 2–0 suture was available (instead of normal, thinner 5–0 or 6–0); instruments proved bulky and unwieldy for delicate operations. But they persisted and began performing primary anastomoses and vein grafts in American soldiers and marines. They soon established a reputation as a "vascular center," and surrounding hospitals would send all their cases to the 8076th. From their start until Apel rotated home in August 1952, the unit reportedly performed more than two hundred arterial repairs while also teaching the technique to surgeons stationed nearby. In an unpublished series, they achieved successful revascularization with palpable pulses on discharge in 90 percent of their cases.[57]

Initially, the military medical leadership was less than thrilled about this development, as Apel indicated with the chapter title "We're Going to Be Court-Martialed" in his memoir. Concerned over the possible command response, Apel and Coleman did not even record their early efforts in patients' charts. They received several orders from senior officers to return to ligation, but "we thought that our failure to use vein grafting on soldiers who needed it violated the Hippocratic Oath that we took when we became doctors," and they continued to suture torn vessels.[58] He noted that it was his and Coleman's youth and lack of indoctrination that provided the intellectual flexibility and courage to branch out into new operations.[59] By the time Apel left Korea in mid-1952, the army had accepted and advocated for arterial repair, although it never credited Coleman or Apel.

Frank C. Spencer, the third example, similarly eschewed ligation for arterial repair. Like Grillo and Apel, he participated in the V-12 program as a medical student at Vanderbilt, graduating first in his class in 1947.[60] He matriculated into Johns Hopkins's surgical residency just after Alfred Blalock, chair of the Department of Surgery, achieved worldwide fame for performing the blue baby operation described in the previous chapter. Hopkins had become the epicenter for cyanotic babies. As an intern, Spencer did little more than hold retractors, but he recalled in a later interview, "The atmosphere was dominated by the success of the blue baby operation, [which] . . . had captured the imagination of the entire country."[61] He estimated that Blalock performed four to five of the procedures a week, and it clearly affected Spencer's career trajectory. The pyramidal system at Hopkins deposited Spencer into a laboratory for his second year in Baltimore, which he left to complete his clinical training at UCLA, but the onset of the Korean War and the Doctor Draft roped him into the navy a year after moving across the country. Of his two years in uniform, he spent a crucial twelve months in the laboratory of Oakland Naval Hospital. There, based on his prior experience with the blue baby operation, Spencer began reading about vascular surgery and practicing vessel anastomoses on dogs—knowledge and skills that undergirded his pioneering efforts in Korea.

Spencer, like Grillo and Apel, refused to ligate traumatically damaged arteries and insisted on repair.[62] He arrived in Korea in August 1952, by which point the army had already deployed its vascular surgery team and had begun training other surgeons, including those in the navy.[63] However, ligation remained the officially sanctioned treatment. Spencer was assigned to Easy Medical Company (analogous to Dog Company where Grillo served) where as chief surgeon (with two years of clinical postgraduate training) he cared for hundreds of wounded marines under challenging conditions (figure

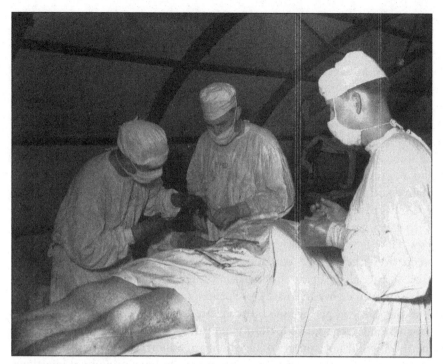

Figure 5.2. Frank Spencer (*center*) operating in Easy Company; note the full surgi-cal garb and semipermanent framing supporting the tent, reflecting practice later in the war after the stabilization of lines. United States Marine Corps Photo A164811 by SSGT Riley, in U.S. Navy BUMED Library and Archives 09-7959-032. Thanks to Mr. Michael Rhode for locating this photograph.

5.2). In an interview late in life when he declared repairing arteries in Korea "the most useful thing that I did in my entire career," Spencer recalled the instigating episode:

> One of the first persons I saw was an 18-year-old boy with a dead foot that we're going to amputate in about three days . . . He had a little wound . . . in the artery in the leg. And I asked . . . why didn't you fix it? And I was told that was contrary to military orders. . . . Do I violate orders and fix the leg, or take the leg off when I could fix it and follow orders? I thought, well, I couldn't live with myself if I took a leg off and knew how to fix it.[64]

Similarly under risk of court martial, Spencer began a policy at his hospital of repairing arterial damage, using the inspiration of the blue baby opera-tion and the technical skills he taught himself in the laboratory. To aid in his work, he founded one of the first artery banks in Korea.

Spencer also started training fellow physicians in the technique. The unit had a few other physicians, none of whom had completed surgical residency. Their early efforts in vascular repair, based on didactic lessons, failed miserably, and Spencer came to recognize the need for practical instruction.[65] "I put out a rule . . . that you had to practice with arteries from dead people . . . then come up and show me your techniques. And it . . . became known as the sewing lessons. And I'd watch how they would do it . . . [and say] 'No, that's terrible. Go practice some more. Come back in three days.'"[66] Eventually the other surgeons mastered the technique and began applying it to their patients. Ray V. Grewe, another young drafted surgeon who had worked with Spencer at the Oakland Naval Hospital, began repairing arteries at neighboring Dog Medical Company.[67]

In 1955, Spencer and Grewe published their results in the *Annals of Surgery*. They (and particularly Spencer) garnered significant recognition and credit from the surgical community for conclusively establishing the efficacy of arterial repair in the literature.[68] Documenting ninety-seven arterial injuries in eighty-five patients, Spencer and Grewe set out to determine, first, the safety of performing intricate arterial surgery on severely wounded patients, and, second, its superiority to ligation. With six deaths in the series, the therapy did not appear to increase marine mortality.[69] The authors discussed employing the Carrel-Guthrie suture technique, using local injections of heparin to prevent thrombus and providing sympathetic blocks postoperatively.[70] If the damage to the artery extended so long as to prevent tension-free anastomosis, Spencer and Grewe left collateral circulation intact and inserted a graft, mostly arterial homografts from their homespun artery bank. (Homografts are tissue from the same species—other humans in this case—but a different individual from the patient.) Ligating less than 10 percent of the ninety-seven injuries, the duo declared arterial repair a far superior therapy and demonstrated such by comparing their results to DeBakey and Simeone's from World War II (see table 5.3, Spencer and Grewe). Long before they published their data in 1955, however, surgeons from Walter Reed had already proven the point and initiated a countrywide program to change practice.

Grillo, Apel, and Spencer were hardly the only three surgeons who experimented with arterial repair early in the Korean War—Richard Hornberger, author of the novel *MASH*, was another—but they serve as representative samples.[71] Significant similarities link these individuals. All were young men, naïve to medical traditions with a willingness and courage to try new procedures. None anticipated remaining in the military, lessening potential consequences any disciplinary action might bring. All fiercely prioritized their patients over policy. Most notably, all three had completed several years of a formal surgical residency, and they credited this experience with providing the inspiration and technical capacity to start repairing arteries in Korea. Sculpted by academic programs, they arrived with a healthy skepticism of extant practices and a faith that clinical research had the potential to improve the status quo. The incalculable benefit of this training distinguished these men from their Second World War forbearers and provided the key difference that allowed them to innovate successfully.

Walter Reed Team in Korea

The above-described rogue surgeons demonstrate the evolution of surgery in wartime, but they do not explain the widespread adoption of arterial repair in the Korean War. Indeed, while Apel and Spencer met great success, other surgeons routinely failed.[72] Until mid-1952, official army documents continually criticized efforts to repair arteries: "Attempts at repairing damaged arteries . . . have usually been fruitless and unwise," commented the *Surgeon's Circular Letter*, a publication distributed to medical units in Korea, that went on to argue that vascular repair violated the fundamental principles of military triage by requiring too much time and too many resources to save a limb when lives were at stake.[73] Rather, it was the auspicious results at Walter Reed, Simeone's 1951 report highlighting the potential for improvement, and the success of the research teams in Korea that changed official surgical practice in the war. After reviewing the positive outcomes from Walter Reed and Simeone's report, the army dispatched a surgical research team to the Far East to perform arterial repairs and analyze their results.[74] Interestingly, the team was as yet unaware of the work of the rogue surgeons.[75]

John Howard led the research team. Howard had attended the University of Pennsylvania medical school and, in 1950, completed his surgical residency there under the highly regarded Isidor S. Ravdin, who had commanded the 20th General Hospital in Burma during World War II.[76] Thereafter, Howard went for further training at Baylor Hospital in Texas with Michael E. DeBakey, who was actively researching arterial anastomosis in trauma victims. While the army drafted Howard within a year, his time with DeBakey provided him with exposure to and practice with performing operations on blood vessels.[77] When he arrived in Korea, he believed himself one of only two fully trained, board-certified surgeons on the peninsula.[78] Edward Jahnke, a surgical resident at Walter Reed who had worked on vascular cases there, joined Howard in 1952 after completing his training. Carl W. Hughes was the third member of the team.[79] Hughes had graduated from the University of Tennessee medical school in 1944 and immediately entered military service. After the Second World War, he completed a surgical residency at Walter Reed under future surgeon general Leonard D. Heaton, where he participated in the early vascular trials with Seeley and Jahnke. He later took command of the surgical research team in Korea after he finished his residency and Howard had rotated home.

By April 1952, Howard initiated vascular research at the 43rd MASH, long after the front lines had stabilized into static warfare.[80] The team initially met deep skepticism from the Surgeon of the 8th Army, who did not believe arterial repair appropriate for widespread use in Korea.[81] Contrary to these instructions, team members began treating every vascular wound that came through their doors and carefully documented their results. By the end of the war, they had published numerous accounts of their experiences in leading surgical journals and presented their findings at various national meetings.[82]

A study of the first nine months of 1952 revealed an incidence of arterial injuries of 2.4 percent, a figure significantly higher than DeBakey and Simeone's value of 0.96 percent in World War II, although that increase more likely reflected better identification and reporting than a true rise in frequency.[83] Anatomical variation paralleled that of World War II (table 5.1). Fragmentation from artillery or mortar shells, hand grenades, and mines caused the vast majority (>85 percent in all series) of the injuries.[84] This mechanism is significant because it rarely resulted in solitary wounds, and the spray of fragments into an arm or a leg was likely to destroy collateral circulation. The annihilation of the collateral vessels made arterial repair all the more essential for saving limbs. The fragments usually lacerated or, less often, severed vessels, although surgeons noted that near misses could result in contusions serious enough to thrombose the artery and require repair.

To obviate accusations of cherry-picking ideal cases, the team attempted to repair every major arterial injury that arrived at the facility, a policy they effected with very few exceptions and one that epitomizes their effort to conform to standard experimental protocol.[85] The team defined "major" as the carotid, axillary, iliac, femoral, or popliteal arteries since these vessels had minimal collateral circulation and thus posed the highest risk of amputation post-ligation. They primarily tied off damaged minor arteries. They did not ligate the concomitant vein unless it was already damaged, and they rarely repaired venous injuries.[86]

Surgeons throughout Korea approached these cases similarly. Most vascular patients arrived at a MASH bleeding, and controlling hemorrhage was the first priority. Carefully and extensively debriding the wound, the second

Table 5.1. Anatomic variation of vascular wounds in Korea. Vascular wounds occurred all over the body, with the distribution relatively conserved over the different series.

	Jahnke and Howard		Jahnke and Seeley		Inui, Shannon, and Howard		Hughes (a)		Spencer and Grewe		Total	Total %
Common carotid	3	5%	1	3%	5	5%	7	4%	0	0%	16	3%
Axillary	7	12%	5	14%	8	8%	13	6%	4	5%	37	8%
Brachial	16	28%	12	34%	31	31%	68	33%	21	25%	148	31%
External iliac	2	4%	1	3%	3	3%	2	1%	2	2%	10	2%
Common femoral	2	4%	1	3%	12	12%	12	6%	4	5%	31	6%
Superficial femoral artery	13	23%	8	23%	16	16%	68	33%	29	35%	134	28%
Popliteal	14	25%	7	20%	23	23%	37	18%	24	29%	105	22%
Total	57		35		101		207		84		484	99%[1]

Sources: Jahnke and Howard, "Primary Repair of Major Arterial Injuries," 648. They also recorded an injury to the subclavian vessel. Jahnke and Seeley, "Acute Vascular Injuries in the Korean War," 161. They also recorded an injury to the external carotid, five to the deep femoral artery, thirteen to the radial and/or ulnar arteries, and twenty-three to various arteries of the lower leg. Inui, Shannon, and Howard, "Arterial Injuries in the Korean Conflict," 851. They also report two injuries to the subclavian artery and one to the internal iliac. Hughes, "The Primary Repair of Wounds of Major Arteries," 299. He also recorded one injury to the aorta and three to the common iliac arteries. This publication appears to incorporate all the data he previously published in "Acute Vascular Trauma in Korean War Casualties." Spencer and Grewe, "Management of Arterial Injuries in Battle Casualties," 305. They also reported injuries to the subclavian (one), radial and/or ulnar (two), deep femoral (three), and tibial (six) arteries. Publications do not explicitly deny overlapping of series, a possibility since all authors functioned as members of the same surgical team.

Note:
[1] Sum does not equal 100% because of rounding.

step, held particular importance given the risk of infection that threatened any anastomosis. Surgeons usually could repair small lacerations of less than one-third the vessel circumference with a few simple stitches. More severely damaged arteries required resection and reanastomosis. Discussion arose regarding how much artery to resect. Jahnke argued that cavitational forces from the projectile microscopically damaged arteries beyond the limits of visual destruction, an assertion he substantiated with histological evidence. He arbitrarily removed an additional centimeter proximally and distally from the visible injury.[87] This modification had consequential implications, as it created a wider gap that surgeons now had to bridge, limiting the ability to apply tension-free end-to-end anastomosis.

Operations proceeded along the Carrel-Guthrie method. Surgeons relied on either the two- or three-guy-wire technique to appose the ends of arteries, 5–0 silk on curved atraumatic needles, and either a horizontal mattress or a simple over-and-over suture to secure the connection.[88] Both interrupted and continuous suture technique were used, although the latter proved more common. The procedure hardly differed from what Carrel and Guthrie had published nearly fifty years earlier.[89]

The operations critically departed from the World War I and World War II philosophy that judged repair to be a risky ideal; Howard and his team of surgeons believed arterial repair should be the standard intervention and saw ligation as failure. Such commitment became evident when Jahnke published a description of his technique: "The artery was freed proximally and distally so that approximation could be made without tension. *Collateral circulation was sacrificed, as necessary, to permit attainment of this goal.*"[90] In the same paper, Jahnke discussed stripping the collateral branches up to *ten inches* away from the site of union in order to create a tension-free anastomosis.[91] This decision represented a titanic departure from previous practice, which sought to conserve collateral circulation at all costs. The sacrifice of collaterals made it an "all-or-none" procedure—failure would essentially guarantee amputation. The willingness to gamble indicates their faith in the operation and in their own ability to perform it.

Jahnke's quote, as well as statistical data from the other surgeons, reveals a strong preference for anastomosis over grafting (table 5.2). End-to-end anastomoses constituted more than two-thirds of the army team's vascular operations. When they did require grafts, they chiefly relied on veins. No official military artery banks existed in Korea in early 1952 when Howard and Jahnke first deployed. DeBakey had assured the army that "the establishment of blood vessel banks . . . [is] of dubious value."[92] Later in the war, army surgeons did experiment with arterial homografts (Hughes [a]), but

Table 5.2. Types of surgical operations on blood vessels in Korea. Note the rarity of ligation, not only in the "Total" column but also in each of the individual series. Never more than 8 percent, this figure was substantially lower than the 92 percent DeBakey and Simeone documented in the North African and European theaters of operation or the nearly 100 percent rate of ligation in the Pacific. End-to-end anastomosis was the most common procedure in all series except Spencer's, where he favored arterial grafts.

	Jahnke and Howard		Jahnke and Seeley		Inui, Shannon, and Howard		Hughes (a)		Spencer and Grewe		Total	Total %
Ligation	2	3%	0	—	0[166]	—	3	2%	8	8%	13	3%
Suture repair	2	3%	3	9%	13	17%	19	10%	18	19%	55	12%
End-to-End	48	80%	28	80%	46	62%	125	65%	24	25%	271	59%
Venous Graft	8	13%	4	11%	16	21%	28	15%	3	3%	59	12%
Arterial Graft	0	—	0	—	0	—	11	6%	44	45%	55	12%
Other[1]	0	—	0	—	0	—	7	4%	0	—	7	2%
Total Number of Operations	60		35		75		193		97		460	100%

Sources: Jahnke and Howard, "Primary Repair of Major Arterial Injuries," 648. Jahnke and Seeley, "Acute Vascular Injuries in the Korean War," 161. Inui, Shannon, and Howard, "Arterial Injuries in the Korean Conflict," 854. They recorded their ligations in a separate series. Hughes, "The Primary Repair of Wounds of Major Arteries," 299. Spencer and Grewe, "Management of Arterial Injuries in Battle Casualties," 305. Publications do not explicitly deny overlapping of series, a possibility given that all authors functioned as members of the same surgical team.

Note:

[1] Includes conservative management, thrombectomy, and spasm release.

that procedure never overtook venous autografts. In contrast, Spencer, as part of a naval unit and with personal experience storing arteries while stationed in Oakland, founded his own artery bank shortly after arriving in Korea.[93] He noted that donations existed aplenty among marine dead and that he rarely had to store grafts very long before another casualty was in need, and thus he primarily relied on arterial grafts for his patients.[94] This variation in technique highlights both the importance of very local factors in determining patient care as well the freedom combat surgeons had to determine the details of their practice.

With one notable exception of the atraumatic Potts clamp, surgeons in Korea had access to the same technology as their World War II predecessors had. Arteriograms again did not appear on the front lines, although investigators at Walter Reed used the technology to follow up on casualties and assess the efficacy of the repair. Heparin use also remained limited and variable by practitioner preference, although no one systemically heparinized the battle casualties for fear of them bleeding to death. Sympathetic interruption again proved more controversial. In obvious instances of spasming arteries, Jahnke and Howard would wrap a sponge soaked in papaverine (an antispasmodic opioid) around the narrowed portion that temporarily eliminated local sympathetic input; they refrained from any formal sympathectomies.[95] Other surgeons routinely used the therapy, and a novel way of delivering continuous lumbar sympathetic blocks was developed in Korea.[96] By the end of the war, anecdotal evidence had produced a consensus for the inefficacy of sympathetic interruption in the management of acute vascular trauma.[97] More importantly, the now-standard practice of repairing the main arterial channel rendered sympathectomies—used to vasodilate and improve collateral circulation—less relevant.[98]

Korean War–era surgeons did benefit from the introduction of one new surgical instrument in late 1952, the Potts clamp, which greatly facilitated arterial repair. Vascular operations require the surgeon to clamp the artery both above and below the injury site to prevent bleeding during the repair. The Goldilocks approach applied here: clamp too gently and blood could still course through the artery and into the surgical field; clamping too aggressively damages the walls of the artery, compromising the anastomosis. Until the Potts clamp, no commercially available device fulfilled this role. Clearly, arterial repair proceeded anyway. Surgeons employed a variety of improvised methods to occlude vessels temporarily, including tourniquets, vessel loops, imperfect clamps, and jury-rigged instruments.[99] In Korea, Spencer used rubber-shod bulldog clamps (see cover image, left); Apel and Coleman used vessel loops until their R&R trip to Japan, where they commissioned a silversmith to cast a homemade device.[100] Howard initially relied on old-fashioned hemostats that macerated the artery wall and often led to failure.[101] The Potts clamp promised a solution: rapid, secure occlusion that did not damage the artery.

Willis J. Potts invented the instrument to facilitate a different operation, division of the patent ductus arteriosus.[102] Robert E. Gross, the pediatric heart surgeon highlighted in the previous chapter for promoting tissue-culture grafts, reported the first successful surgical ligation of a patent ductus arteriosus in 1939.[103] By the 1940s, the procedure extended to academic centers throughout the United States and gave rise to a debate between simply ligating the ductus versus surgically severing it.[104] Prior to World War II, surgeons had conclusively recognized that dividing and ligating arteries produced outcomes superior to ligation in continuity, but technical difficulties inherent in this operation complicated the application of that principle. Specifically, the short length and wide breadth of the ductus complicated efforts to secure and maintain control of it during the operation. As Potts commented, "Without question, the only obstacle to universal acceptance of division and suture of a ductus is the well-founded danger of uncontrollable hemorrhage due to slipping clamps."[105] Potts solved that problem with his eponymous clamp in 1948 (figure 5.3 and cover image). It had fine teeth, pointed enough to grasp the vessel but too dull to puncture it. The manufacturer, Brüno Richter, compared the tooth density (forty teeth per inch) to a bed of nails on which a fakir sleeps, in that it distributed pressure among so many points that each individual tooth exerted minimal force on the artery wall.[106] Narrow jaws provided surgeons more room to work. Most importantly, the clamp included a hub that blocked the interdigitation of the teeth, keeping them from pulverizing the artery. The Potts ductus clamps greatly facilitated not only ductus ligation but also peripheral arterial surgery, and it came into high demand.

While invented in 1948, the instrument did not appear in Korea until late 1952. As a brand-new device utilized primarily in an esoteric surgery performed only at elite academic centers, it was unlikely to appear on standard Army Tables of Organization and Equipment; few surgeons in Korea even knew it existed. When Jahnke arrived in 1952, he brought a single Potts clamp from Walter Reed.[107] Howard (and every other surgeon) immediately appreciated the ability of the new accoutrement to facilitate arterial repair and demanded more of them. However, the medical supply company told Howard that it would take several months to deliver the instruments, as they were backordered because of their popularity for the patent ductus operation. The commander of the research team in Korea subsequently informed

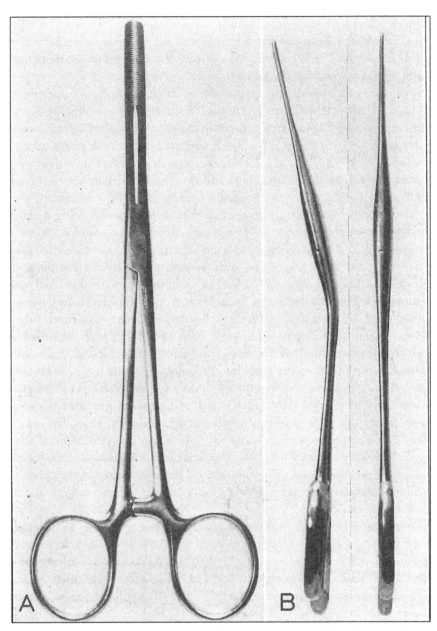

Figure 5.3. Potts ductus clamp. Note the opposing but not interdigitating teeth on the left image. *Archives of Surgery* 58, no. 5 (1949): 612–22. Copyright © American Medical Association. All rights reserved. Reproduced with permission.

the manufacturer that it had two weeks to deliver six clamps before the army broke the patent and produced its own; seven promptly materialized for military use.[108] One went to each MASH unit and another to Spencer with the marines. By the end of the war, the clamp appeared in standard military surgical sets, like the one featured on the cover.[109] The widespread demand for the instrument in Korea indicates the prevalence of advanced vascular surgery among the various military hospitals.

The Potts clamp itself did not lead to arterial repair in the Korean War. Rather, its use both reflected and resulted in the expansion of such operations.[110] Without early efforts to repair arteries in Korea, no need for the clamp would have existed. At the same time, the clamp so facilitated the steps of the surgery that the instrument catalyzed the dissemination of repair throughout Korea. In a 1953 journal article, Hughes wrote how "the Potts ductus . . . clamps contributed immensely to the success of the entire vascular surgery program."[111] Its ability to simplify the operation certainly made it much easier for the experts to train neophytes, a role that came to encompass a growing task of the research team in Korea.

Teach a Man to Fish

Teaching other surgeons became the primary mission of these new vascular surgeons in the latter portion of the war. The surgical research team had clearly demonstrated both the superiority and feasibility of forward arterial repair, but they alone could not care for every vascular patient in Korea. Having a broad network of surgeons trained in these techniques held particular importance given the significance of time lag to successful treatment. The wider the geographic distribution of such practitioners, the more likely wounded soldiers could reach a capable operator in time.[112] By 1953, the army established the goal of having at least one surgeon trained in arterial repair techniques at each MASH.[113] The navy also sent its medical officers to learn these skills and apply them to wounded marines.[114] Because army and navy surgeons rotated home after serving year-long tours in Korea, the instructional program ran repeatedly to train new personnel.[115]

The courses involved a variety of heuristic methods. Didactic lessons included lectures on the value and methods of arterial repair. Crucially, trainees had a chance to practice: the army sent all stray dogs to the 8055th MASH to serve as educational material. "Obtaining dogs in the war-ravished country was not an easy task," recalled Howard, reflecting on the Korean's taste for consuming canines, particularly in this period of mass penury.[116] Students would perform between four and eight operations, repairing the femoral and iliac arteries of anesthetized animals. Depending on what casualties arrived during the multi-day class, some pupils had the opportunity to apply their new skills to human patients under the supervision of an expert.[117] This model hewed closely to standard surgical education at the time and again emphasized the importance of practical instruction for teaching how to perform operations.[118] It also depended on students arriving with a certain level of technical ability, skills that general medical officers who populated World War II hospitals lacked. By the Korean War, most surgeons had completed some postgraduate training. As consultant Paul Sanger averred, anyone "who is capable of suturing intestine and who knows the necessity and understands the delicate handling of tissue . . . can easily be trained to anastomose blood vessels."[119] Most of the early drafted doctors in Korea had undergone at least a few years of residency, appreciated these principles, and came with the basic technical ability to learn how to repair arteries.

Teaching proliferated in trickle-down fashion, with Howard, Jahnke, and Hughes at the 8055th/43rd MASH on the summit. Jahnke also traveled to other hospitals, like the 121st Evac, to instruct medical officers.[120] Surgeons who took these quasi-official courses then returned to their home unit and taught operators there. This secondary schooling normally occurred on an ad hoc basis (analogous to Spencer's "sewing lessons"), but the 11th Evacuation Hospital established formal educational activities. After sending some of its staff to 8055th MASH for vascular training in June 1952, the 11th Evac held its own four-day postgraduate course in July that "included lectures, lantern slides, motion pictures and practical experience operating on live anesthetized dogs."[121] Incorporating both practical training and the technology of motion pictures cost the army substantial sums of money and time. Its willingness to dedicate these resources demonstrates the value it placed on improving the care of vascular patients.

Continuing medical education in Korea covered a wide range of topics; however, arterial repair "brought forth greater periodic teaching efforts than for any other type of injury," presented Colonel John Salyer, MC, in a 1954 conference reviewing military medicine from the recent war.[122] Multiple reasons explain this emphasis. First, vascular surgery genuinely made a difference in the care of casualties. Physicians faced many medical challenges in Korea, and some proved intractable to their best efforts. For example, courses on Korean hemorrhagic fever could teach young doctors about the disease, but, with no known cure, such knowledge served little more than academic purposes. Conversely, repairing arteries demonstrably saved limbs.

Second, arterial repair, unlike some other advances, required extensive hands-on training, again distinguishing surgical from medical innovations. *P. vivax* malaria also posed problems, and the new drug primaquine provided an effective response, but a simple order of "you shall give this pill to all soldiers" sufficed for physician education. By comparison, suturing vessels required time consuming minischools with practical instruction as discussed above. Third, repairing arteries had the potential to prevent hundreds of soldiers from becoming amputees, an applicability far broader than some other medical developments, such as dialysis. Unlike the prior two examples, hemodialysis both saved the lives of patients in acute renal failure and required extensive training to use properly. However, the single artificial kidney in Korea limited its impact and required only a handful of competent specialists. In contrast, providing broad access to vascular surgery required training dozens of surgeons: each of the six MASHs required at least one, and the rotation system ensured that none remained for longer than a year. Finally, one cannot discount the excitement of the cutting edge. Courses on proper abdominal or thoracic surgery may well have been of great (or greater) benefit to wounded soldiers and marines, but surgeons had established the fundamental principles behind those operations long ago. Arterial repair was new, and teachers and students alike reveled in the adventure of that novelty.

Were the courses effective in training young doctors how to anastomose vessels? Contemporary opinions varied. Francis Moore, chief of surgery at Brigham Hospital in Boston and a consultant to the Far East Command in Korea, complimented the vascular work of the research team members in a report to the surgeon general, but he did "not feel that this [arterial repair] is an area of surgery which can at present be considered as 'released' for general use by all the young surgeons in a MASH unit" because of their inexperience.[123] Another consultant, while praising Jahnke's efforts, believed "many of the general surgeons who are doing the forward surgery are not equipped to manage the demanding work required" of arterial repair.[124] However, other itinerant experts saw value in the ad hoc training and improvement in vascular care, especially by the end of the war. One consultant in 1953 remarked, "The recognition of arterial injuries in the Surgical Hospital is notably on the increase. The surgeons have become vascular conscious," and credited the courses with creating that awareness.[125] Unfortunately, no data confirm or refute these impressions. The average MASH physician did not replicate, or at least did not publish, statistics on the prevalence of his arterial repairs, success rates, or any other information that might elucidate the effect of teaching advanced vascular surgery to semitrained surgeons in an abbreviated course.[126] Ultimately, whether or not the grafts stayed patent is less relevant historically than their attempts, which demonstrated a commitment to repair. Clinically, a clotted graft or anastomosis rarely resulted in outcomes worse than ligation,

Table 5.3. Comparison of amputation rate by artery for vascular wounds in Korea and World War II, demonstrating significantly lower amputation rates in Korea compared to World War II across all series and all arteries

	Jahnke and Howard	Jahnke and Seeley	Inui, Shannon, and Howard	Hughes (b)	Spencer and Grewe	Total	WW II[1]
Common carotid[2]	0%	0%	0%	0%	n/a	0%	30%
Axillary	0%	0%	0%	33%	0%	4%	43%
Brachial	0%	0%	0%	0%	5%	1%	27%
External iliac	50%	0%	33%	0%	0%	22%	47%
Common femoral	0%	0%	0%	66%	25%	16%	81%
Superficial femoral artery	15%	13%	8%	0%	21%	12%	55%
Popliteal	21%	29%	18%	25%	38%	27%	73%
Total[3]	11%	9%	7%	10%	20%	12%	50%

Sources: Jahnke and Howard, "Primary Repair of Major Arterial Injuries," 648. The one subclavian repair did not result in amputation. Jahnke and Seeley, "Acute Vascular Injuries in the Korean War," 161. Inui, Shannon, and Howard, "Arterial Injuries in the Korean Conflict," 851. The data in the table reflect only those patients treated after Jahnke arrived. Hughes, "Acute Vascular Trauma in Korean War Casualties," 92. Spencer and Grewe, "Management of Arterial Injuries in Battle Casualties," 305. Amputation rates for Spencer and Grewe's series are higher than the others because they included cases of arterial ligation, which the other authors excluded. Publications do not explicitly deny overlapping of series, a possibility given that all authors functioned as members of the same surgical team.

Notes:

[1] DeBakey and Simeone, "Battle Injuries of the Arteries in World War II," 534–79.

[2] "Amputation" for the carotid artery refers to permanent, major neurological deficits.

[3] Total amputation rate determined by dividing the number of limb amputations by the total number of major arteries injured. The percentages differ from the values given by the articles, as the articles include data on minor arteries that this table ignores.

the alternative. Significantly, the teaching exposed dozens of surgeons to the technical and curative possibilities of arterial repair that had the potential to benefit not only wounded soldiers and marines in Korea but also civilian victims of car accidents and violence in America.

Saving Arms and Legs:
The Effects of Repairing Arteries in Korea

The adoption of arterial repair dramatically reduced the incidence of amputation among vascular casualties in the Korean War compared with World War II (table 5.3). For all major arteries, amputation rate dropped 75 percent (from 50 percent to 12 percent) in cases managed by Howard's and Spencer's teams. On the basis of these results, by 1953 the 8th Army adopted vessel repair as the official policy for vascular injuries in Korea.[127]

The particular operations surgeons used significantly influenced outcomes.[128] In general, success correlated with the difficulty of the procedure, although more devastating wounds tended to require operations of increased complexity, denying a facile correlation. Simple suture repair of tears in the vessels routinely returned the most favorable results, with amputation rates in the low single percentages—an unsurprising conclusion given the comparatively minor nature of these wounds. End-to-end anastomosis followed, with series documenting that around 10 percent of cases resulted in limb loss. Vein and artery grafts met with less success. Numbers fluctuated among different investigators and by blood vessel, but venous autografts resulted in amputation rates hovering between 15 percent and 30 percent; arterial homografts, 25 percent to 33 percent. Critically, amputation following either venous or arterial grafts still remained far less frequent than after ligations in World War II.

Arterial repair led to unexpected challenges, notably the identification of what physicians now call reperfusion injury. This occurs when an area of the body bereft of blood for a length of time suddenly regains circulation, a scenario that by definition occurred after repairing wounded arteries. The rapid reoxygenation of ischemic tissue results in cellular damage and edema, or swelling. When this swelling takes place in confined fascial compartments, it can compress the vasculature and interrupt blood flow, resulting in gangrene.

While never calling it reperfusion injury, physicians and surgeons identified the pathology in Korean War casualties and developed effective therapies. Scientific investigators previously had noticed the tendency of reperfused tissue to swell, but they initially attributed the excess fluid to the interruption of lymphatic flow that would accompany any major trauma.[129] Later studies reported a clear link between the length of ischemic time and the degree and duration of edema upon restoration of vascular flow.[130] Given the rarity of arterial repairs before the 1950s, few clinicians or scientists noticed or commented on this relationship. By the third year of the Korean War, where for the first time arterial repair became the expected mode of treatment, the sheer volume of cases made the condition apparent, highlighting the potential for new therapies to create new diseases.[131] Physicians quickly realized the importance of prompt and prophylactic fasciotomy to obviate the condition.[132] After the war, prophylactic fasciotomies following arterial repair became part of the standard education for military medical officers.[133]

Unlike previous conflicts, the limited nature of the Korean War allowed investigators to follow their patients long term. In a 1958 study, Jahnke identified 115 patients who had their arteries repaired in Korea and who did not subsequently require amputation.[134] He relied on arteriograms to assess patency, which by then had become the gold standard methodology. The results surprised Jahnke: 33 of 115 patients (29 percent) had thrombosed their artery at the site of repair.[135] Complete clinical records allowed Jahnke to break down the failures more specifically. He found that fewer than 20 percent of end-to-end anastomoses failed, but nearly half (47 percent) of venous grafts did. Surprisingly, nearly 45 percent of lateral suture repairs clotted, resulting in Jahnke recommending surgeons avoid that operation in favor of resection and anastomosis. An exorbitant 71 percent of arterial homografts eventually thrombosed.[136] Given the laboratory success of arterial homografts, their failure in traumatic vascular wounds remained ill understood at the time, but the statistics nonetheless warned against their further use in this capacity. In reviewing these data, Jahnke reminded the reader that, while far from achieving ideal results, this series still demonstrated the ability of arterial repair to save limbs, calling vascular surgery "one of the most outstanding achievements in war surgery."[137] However, he was quick to note the "greatest value [of the data] is that they demonstrate that the results have not been perfect and much additional experimental and clinical investigation still needs to be done."[138]

Why Arterial Repair Finally Took Hold in Korea

In the Korean War, repairing arteries finally became standard operating procedure. The widespread adoption of these techniques came fifty years after Alexis Carrel won his Nobel Prize for their invention. How, then, did the Korean War differ from earlier times to permit and even encourage the advancement of vascular surgery? A multitude of influences converged at the right time in the right place to revolutionize practice.

Military

The war itself was one critically important ingredient. Combat provided the thousands of patients required to collect adequate statistical proof of reliability and efficacy of arterial repair. Just any war would not suffice, as evident by the lack of routine vascular repair in the two world wars. The limited nature of the "police action" allowed the United States to concentrate its resources on a relatively small battlefront. In a volume impossible in the larger world wars, America supplied instruments, shipped blood, deployed nurses, evacuated casualties, and generally provided magnanimous logistical support. The war capitalized on a growing medical-industrial complex that helped provide this matériel.

The nature of the fighting enabled surgical experimentation. One can broadly divide the Korean War into two segments: mobile warfare (June 1950–spring 1951) and static warfare (spring 1951–July 1953). In the first portion, US troops moved constantly: they started by retreating some two hundred aerial miles to the Naktong River. After the breakout from the Pusan Perimeter, they advanced more than four hundred miles, only to retreat another two hundred or so after the Chinese intervened. In the span of eight months, US forces traveled well over one thousand road miles. Hospitals struggled to stay close to the fighting and not get left behind during retreats; the 8055th MASH, for example, moved four times in twenty-two days in October 1950.[139] Constantly relocating, it could not accumulate any extra equipment or material. Lacking the ability to hold and monitor cases postoperatively, MASHs evacuated nearly every patient they admitted, usually directly to Japan via airplane. Aeroevacuation was so readily available that clinicians after the war criticized "the emphasis on *transportation* at a certain expense of *treatment*."[140]

With enemy action rarely abating, especially during the retreats, casualties swamped the hospital. During one six-day period in the course of the North Korean counterattack, the 8076th MASH received 1,836 patients, with 661 admitted in a twenty-four-hour span. "The patients were arriving in such large numbers," documented the unit official history, "that there was no place to put them inside the hospital tents. When the ambulances arrived, patients would have to be left lying in the snow, where some froze to death before they could even be admitted."[141] The triage situation combined with constant mobility did not lend itself to experimental medicine or intricate, time-consuming vascular repair.

By contrast, stabilized front lines characterized the final twenty-seven months of the war. MASHs became permanent fixtures—only two of the six MASHs moved at all in 1952.[142] Tents became buildings, dirt floors wooden, and both the quantity and the sophistication of medical equipment increased.[143] Without having to worry about sudden retreats, hospitals could position themselves ever closer to the front lines. Total air superiority permitted the construction of aboveground, bulky structures that never would have survived the bombing raids that had tormented medical units in World War II.[144] Casualties came in spurts, corresponding with UN or enemy efforts to take a position, rather than the continuous deluge earlier in the war. Whereas in 1950 there were 1,200 hospital admissions for trauma per 1,000 troops, by 1952 it had fallen by an order to magnitude, nadiring well below 100.[145] This situation allowed for medical and surgical research, advanced facilities, better communication among various hospitals, and the opportunity for surgeons to attend continuing medical education sessions.

Two new military technologies had the potential to catalyze arterial repair: body armor and helicopters. Returning to the battlefield for the first time since knights on horseback, body armor in the form of protective vests had the potential to redirect wounds away from the chest and abdomen and toward the extremities, with their susceptible blood supply.[146] However, careful statistics proved no such redistribution occurred, and the vests did not influence the practice of vascular surgery in Korea.[147]

Helicopters, with the ability to evacuate patients rapidly, offered even greater promise. Able to take off and land on the battlefield, these rotary-wing aircraft could theoretically bring casualties directly from the fighting to the MASHs within minutes instead of the hours ground transport required. Sources ranging from rogue surgeon Frank Spencer to contemporary military reports to later histories of surgery all credit helicopters and the associated decreased transit time as a crucial factor in the adoption of arterial repair.[148] Seeing patients more quickly meant doctors had a chance to revascularize limbs before tissue died from lack of blood flow.[149]

Despite this potential, helicopters did not affect vascular surgery in Korea.[150] There were relatively few functioning aircraft: in July 1953, at the end of the war and at peak buildup, the army had only sixteen dedicated helicopter-ambulances, with rarely more than ten flyable on any given day (mechanical problems grounded the remainder).[151] Fragile technology prevented flying at night or in inclement weather and dictated pilots retrieve patients behind the lines, at battalion or even division aid stations, to protect them from enemy fire. This limitation negated much of the time advantage aircraft offered since it required hours to transport casualties through mountain passes under fire to the safety of a medical facility.[152] As such, the lag between wounding and surgery—seven to ten hours—hardly differed from that of World War II.[153] Furthermore, in a distinct departure from prior practice and in an effort to prove the efficacy of arterial repair, surgeons operated regardless of the delay. "Under the conditions in Korea," remarked one newly minted vascular surgeon, "a prolonged time lag was not a con-traindication to repair."[154] Every M*A*S*H episode on television begins with physicians and nurses racing to a landing pad as a chopper laden with wounded soldiers swoops in to deliver its human cargo, seemingly moments away from death, saved by the Bell H-13 helicopter. This scene is fiction. Helicopters evacuated approximately 5 percent of combat casualties, did not appreciably shorten the time between wounding and surgery, and did not affect the practice of arterial repair.[155]

Medical

The medical milieu also contributed to an environment conducive to chang-ing the practice of vascular surgery. Coming just seven years after VJ Day, Korea benefitted from World War II. While the arterial repair lessons of the aux groups and vascular centers went unheeded, almost all the senior mili-tary and medical officers had fought in the Second World War. Develop-ing an efficient, effective military medical system with evacuation chains, echelons of care, and supporting hospitals was not just conceptual for them but recent, lived experiences. Both clinically and organizationally, medicine in Korea was a continuation of previous efforts, which facilitated preparing patients for vascular surgery. Better-trained anesthesiologists felt more com-fortable managing critically wounded patients on the operating table. More professional nurses provided superior postoperative care, including the regu-lar pulse checks necessary to assess the patency of vascular repairs.[156] Enor-mous blood transfusions that became common in Korea kept soldiers alive and perfused limbs. New antibiotics stymied infection. Without this envi-ronment, arterial repair could never have flourished, yet it still required the introduction of proper vascular techniques to MASH surgeons. A fortuitous set of circumstances at the 46th MASH provides compelling evidence for the importance of both elements.

This hospital emerged as a test case for exploring the factors prompting arterial repair. In the first four months of 1952, surgeons there practiced liga-tion, as in World War II. Howard arrived in April and thereafter began a policy of arterial repair. The 46th MASH thus performed a de facto clini-cal trial, inadvertently (but helpfully) controlling for variables like surgeon competence, physical plant, nursing care, anesthesiology, and other factors. The differences between these two periods are striking. The amputation rate when the hospital performed ligations was 62 percent but fell to 7 percent following the adoption of arterial repair.[157] This transformation could not—and indeed did not—occur outside this specific environment, yet it simultaneously proves the seminal importance of the surgeon's technical ability.

It also demonstrates how these young surgeons were willing to buck authority. Entering Korea, ligation remained the dominant and recommended procedure. Harvard vascular specialist Richard Warren, visiting Korea as a consultant, asserted that "venous grafts should be discouraged" and recommended conservative therapy instead.[158] A 1953 military surgery textbook espoused similar recommendations.[159] Even adamant proponents of arterial repair in civilian life like Simeone strongly doubted military doctors could apply it to war casualties, leading to a reluctant recommendation to ligate.[160]

Young surgeons refused to accept practices they deemed outmoded and harmful.[161] In Washington, Seeley and his team followed their clinical results when they contradicted Elkin's recommendations. Some operators in Korea, like Apel and Spencer, risked being court-martialed to proceed with arterial repair, convinced their operations provided better care to the wounded Americans they treated. When Howard and Jahnke arrived in Korea, they too faced a skeptical medical establishment that remained wedded to ligation, forcing the team to prove the supremacy of anastomosis and grafting. In all these cases, compelling data ultimately overpowered tradition, seniority, and established patterns of practice. The army deserves credit for acknowledging and accepting these conclusions, changing its policy mid-war, and instituting an intra-theater educational program for surgeons.

This flexibility largely resulted from relying on young, drafted surgeons whose recent residency exposure provided them both the intellectual and manual skills that not just enabled but encouraged them to suture and anastomose vessels. These same conscripted surgeons, soon discharged from military service, returned to their residencies and hospitals in the United States not only vividly aware of the potential of arterial repair to save lives but also exceptionally capable of performing the procedure, having gained more experience in their year-long tour of duty than even their most senior colleagues had attained over a career. They brought this knowledge and skill to operating rooms across America, driving the dissemination of arterial repair around the country.

Chapter Six

Bringing It All Back Home

The emergence and propagation of arterial repair in the Korean War proved both its superiority over ligation for vascular trauma and, as important, the ability of average, residency-trained surgeons to perform the operation with success. If the procedure worked on severely injured patients in the austere, resource-limited environs of Korea, then its application in the comparatively stable, well-equipped operating rooms of the United States seemed the logical next step. This chapter demonstrates the rapid increase in the practice of arterial repair in the United States from the early 1950s until 1960, by which time it had been established as a common, standardized procedure in hospitals around the country. Presentations and publications from the Korean War experience provided data proving its potential. Individual drafted surgeons learned the techniques overseas and brought them home to stateside hospitals. There, they taught a new generation of residents the intricacies of this operation while demonstrating its superiority for patients.

Over the course of the 1950s, the indication for arterial repair expanded from trauma (both military and domestic) to atherosclerotic arterial disease. Long identified in the medical literature, atherosclerosis gained prominence in the 1950s as part of the general epidemiological shift from infectious to chronic diseases. Cholesterol-clogged arteries, supplying logarithmically more patients then trauma ever would, partly emerged as a prominent medical problem because of the curative potential of arterial repair. It simultaneously helped to develop the specialty of vascular surgery, which took increasing responsibility for the millions of Americans suffering from this condition.

The Rise of Arterial Repair in the United States

Between the end of the Korean War and 1960, arterial repair went from being a rare operation practiced almost exclusively at elite, academic hospitals by a

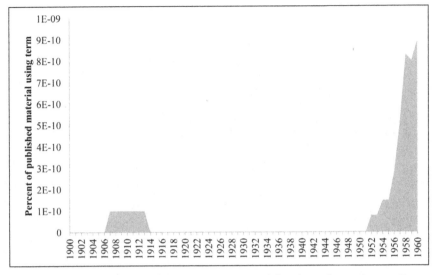

Figure 6.1. Google Ngram depicting rise in usage of the phrase "arterial repair."
Note the dramatic spike starting in 1953, just as surgeons in the Korean War started
publishing their results.

few experts to a common one that every American surgeon was expected to
perform. A review of the published literature reveals an explosion of people
discussing the procedure. Google Ngrams, which track the appearance of
words in written material, shows that usage of the phrase "vascular surgery"
leaped fourfold between 1951 and 1960.[1] The term "arterial repair" similarly
surged more than twentyfold over those same years (figure 6.1).[2] While writing about this method does not provide direct evidence of its performance, it
does show an increasing level of interest.

Much of this discourse took place at formal academic conferences. In the
fall of 1951, Sam Seeley, Francis Cooke, Carl Hughes, and Edward Jahnke
presented their positive results using arterial repair at Walter Reed to the
Clinical Congress of the American College of Surgeons, the largest surgical meeting in the country, hosting an average of 6,200 surgeons a year.[3]
Between 1951 and 1957, presentations on arterial repair at Clinical Congresses quintupled and broadened to cover topics like vessel banks, preferred
graft material, and new management strategies for vascular disease and
trauma.[4] In 1953, Jahnke collaborated with Harris B. Shumacker to teach
anastomoses to conference attendees in a hands-on wet lab at the Clinical
Congress.[5] Other surgeons taught their colleagues at local medical meetings,
like the 1951 course at the Annual Medical Meeting of Wisconsin.[6] These

sessions again emphasize the importance of practical education in the dissemination of surgical technique.

At the smaller, more specialized Society for Vascular Surgery meeting, a similar trend was evident. Papers on arterial repair, making up fewer than 10 percent of all presentations in 1950, more than tripled to greater than a third of the entire program by 1955 and included talks by Korean War veterans like Seeley, Cooke, and Hughes.[7] Data analyzing the introduction of novel antibiotics have demonstrated that those physicians attending conferences were more likely to use the new drugs and prescribe them correctly as compared with colleagues who remained home. These studies cited attendees being more open to change, abreast of current developments, receptive to opinion leaders, and benefitting from the interpersonal connections and communication that occurs at these events.[8] Extrapolating these conclusions to medical innovations more generally suggests the repetitive presentations on the success of arterial repair combined with hands-on teaching sessions at conferences around the country stimulated its adoption.

The value of this new vascular surgery also appeared in the written literature. Reviewing the four main general surgical journals of the era from 1940 to 1961 demonstrates a surge in publishing on arterial repair.[9] Whereas in 1949 only 2 percent of articles discussed this technique, in 1958 almost 10 percent did—a fivefold increase (figure 6.2). This trend was predictably most pronounced in *Surgery*, which served as the official periodical for the Society for Vascular Surgery in these years, but the prominence of articles in other general surgical journals indicates both the practice of the technique by general surgeons as well as the emphasis editors placed on the topic when selecting what to include in their monthly issues. The flurry of studies partly resulted from the increasingly magnanimous support the National Institutes of Health (NIH) provided. In the post–World War II years, political maneuvering by the NIH positioned it to assume control over federally funded biomedical research.[10] Budgetary growth reflected its new position of power, with Congress increasing its appropriations from $707,000 in 1940 to almost $400 million by 1960, a 546-fold raise.[11] This money helped support vascular research and the salaries of the faculty conducting it.

Not only did the quantity of articles on vascular surgery change over the course of this decade, but so did their content. Whereas publications in the 1940s and early 1950s tended to present either laboratory experiments in animals or exciting but rare case reports, after the Korean War the literature encompassed a more clinical orientation and featured series of dozens or even hundreds of patients.[12] Commenting on a 1957 study of vascular trauma among civilians, Stanford chief surgeon Carleton Mathewson reminisced,

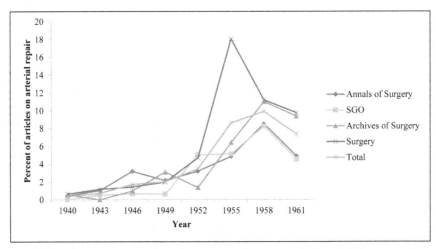

Figure 6.2. Rise in percent of articles on arterial repair in the surgical literature, 1940–61. Again, note the spike following the Korean War, with *Surgery* the highest due to its formal affiliation with the Society of Vascular Surgery. By the late 1950s, the initial excitement surrounding the success of arterial repair was fading, hence the decline in articles on the subject.

"In 1941, I believe it was important enough to report a single successful end-to-end suture of the brachial artery," but today "Dr. [George C.] Morris has now recorded 93 repairs, with a restoration of function of 86 per cent. This, indeed, is evidence of the tremendous advances in this field of surgery in the past fifteen years."[13] Other articles focused less on numbers or novelty but, in sections like "Surgeon at Work" (published in *Surgery, Gynecology, and Obstetrics*), served as instructional how-to manuals for the technique.[14] Language within articles changed. A 1951 description of treating Korean War casualties discussed using a "vein graft," putting scare quotes around the term to connote the tentative, experimental nature of the procedure.[15] Later authors expressed no such hesitation when describing what had become a standard technique. By the end of the decade, surgeons were investigating long-term complications of arterial repair with grafts, a topic inconceivable in 1950 since almost no patients existed who would have developed such sequelae.[16]

These advances in the research literature altered expectations for the practice of surgery. In 1954, the Committee on Trauma for the American College of Surgeons published its text *Early Care of Soft Tissue Injuries*. This popular volume sold more than twenty thousand copies, including one for every ship in the US Navy, which used the book to educate its medical officers.[17] The chapter on vascular injuries, written in the midst of the Korean War by Harris B. Shumacker, reflected contemporary uncertainty on the feasibility or value of arterial repair. "The choice between ligation . . . or repair . . . rests principally upon the experience of the surgeon and the availability of proper facilities," as Shumacker emphasized the prioritization of saving life, then the limb itself, then the functionality thereof as only a tertiary concern.[18] When the second edition came out in 1960, the text clearly recognized that "recent advances in vascular surgery have brought about a transformation in our attitude towards injuries of blood vessels." In contrast to Shumacker's earlier recommendation, it averred that the surgeon's "responsibilities have thus been immensely extended beyond the time-honored methods of ligation or amputation" and insisted that "restoration of blood flow, not merely [sic!] saving of a life, is now the prime consideration."[19] Several pages of detailed instructions complete with diagrams followed to assist young clinicians perform vascular anastomoses.

This shift in expectations also appeared in general surgical textbooks intended for medical students and residents. In 1936, Frederick Christopher published his single-volume *A Textbook of Surgery by American Authors*, which quickly became the standard reference for the subject.[20] Emile Holman, former Halsted resident and chair of surgery at Stanford, wrote the sections on arterial disease and trauma.[21] While he acknowledged that suturing wounds of the arteries was theoretically preferable, the seven lines he dedicated to this treatment paled in comparison to the thirty-five lines he spent describing proper ligation procedure, itself a far simpler operation. He continued to recommend the Matas operation for the treatment of aneurysms and never discussed bypass grafts or other mechanisms of repair. Subsequent editions in 1942 and 1949 changed minimally and continued to recommend ligation.[22]

In 1956, a new edition was issued strongly favoring arterial repair. Authored again by Harris Shumacker, this chapter benefitted from the lessons of the Korean War and instructed students to make "every effort . . . to preserve or restore the continuity of the damaged artery" via lateral suture, end-to-end-anastomosis, or venous grafting.[23] He followed this assertion with detailed prose and diagrams to teach students how to perform the operation, writing that repair is not just for elite surgeons or unique cases but "is ordinarily possible." This same transformation appeared in more specialized vascular surgery textbooks as well: the 1955 edition of *Peripheral Vascular Disease* featured entire chapters on arterial repair that were absent from its 1946 predecessor.[24] Textbooks, less responsive to the vagaries of a field than oral presentations and journal articles, represent expert opinion and accepted wisdom.[25] The transition away from ligation in their pages confirmed that arterial repair had arrived. Moreover, by 1956 at the latest, the American College of Surgeons required that all graduating residents demonstrate competency in vascular surgery operations including peripheral arterial repair and venous grafts for aneurysms, disease, or trauma.[26]

Evidence for increased *practice* of arterial repair comes not only from the aforementioned publications describing hundreds of patients but also through the expansion and greater utilization of blood vessel banks. Initially established in the late 1940s to provide material for cardiac and aortic cases, banks widened their mission to encompass peripheral arterial repair in the 1950s. The institutions themselves proliferated in the early 1950s, as repositories appeared in cities with major medical centers including Boston, New York City, Chicago, Washington, DC, Baltimore, Miami, Madison, and Houston.[27] The facility the US Navy established in Bethesda, Maryland, was the largest tissue bank in the country and exemplified the growing national attention to peripheral arterial repair.

The US Navy led the nation in supporting tissue banks through both grants to outside institutions as well as research conducted in its own world-class facility.[28] Given the dramatic success of stored blood in World War II, the military envisioned extending this technology to create a stockroom of spare tissues and organs that surgeons could take off the shelf and use to repair the wounded. This goal fit the prevailing notion of the body being composed of replaceable parts, as demonstrated by the contemporary article "Spare Parts for People" in *Harper's Magazine* that described the program at Bethesda.[29]

Founded in 1949 as the first free-standing tissue bank in the world, the naval institution initially focused on freeze-dried bone.[30] By the summer of 1952, it branched out to other types of tissue, including preserved arteries.[31] "The use of arterial grafts seems to offer particularly favorable possibilities, and additional supplies of arteries are especially needed," noted a 1953 memorandum.[32] Rejecting a quarter of submitted specimens for disease, inadequate length, or poor tissue quality, the bank always lacked sufficient samples. By 1955, it had collected 103 arteries, deemed 27 as unsuitable, used 33 in patients, and devoted 14 to research.[33] Both the investigative effort and the sheer volume of material—no other bank in the world accumulated as many specimens—catapulted the Navy Tissue Bank to become the vanguard of the field. Civilian hospitals sent their personnel to Bethesda to learn preservation techniques in order to construct analogous facilities at home.[34]

Following the Korean War, civilian surgeons also petitioned the navy for preserved arteries to use in their patients. For example, a forty-three-year-old woman in Washington, DC, was diagnosed with Leriche syndrome, or occlusion of the lower aorta. Surgeons at George Washington University Hospital obtained a graft from the navy bank and successfully implanted it, curing the patient.[35] The bank had far more requests than its inventory permitted it to fill.[36] Repeated requests, though, clearly indicate doctors were repairing arteries, and at hospitals away from the large academic facilities that managed their own repositories. With the navy unable or unwilling to share its own arteries and with banks expensive to establish and maintain, consortia of surgeons paid the navy to store vessels for them, which they could then request as needed.[37] This arrangement reflected not just the repair of trauma but also the frequent practice of elective operations on diseased arteries, an indication that grew in importance over this decade.

The Korean Connection

The spreading practice of arterial repair resulted from its successful application in the Korean War. Knowledge transfer partly resulted from statistics and reports enumerating the Korean War experience. While not every doctor in Korea recorded his results, others, like Frank Spencer, came from academic residencies and aspired to professorial careers. They recognized the novelty of their practice and both the scientific and professional benefits to publishing their methods and outcomes.[38] The Walter Reed research team was especially aggressive in reporting their results. They presented preliminary data via posters and talks at conferences before ultimately authoring more than a dozen articles that appeared in surgical journals.[39] These papers and presentations exposed the surgical community to the success of arterial repair.

The subsequent vascular surgery literature produced in the United States almost universally acknowledged data from the Korean War as catalyzing a change in practice. Holman, the Stanford chair and vascular expert who, during World War II, adamantly opposed arterial repair in wartime trauma and only tepidly favored it for civilians, published the aptly titled book *New Concepts in Surgery of the Vascular System* in 1955. "Experiences reported recently from the Korean War demonstrate beyond question that some of the old concepts regarding the surgical care of vascular injuries . . . have become radically, basically and permanently altered," wrote Holman.[40] Surgeons ought to "abandon" ligation and instead apply the techniques of arterial repair that Spencer, Jahnke, and Hughes had demonstrated in Korea.[41]

Similarly, Michael DeBakey, who had initially discounted repairing blood vessels in combat after World War II, changed his approach to arterial trauma. Following the war, DeBakey had assumed the chairmanship of Baylor College of Medicine in Houston, Texas, where he started a cardiovascular research program that attained global acclaim over the ensuing decades. In a 1957 article citing the work of Jahnke, Howard, Hughes, and Spencer, DeBakey noted that "the Korean conflict . . . demonstrate[d] conclusively the feasibility and efficacy of primary repair of acute vascular wounds."[42] Tracking 136 consecutive patients with acute arterial injuries in Texas over seven years, DeBakey and colleagues noted a distinct trend from ligation (50 percent of cases in the first 3.5 years of the study) to repair (76 percent of cases in the final 3.5 years). Most of these trauma patients presented to the community hospital, where the resident staff performed the surgeries. Their involvement demonstrates both that residents did learn how to repair arteries during their education and that operators with even limited ability and training could perform the procedure, with practice and instruction. Additional articles followed, consistently crediting the Korean War for providing the proof needed to change practice in the United States.

Reports from the Korean War furnished promising data, but papers and presentations could not teach how to repair arteries. Other surgeons could—especially the hundreds of drafted doctors who had deployed to Korea and observed the appropriate technique and favorable results in a MASH unit. They proved instrumental in the transmission of knowledge.[43] Many of them settled into a life of private practice and never wrote about their experience, challenging historical analysis. But the importance and effect of interpersonal communication for disseminating an innovation, repeatedly demonstrated in other fields, emphasizes the value of this pipeline of new experts in the adoption of arterial repair in America.[44]

The three previously discussed rogue surgeons exemplify this effect. Hermes Grillo returned to Boston after his tour, finished his surgical residency there, and eventually became chief of thoracic surgery at Massachusetts General Hospital. While not a vascular surgeon, he relied on similar anastomotic techniques in the tracheal and esophageal operations for which he became famous; importantly, as an academician, he taught dozens of housestaff how to practice surgery, including arterial repair.[45] Otto Apel became a private practice breast surgeon after finishing his residency and did little vascular work himself, but one of the other doctors he taught at the 8076th MASH in Korea was Albert Starr. Continuing cardiovascular work after returning home to Oregon, Starr later achieved global fame for his invention of a successful artificial heart valve. As a professor at the University of Oregon's medical school, he taught the techniques he learned in Korea to hundreds of residents and fellows.[46]

Frank Spencer rotated back to the United States and not only practiced vascular surgery but also influenced the trajectory of the young specialty.[47] After his tour in Korea, he returned to Baltimore and completed his residency at Johns Hopkins Hospital, which hired him upon his graduation in 1955 to take charge of its peripheral vascular surgery section. Spencer helped manage its vessel bank, operated on the majority of peripheral vascular cases, and participated in teaching the residents. Recruited by his friend Ben Eiseman in 1961 to the University of Kentucky, he started its cardiac and vascular surgery program before leaving to assume the chair at New York University.[48] Spencer simultaneously leveraged his vascular work in Korea to launch his career while also disseminating the technique through his leadership roles at three different institutions, coediting the seminal textbook on vascular trauma surgery, and training hundreds of surgical residents.[49]

Other army surgeons similarly applied the arterial repair they learned to their later practices. Keith Reemtsma, another V-12 graduate, deployed to Korea in the midst of his residency and worked with Spencer at Easy Med. He returned to have an illustrious academic career, relying on his introduction to anastomoses in the military to develop the field of xenotransplantation. Later chairing the departments of surgery at the University of Utah and Columbia Presbyterian Medical Center, Reemtsma advocated for the importance of advanced vascular surgery.[50] Korean War surgeon Russell Nelson eventually moved home to Salt Lake City, performed the first open heart surgery in Utah, and subsequently rose to preside over the Society for Vascular Surgery in 1975.[51] Carl Hughes, exposed to anastomosis and vessel repair while at Walter Reed Hospital and in Korea, stayed in the army and established the first military vascular surgery fellowship program at Walter Reed in 1966, taking Norman Rich as his inaugural student.[52] John T. Phelan, a flight surgeon in the Korean War, started his academic practice at the University of Wisconsin–Madison, where he used his Korean experience to found an artery bank there and publish more than a dozen articles studying various aspects of vascular surgery, such as testing novel suture materials and different methods of anastomosis.[53] Many of these publications appear in the *Wisconsin Medical Journal*, a state periodical with review articles like "Newer Aspects of Peripheral Vascular Surgery" that served to educate local doctors rather than to announce original discoveries.[54]

Francis N. Cooke also took his newfound expertise to the civilian community. He assisted in the development of the army's first artery banks at Walter Reed and had participated in some early studies on definitive arterial repair in Korean War wounded.[55] After doffing his uniform, Cooke assumed a faculty position at the University of Miami, where he applied his military research to establish a blood vessel bank at Jackson Memorial Hospital and promote the repairing of arteries there.[56] As a professor of surgery, he taught these techniques to residents; Cooke's most famous trainee, Thomas Starzl, proceeded to use the principles of vessel anastomosis to perform the first liver transplants in the world.[57]

The rogue surgeons and Starr, Hughes, Nelson, Phelan, and Cooke provide just a few examples of those who served in Korea and brought new vascular ability home. Because of the Doctor Draft, they were all young men deferred from World War II programs, most in the middle of residency, who subsequently spent decades in the field practicing and teaching surgery. Multiplied hundredfold across cities and hospitals throughout the United States, these military medical veterans provided personal attestations to the data presented in the literature, taught the technique to colleagues and students, and served as agents of change that actualized the widespread implementation of arterial repair.

Assaults, Automobiles, and Atherosclerosis

The rapid expansion of vascular surgery in the 1950s depended on the experiences gained in the Korean War, but it was also driven by an exponential increase in the number of patients who required arterial repair to preserve their arms and legs. This demand stemmed partly from trauma: urban crime and especially motor vehicle accidents climbed precipitously in this decade. But, far more importantly, new attention to atherosclerotic peripheral vascular disease created a potential patient population of millions of sufferers who, by 1960, could look to vascular surgery to assuage their symptoms.

Social and demographic shifts of the postwar era contributed to a rise in traumatic injuries to arteries that surgeons in the United States had to address. Violent crime beset cities as the murder rate rose and the number of aggravated assaults nearly doubled between 1937 and 1957, filling operating rooms with patients bleeding from torn vessels.[58] The penetrating nature of criminal injuries—typically stabbing or shooting—made vascular lacerations more likely.[59] Surgeons in trauma centers like Houston, Texas, St. Louis, Missouri, and Atlanta, Georgia, documented the rise of these injuries through the 1950s and their increasing commitment to address them through modern techniques of arterial repair.[60] Surgeons at Emory, for example, transitioned from repairing under 10 percent of vascular wounds in 1950 to 80 percent in 1959.

Automotive trauma stemmed from some of the same societal forces. Americans fled cities for suburbs after World War II.[61] This geographic shift, combined with President Eisenhower's interstate system for military-economic transit, led to a network of roads and highways imbricating the United States.[62] Car ownership more than doubled from 1950 to 1958 to greater than sixty-seven million vehicles. Millions of miles driven by Americans also doubled from fewer than forty thousand in 1948 to more than eighty thousand by 1962.[63] Engineering technology from World War II created more powerful cars capable of higher speeds and faster acceleration while decorations like fins and chrome led to a prominent car culture of the 1950s.[64]

More driving meant more crashes. While fatalities per mile driven decreased, in a testament to the billions of miles odometers logged, the absolute numbers of deaths rose from fewer than twenty-five thousand per year in 1945 to thirty-five thousand by the end of the decade.[65] By 1960, traffic accidents were the third-most-common cause of death in the United States, behind only cardiovascular disease and stroke.[66] Nonfatal injuries did not receive the same actuarial attention, but in 1955 automobiles wounded more than 1.35 million Americans.[67] These casualties partly resulted from unsafe vehicles: for example, in 1956, fewer than 5 percent of car models came with seatbelts as a standard feature.[68] Physicians and particularly surgeons helped lead public health efforts to change car designs, outlaw drunk driving, establish a national system of 911 call centers, and certify trauma hospitals.[69]

When prevention failed, the human wreckage required surgeons to repair the damage. The profession acknowledged and embraced this responsibility, as indicated by Robert Zollinger's article "Traffic Injuries—a Surgical Problem" in 1955.[70] These injuries often afflicted the vascular system. As early as 1951, surgeons explicitly linked the Korean experience to automotive trauma in the United States: "We not only have war casualties to treat," commented Frank Gerbode, who was patching up war wounded in California as they returned to the United States, "but we have vascular problems resulting from automobile accidents."[71] The vascular techniques learned in Korea and, later, residency applied analogously whether the injuring agent was an enemy mortar shell or a Ford Thunderbird. Yet even the tens of thousands of victims of car crashes and urban crime paled in comparison to the millions of Americans suffering from atherosclerosis, or cholesterol-clogged arteries.

Atherosclerosis became the subject of increased attention in the 1950s as both its prevalence and treatment options rapidly expanded. Scientists had been studying the pathology since the nineteenth century, with Jean-Frederic-Martin Lobstein coining the older term, "arteriosclerosis," in 1833.[72]

Clinical interest increased in the twentieth century, with much of the research dedicated to atherosclerotic plaques in the coronary arteries supplying the heart that presumably caused heart attacks.[73] Plaques in the peripheral circulation similarly limited blood flow. These patients with peripheral vascular disease complained of severe leg pain and an inability to walk, with many ultimately developing gangrene and requiring amputation.

The rise in incidence following World War II reflected a general epidemiological shift in developed countries as chronic diseases proved more deadly than infectious ones. This transition largely resulted from improved public health efforts like clean water and vaccinations. Antibiotics aided in the treatment of bacterial and parasitic diseases.[74] Other medical advances actually increased the incidence of atherosclerosis. Insulin, heralded as a major triumph in the early twentieth century, effectively treated diabetes, but, as patients with the disease began to live years after their diagnosis, doctors recognized that the majority suffered from severe arterial blockages, as well as other comorbidities.[75]

Developments like new "miracle drugs," insulin, and exciting surgical operations drove a robust postwar popular confidence in the medical profession.[76] Television shows like *Medic* and *Ben Casey* and repeated photo essays in *Life* magazine reflected these attitudes.[77] Americans' willingness to submit their children to polio vaccine trials epitomized their faith in modern medicine.[78] This trust later encouraged patients to seek surgical cures for their chronic limb pain.

At the same time, Americans increasingly purchased health insurance or received it through their employment, making medical and surgical care more affordable. Prepaid insurance plans like Blue Cross emerged to provide access to lower-income, working-class patients in the early twentieth century and expanded rapidly after World War II.[79] In 1940, Blue Cross had six million members; in 1950, it had forty million—a quarter of the US population—and these numbers reflected only workers, not the dependents who also benefitted.[80] By the mid-1950s, private companies like Prudential began offering health insurance as well.[81] These plans provided patients the financial ability to consult doctors and receive otherwise unaffordable treatments. Moreover, insurance resulted in fiscal abdication to a third-party payer, increasing patients' willingness to undergo a now free/low-cost elective operation.[82]

The American lifestyle also changed. White collar jobs slowly replaced manual labor, and sedentary lifestyles became more common. Smoking rose dramatically following World War II, with over 50 percent of American men addicted to cigarettes in the 1950s.[83] Doctors had long linked tobacco use to worsening peripheral vascular disease via vasoconstriction and other mechanisms. Increased affluence led to different dietary habits, as people consumed more processed and fast food, raising cholesterol levels.[84] Individuals lived longer, with the number of Americans over the age of sixty-two rising from four million in 1900 (5 percent of the US population) to almost twenty-one million (11 percent) in 1960.[85] Surgeons repeatedly commented on the rising age of their patients and the corresponding increased prevalence of arterial disease. Older patients not only presented with peripheral vascular disease but also suffered from a host of comorbidities like heart conditions, difficulty breathing, and kidney problems that placed them at higher risk of developing complications; compromised immune systems predisposed them to wound infections and pneumonia. Their involved medical history and general frailty required an expertise in anesthesia and postoperative care not always necessary for otherwise healthy eighteen-year-old soldiers. Thus, the coeval, continuous development of anesthesiology, intensive care units, new antibiotics, hemodialysis, and other medical technologies in the 1950s and 1960s proved critical to enabling safe operations on an aging population.[86]

But atherosclerosis did not just affect the elderly: in 1953, a trio of military pathologists published a landmark study in the *Journal of the American Medical Association* documenting severe disease in 77 percent of the hearts of three hundred American soldiers killed in the Korean War. The average age: 22.1.[87] This report, confirming autopsy results from World War II, jolted the medical and lay belief that associated the disease with old age.[88] It drew renewed attention to a condition now seen as endemic to American society and, subsequently, to the therapeutic options to treat it.

Doctors tried to help their patients suffering from pain and limb loss, but, before arterial repair became common, they had little to offer. The paltry operative options are reflected in the inaugural membership of the Society of Arteriosclerosis, which first met in 1948 and had only three of eighty-five members identify as surgeons.[89] Doctors tried various drugs like histamine and even drinking whiskey in an effort to dilate blood vessels; none proved particularly successful.[90] Sympathectomy remained the most common surgical therapy into the early 1950s.[91] When that failed and patients developed gangrene, surgeons all too often had to amputate.

In the decade between 1950 and 1960, arterial repair became the definitive treatment for peripheral vascular disease. "I began in July 1955 to employ exclusively by-pass grafts in all patients operated on for acquired segmental occlusion of the major arteries of the lower extremities," wrote Ralph Deterling at the time.[92] Hundreds of publications in the surgical literature confirm that transition, discussing indications for operating, debating the safest material to use for bypasses, and describing permutations of the technique (see figure 6.2). In 1958, for example, the year the greatest number of articles on arterial operations appeared in *Annals of Surgery*, 90 percent addressed elective procedures, with titles like "Direct Surgery of Arteriosclerosis."[93] State medical journals evidence a similar trend.[94] Centers amassed hundreds of cases, quickly outnumbering traumatic injuries.[95]

In addition to bypasses, doctors also used a new operation called endarterectomy, a procedure in which the surgeon opened a diseased artery, removed atherosclerotic plaque from the inside, then sewed closed the rent made in the vessel. João Cid dos Santos first performed the technique in 1946, and it became increasingly popular in the mid-1950s as the patient population for this "roto-rooter" operation expanded exponentially.[96] As a potentially less morbid option than bypasses, endarterectomies represented the ongoing exploratory efforts to treat atherosclerotic vascular disease in the 1950s.

This shift toward surgical management of atherosclerosis—both bypass and endarterectomy—also relied upon the improving technology of arteriograms.[97] Developed between World War I and World War II, this imaging modality provided crucial information localizing the disease. While X-ray images helped with aneurysms and trauma, doctors were grossly able to identify those focal pathologies via physical exam and operative exploration. However, atherosclerotic vascular disease patients usually complained of diffuse leg pain without much external indication of where or which artery was diseased. This anatomical uncertainty limited surgery, which is an inherently local therapy focusing on a specific place in the body. Until surgeons could precisely locate which artery was blocked and where, they could not intervene. Arteriograms provided them that ability.

The increased utilization of arteriograms led to improvement in the technology, which subsequently facilitated greater use, in a positive feedback loop. By the mid-1950s, doctors reported performing hundreds of these tests per year.[98] The Thorotrast that Egas Moniz developed in the 1920s remained a standard dye, although ongoing experimentation produced contrast agents like diodrast that provided a more precise picture with less-noxious side effects.[99] More significantly, the technique of performing an arteriogram changed. For most of the early twentieth century, surgeons either inserted a long needle through the patient's back directly into the aorta or took the patient to an operating room to expose the femoral artery via surgery. Both these options are invasive and carry major risks. In 1953, Sven Seldinger pioneered a new method: he used a small IV needle to access the desired artery, threaded a guidewire into the vessel, then utilized that wire to advance a thin plastic tube into the artery through which he could inject contrast.[100] The

Seldinger technique allowed physicians to direct the exam to a specific artery, limiting the dye load and avoiding potentially unnecessary operations. Its comparative ease, safety, and broad applicability promoted its adoption by physicians around the world.

Michael DeBakey was one of those physicians, relying on arteriograms for both the care of patients and in research projects. His postwar investigative efforts began by trying to mimic the injuries he saw in combat, shooting anesthetized dogs with a .22 rifle in the hind leg and perfecting methods to repair the arterial damage.[101] While he applied these findings to traumatically wounded patients in Houston, his vascular practice remained inherently limited until he began performing elective cases for atherosclerotic disease and, later, aneurysms. This shift in the mid-1950s drew thousands of patients. DeBakey recorded completing at least 2,500 vascular operations between 1950 and 1960, with the majority treating cholesterol-clogged arteries.[102] (In stark contrast, he performed two in 1948, neither for peripheral vascular disease.)[103] When district judge R. Jasper Smith wrote to his friend about his 1959 femoral bypass operation, he described how his family doctor referred him to DeBakey based on symptoms of leg pain. DeBakey shot an arteriogram, confirmed the blockage in both femoral arteries, and treated the occlusion with bilateral femoral to popliteal bypasses using Dacron. Pronouncing himself "entirely happy and satisfied" with the outcome, Smith boasted that these procedures were "just routine" for the Houston surgical team.[104]

Smith's letter not only demonstrates the routinization of peripheral vascular surgery but also shows the widespread exposure of the therapy both to family practitioners and to the lay public. While medical practitioners could learn about new techniques through journals and conferences, the average American patient relied on mass media. Newspapers, magazines, and TV covered the subject, starting with developments during the Korean War. Articles described the ability of arterial repair to save lives and limbs both at Walter Reed Hospital and on the front lines.[105] This reporting continued for elective repair in the 1950s, with the CBS show *March of Medicine* featuring DeBakey's work in 1954.[106] Newspaper articles from around the country highlighted the drama associated with these procedures, including medical advice columns telling patients "clogged arteries [are] remediable."[107]

This news coverage not only reported on operations to repair trauma and occlusive disease but also featured exciting work on aortic aneurysms. Dramatic, potentially lethal, and often treatable via ligation, aneurysms had long provided surgeons an opportunity to demonstrate their ability to heal patients. However, aneurysms of the aorta, the largest artery in the body, defied this paradigm. Despite some of the most brilliant surgeons in the world creatively proposing cures—including ligation, gelatin injections, and electrocution, among others—this disease remained invariably deadly.[108] Rapid innovations in the science and practice of arterial repair in the middle of the twentieth century appeared to provide a surgical solution.

Successful treatment of aortic aneurysms in part resulted from the same epidemiological shift that changed the character of arterial disease in the mid-twentieth century. Syphilis, which infected an estimated 10 to 20 percent of Americans in 1920, had caused the majority of nontraumatic aneurysms in earlier generations.[109] In a series of 119 cases in nontrauma patients between 1905 and 1934, Rudolph Matas linked 80 percent to syphilis, a percentage confirmed by thousands of autopsies in both England and the United States.[110] But by the 1950s, pathologists found atherosclerosis causing over 90 percent of arterial aneurysms, a transition partly due to penicillin curing venereal disease.[111] This etiologic shift profoundly affected their treatability. Syphilis preferentially affects the thoracic (chest) aorta, where multiple branches to vital organs complicate any attempts at surgical repair. In contrast, atherosclerotic aortic aneurysms preferentially occur in the abdomen, lack major tributaries, and are simpler to remove. Contemporaries recognized this anatomical relocalization and its implications on the possibility of surgical cure.[112]

Already bypassing arteries torn by trauma or clogged with cholesterol, surgeons reasoned they could perform a similar operation on an aneurysmal aorta. This idea dated back to Carrel's work, but for decades no one was willing to try the technique on the largest blood vessel in the body, where any mistake threatened the life of the patient. Additionally, noting the repeated deaths following attempts at aortic ligation, physicians feared the physiological insult of clamping the aorta during the repair, as this act would temporarily eliminate blood flow to half of the body until they sewed the graft in place. Thus, successful aortic surgery depended as much on the ability to support a patient through a major operation, with anesthesia, blood banks, and intensive care units, as it did on the specific surgical technique.[113] In 1951 France, Charles Dubost performed the first modern surgical cure of an abdominal aortic aneurysm, replacing the diseased artery with a homograft.[114] Unaware of Dubost's accomplishment, DeBakey performed the second, and first in the United States, in an analogous fashion in 1952.[115] He later admitted to being "apprehensive" about this first case and the uncharted territory he was entering: "We didn't know, for example, how long we could occlude the aorta without producing serious consequences, we didn't know whether we would need to maintain circulation of the extremities and so on. We were just kind of experimenting in a way on human beings."[116]

Surgical management of abdominal, and later, thoracic, aortic aneurysms expanded in the 1950s and especially the 1960s, transforming from "experimenting on human beings" to a standard procedure offered at most major hospitals. By 1961, more than six hundred cases appeared in the literature.[117] Initially, surgeons depended on cadaveric vessels, which limited the number and type of operations they could perform. "I never was very happy with homografts," recalled DeBakey. "Relying on dead tissue meant you were compromising all the time . . . you had to use what was available for the patient, not what the patient needed."[118] In 1952, Arthur Voorhees invented an artificial artery made from a new fabric called vinyon.[119] His cloth prostheses succeeded where the glass, silver, and Vitallium tubes of Abbe, Tuffier, and Blakemore had failed. Infinitely customizable to patient specifications, comparatively cheap, relatively resistant to clotting, and always available, cloth grafts greatly facilitated the performance of a complex operation. DeBakey and others quickly adopted the concept, proposed novel textiles such as Dacron, and standardized the technology. By 1955, there were eight different materials fabricated into seventeen types of prostheses, a breadth that prompted the SVS to study the assortment and ultimately determine the superiority of Dacron and Teflon.[120] Combining the technical skills of arterial repair, the improvement in ancillary care, and cloth grafts, surgeons began repairing abdominal aortic aneurysms regularly by 1960.[121]

The success of these cases spawned adulation and acclamation both for the surgeons and for the field. "Just as the world had been trying to scale the summit of Mt. Everest, vascular surgery had been struggling to conquer the surgery of the aorta," wrote Rudolph Matas to DeBakey in 1954 upon learning of his successful treatment of an abdominal aortic aneurysm. Comparing DeBakey's achievement with that of Sir Edmund Hillary a year prior, Matas insisted that DeBakey's "conquest of the aorta marked a new era in surgery."[122] Popular accounts echoed Matas's praise, with titles like "Surgeons Can Correct Aneurysms" and "Rare Surgery Feat Saves Life of Man."[123] DeBakey brought considerable attention to the surgery after repairing the aortic aneurysm of the Duke of Windsor in 1964.[124] The "ideal" operation that Goyanes and Lexer performed in 1906/7 using Carrel's techniques expanded not just in volume as arterial repair became a standard operation in the 1950s but also anatomically, to the largest blood vessels in the body. Until heart bypasses became common in the late 1960s, operations to repair aortic aneurysms represented a seminal operation not just for vascular but for the entirety of surgery as they combined intricate technique, novel technology, and a mastery of physiology to cure patients of an otherwise lethal condition.

Conclusion

Just as a single officer charging the enemy cannot by himself win a battle, neither can a single physician, no matter how great, turn the tide of medicine. Change in practice requires an army of practitioners. Both Alexis Carrel and Michael DeBakey were brilliant investigators, technically gifted operators, and forward-thinking pioneers. But whereas Carrel never saw his vascular innovations enjoy widespread use, DeBakey witnessed the regular application of the procedures he invented and promoted. The key differences lay not in the abilities of either man but the context in which he worked. Extraordinary physicians like Carrel and DeBakey are undeniably essential to changing how a society treats patients and diseases. But particularly in a discipline like surgery, where individual practitioners manually apply complex therapies to each patient, these leaders are just that: leaders. They need a bevy of followers to make their discoveries relevant. The 1950s provided that multitude. Multiyear, formalized surgical residencies had become mandatory. The Korean War had proven the feasibility of arterial repair and created both the statistics and the personnel to effect change. Advances in highway infrastructure and rising crime rates led to a higher incidence of arterial trauma. Epidemiologic shifts increased the prevalence and awareness of atherosclerotic disease, manifesting in an exponentially larger patient population. As a result of these factors, arterial repair transformed from an operation isolated in academia into a standard procedure practiced throughout the United States.

Vascular surgery continued to develop after 1960. Surgeons invented different graft materials like PTFE, designed novel operations like William Blaisdell's extra-anatomical bypasses, and perfected techniques and perioperative management to lower morbidity and improve outcomes.[125] By the 1970s, the field had expanded in breadth and complexity such that new trainees required additional vascular fellowship training following their five-year residency. As this field matured into a distinct specialty, leaders in the Society for Vascular Surgery, notably Jack Wylie in San Francisco, created board exams and official certifications to distinguish individuals who had undergone additional years of training and could call themselves vascular surgeons.[126] Unfortunately, political squabbles among general, vascular, and cardiac surgery subsequently arose over who should care for which patients.

More recently, endovascular techniques, where surgeons treat aneurysms and atherosclerotic disease from inside blood vessels via stents, has challenged the dominance of open arterial repair.[127] Part of a general movement toward minimally invasive surgery in the 1990s and 2000s, endovascular therapies offer a new opportunity to explore surgical innovation that is beyond the scope of this work.[128] Yet the core elements of how and why surgery changes—exemplified by arterial repair and outlined further in the conclusion—provides a framework for understanding the process.

Conclusion

Arterial Repair and the Process of Surgical Change

In 1880, no operation to repair or anastomose arteries existed. By 1960, surgeons across the United States were applying these new techniques to arrest traumatic bleeding, keep aneurysms from rupturing, and prevent atherosclerotic vascular disease from irreversibly clogging vessels. Alexis Carrel receives the majority of credit for inventing arterial repair, although, as with most famous names attached to a procedure, Carrel followed and adopted advances established by his predecessors.[1] These pages have explored this process of technical development in depth to unveil unique aspects of surgical culture like the prioritization of practice over theory, the reliance on animals, and the crucial importance of in-person communication for the transfer of knowledge. Despite its promise, arterial repair paradoxically remained confined to textbooks and a handful of elite practitioners for half a century.

While the creation of a potentially curative operation is critical, the trajectory of arterial repair shows that this stage is but one step to understanding surgical change. Demonstrating the broad acceptance of a procedure and exploring how that process transpired are equally important components to the history. Examining that transformation, this book explicitly distinguishes surgical innovations from medical ones by highlighting the manual manipulations unique to operating. These features required a more parallel system of transferring knowledge that demanded prolonged training to acquire the necessary expertise and in-person teaching to convey the specific techniques. Ironically, surgical innovation has received less historical attention than other medical and public health interventions despite the strong historical interest among surgeons.

In a recent review, Christopher Lawrence characterized surgical innovation as a "slippery fish"—examples for individual operations exist, but all-encompassing explanations continue to escape the grasp of historians.[2] The history of arterial repair simultaneously reinforces and rebuts his argument.

The preceding chapters empirically investigated the nuanced evolution of arterial repair, demonstrating the impossibility of understanding the development of any operation without analyzing the elements and environment specific to that case. Yet, at the same time, the example of arterial repair can work as an effective case study to explore universal themes of how and why surgery evolves. This book has emphasized the importance of considering vectors of stasis and change ranging from the broadest social and cultural factors to the most specific technical details. While particular elements will vary on a case-by-case basis, certain tropes are conserved.

Doctors must first identify a clinical problem conceivably amenable to a surgical solution. For arterial repair, traumatically wounded vessels long demanded some form of operative intervention to save patients' lives. The increased incidence of aneurysms following the introduction of syphilis into Europe stimulated interest in that pathology, ultimately leading to John Hunter's ligation procedure. As surgery developed generally, the risks of gangrene and amputation following ligation drove the innovation of new techniques of anastomosis. By the 1950s, these procedures expanded from their original indications of managing traumatic bleeding and aneurysms to treating primarily atherosclerotic vascular disease. Later in the twentieth century, heart bypasses, solid organ transplants, and free-flap tissue grafts came to rely on these same fundamental techniques. This evolution demonstrates how surgeries designed for one pathology are often repurposed to manage others.[3]

Outside of trauma, most indications to operate awaited the localization of pathology in the late nineteenth and early twentieth centuries. Appendectomies made no sense before appendicitis; coronary artery bypasses had no role without a disease model where focal blockages of coronary circulation caused heart attacks.[4] Conversely, when surgeries seemed to alleviate symptoms, their methodology shaped the understanding of disease causation.[5] For example, the apparent success of bypasses in preventing gangrene and myocardial infarctions reaffirmed the etiological presumptions of atherosclerotic occlusive disease.

History presents numerous admonitory instances of doctors, patients, and society too glibly embracing the connection among sickness, surgery, and healing. This enthusiasm prompted support for operating on patients who, in retrospect, ought never to have been inside an OR. Neurosurgeries to cure criminal tendencies, lobotomies to manage insanity, gynecologic extirpations to treat hysteria and nymphomania, sympathectomies for constipation, and nephropexies to resolve vague abdominal pain all represent procedures widely accepted in their day for their curative potential.[6] Since discredited, these examples, along with many others, offer cautionary lessons on the readiness to pick up a scalpel and attempt to cut out all the body's problems.[7] Even medically justified operations, like tonsillectomies, have widely divergent rates of application seemingly explained primarily by physician preference, further demonstrating that what the medical profession and patients believe to be pathological and treatable by surgery varies over time and by region.[8] While scholars like John Wennberg have analyzed contemporary factors causing this disparity, historical investigations remain relatively rare.

Many of these surgeries depend on technology. Even comparatively low-tech procedures like arterial repair or appendectomies required anesthesia and antisepsis to achieve routine success. While heparin, arteriography, synthetic cloth grafts, and new tools like Potts clamps were not absolutely necessary to anastomose arteries, they greatly facilitated its performance and contributed to its rapid adoption in the mid-twentieth century. For other operations, specific instruments or devices are sine qua non. Surgeons rely on orthopedic hardware, bypass machines, and laparoscopes for the actual performance of the operation itself; other tools, such as immunosuppression, are equally important scientific developments used outside of the operating room. Ranging from a knife to the latest genetic manipulations, technology has and will continue to shape the practice of surgery.

Social science breakthroughs, notably the education of surgeons, form a different type of technological advance. The purposeful creation of a group of competent, well-trained surgeons who could successfully execute challenging interventions like arterial repair enabled its movement out of isolated academic centers and into mainstream practice. This residency-based education—followed by a second wave of fellowships in the late twentieth century—provided the foundational expertise that enabled the proliferation of complex operations that have come to characterize modern surgery.

For an operation to receive widespread adoption, it needed a semblance of superiority to existing treatments. Christopher Crenner and David Jones have described the difficulties of assessing the efficacy of surgical interventions, noting interoperator variability in skill, changes in technique over time, the challenges of using placebos, the near impossibility of blinding practitioners or patients, and determining what "effective" even means in different contexts.[9] In retrospect, the restoration of blood flow seems like an obvious improvement over ligation. But legitimate apprehensions concerning the risks of the novel procedure and doubts about the ability of the average practitioner to perform it delayed broad application. Addressing these concerns required the mass casualties and special circumstances of war, where case series and expert opinion provided the justification for adopting this therapy. Thus, what in principle attained universal acknowledgment as

the "ideal operation" in 1907 required another forty-five years before sufficient evidence existed to allow patients to benefit from it routinely.

The definition of operative success varies considerably depending on the
goals of the surgeon and the patient. Pott's prophylactic amputation definitively treated peripheral aneurysms, but by the late eighteenth century the
cost of an arm or leg proved too steep, justifying the riskier but less morbid
Hunterian ligation. The standard of care for 150 years, this procedure often
left patients like Marvin Rynar suffering from symptoms of vascular insufficiency that, by the twentieth century, bypass operations promised to obviate.
Which operation is best depends on the balance between effective management of the pathology and the side effects that both the doctor and patient
are willing to accept. If "cure" means preventing the patient from bleeding to
death from a ruptured peripheral aneurysm, then amputation actually provided the most definitive therapy using the simplest and fastest technique.
What drove the investigation and ultimate adoption of first ligation and later
repair was not improved efficacy at managing aneurysms or arterial trauma
but rather an effort to ameliorate the sequelae of the operation.

This trajectory emphasizes surgery's attention to the patient, not the disease.
Surgery is ultimately a service-based profession, focusing on the care, com-
fort, and, whenever possible, the cure of those who are ill and suffering. This
mission has driven the development of less morbid operations. In some cases
like breast surgery, patient advocacy prompted a shift away from unnecessarily
aggressive procedures. For laparoscopic and robotic operations, a combination
of patient demand, economic incentives, and industry lobbying has stimulated the rapid adoption and application of an entirely new way of operating. Yet whether one removes the gallbladder or appendix via a large incision,
a laparoscope, or a robot does not affect the treatment of acute cholecystitis
or appendicitis—in all cases, you are curing the infection by extirpating the
diseased organ. Minimally invasive techniques can improve the cosmetic outcome, shorten the recovery time, minimize the pain, and reduce the incidence
of certain complications, but, at least in some cases, these benefits come at
the cost of significant side effects or even suboptimal management of the primary pathology. A similar trade-off has appeared in vascular surgery, with the
increasing dominance of endovascular options to treat aneurysmal, atherosclerotic, and even traumatic disease. This emphasis on achieving desired clinical
outcomes while maintaining normal appearance and function is evident in this
history of arterial repair and has especially dominated the practice of surgery
recently through the minimally invasive movement.

These changes—and surgical development generally—depend on the
milieu in which they are invented, adopted, and practiced. What particular

elements of that environment affect which procedures varies tremendously.[10] But, universally, surgery requires quantitative volume to drive clinically meaningful diffusion. Requisite numbers vary by era and procedure, but the relatively rapid, early, and broad adoption of operations like appendectomies or tonsillectomies, for example, partly reflected the tens of thousands of patients who seemingly benefited from its practice, a pattern applicable to arterial repair in the 1950s with the Korean War and atherosclerosis. The repetition not only helped individual doctors build the skills to perform the procedure; it also provided data to analyze its efficacy, compare different techniques, and determine when and on whom surgeons should operate, creating a positive feedback loop where practice begets practice. In contrast, something like a face transplant—an exquisite procedure requiring multidisciplinary teamwork and the latest technology—occurs infrequently and remains confined to an elite few academic medical centers.[11] This rarity inherently limits the accumulation of information with which to evaluate and improve the procedure, constraining its diffusion.

The historical literature has debated the value of battle in fostering conditions amenable to surgical innovation, but the history of arterial repair clearly demonstrates that the particular setting of the Korean War catalyzed the dissemination and rapid adoption of procedures to sew blood vessels together. The comparatively limited military engagements of the later twentieth century, in which one dominant side controlled the air and sea, when smaller battles caused comparatively fewer casualties, and where less desperate circumstances provided greater ancillary support have created more amenable conditions for investigation and innovation than the cataclysmic world wars. More broadly, the evolution of surgery requires an environment open to experimentation, trial and error, and tolerance for the failures that will occur with any new invention. A postwar America, enamored of medicine and flush with resources, facilitated the rapid dissemination of not just arterial repair but also other advanced interventions like heart bypasses, cancer extirpations, and organ transplantation in the 1950s and 1960s. As surgery continues to expand in both volume and complexity, studying whence it came and how it developed carries increasing importance. Arterial repair provides a window into this history, casting light on the process of how surgery changes.

Notes

Abbreviations

ABS Archives	American Board of Surgery Archives, Philadelphia, Pennsylvania
ACS Archives	American College of Surgeons Archives in Chicago, Illinois
AMA Archives	American Medical Association Archives in Chicago, Illinois
Becker Archives	Washington University in St. Louis Becker Medical Library Archives, St. Louis, Missouri
BUMED Library and Archives	US Navy Bureau of Medicine and Surgery Library and Archives, Washington, DC
Countway Archives	Harvard Medical Library in the Francis A. Countway Library of Medicine, Boston, Massachusetts
Georgetown Archives	Special Collections Center at the Georgetown University Library, Washington, DC
JAMA	Journal of the American Medical Association
JHU Archives	Alan Mason Chesney Medical Archives at Johns Hopkins University, Baltimore, Maryland
Mayo Clinic Archives	W. Bruce Fye History of Medicine Library at the Mayo Clinic in Rochester, Minnesota
MHI	US Army Military History Institute at the US Army Heritage and Education Center, Carlisle, Pennsylvania
NARA	National Archives and Records Administration. All citations to NARA herein refer to NARA II, at College Park, Maryland. Documents are cited as follows: author, "title," date, record group/stack area/compartment/row/shelf/box/folder.
NEJM	New England Journal of Medicine
NLM Archives	National Library of Medicine History of Medicine Division, Bethesda, Maryland
SGO	Surgery, Gynecology, and Obstetrics
Tulane Archives	Louisiana Research Collection, Special Collections, Howard-Tilton Memorial Library, Tulane University, New Orleans, Louisiana

Introduction

1. R. Garland, "The Causation of Death in the *Iliad*," 43–60; Adamson, "A Comparison of Ancient and Modern Weapons in the Effectiveness of Producing Battle Casualties," 93–103.

2. For a historiography of surgery, see C. Lawrence, "Democratic, Divine, and Heroic"; and C. Lawrence, "Surgery and Its Histories."

3. Ackerknecht, "A Plea for a 'Behaviorist' Approach in Writing the History of Medicine"; Schlich, *The Origins of Organ Transplantation*, 9. See also Warwick, "X-Rays as Evidence in German Orthopedic Surgery," 1–24, esp. p. 3. Schlich's work on organ transplantation and orthopedic surgery are notable exceptions. For broader concerns about the absence of science in medical history, see Warner, "Science in Medicine," 37–58.

4. For physician written works on vascular surgery, see D. M. Friedman, *A History of Vascular Surgery*; W. F. Barker, *Clio*; and Dale, with Johnson and DeWeese, *Band of Brothers*.

5. Pickstone, introduction, 1–15; Anderson, Neary, and Pickstone, *Surgeons, Manufacturers, and Patients*. For a similar argument in the history of technology, see, for example, Edgerton, "From Innovation to Use," 111–36. The operation need not remain in use. Studying initially popular, later abandoned surgeries can be particularly revealing of the physiological and social beliefs in a given era, as Jack Pressman has demonstrated in *Last Resort*.

6. Schlich, *Surgery, Science and Industry*.

7. Effective surgical management required the localization of the pathology, which for many conditions like appendicitis depended on a germ theory of disease. D. C. Smith, "Appendicitis, Appendectomy, and the Surgeon," 414–41; D. C. Smith, "A Historical Overview of the Recognition of Appendicitis." For more on the importance of germ theory and localization for modern surgery, see Kernahan, "Franklin Martin and the Standardization of American Surgery," especially chapter 2; and Schlich, "The Emergence of Modern Surgery," 61–91.

8. See, for example, Grob, "The Rise and Decline of the Tonsillectomy in Twentieth-Century America," 383–421. The seeming technical simplicity of operations like the tonsillectomy concerned surgical leaders at organizations like the American College of Surgeons who worried that while doctors might be able to perform the steps of these cases adequately, they lacked the training and experience to know when to operate and how to manage the patient after the surgery. Nonetheless, many general practitioners perceived themselves capable and performed cases like tonsillectomies and appendectomies in large numbers.

9. For an overview of technology in surgery, see Schlich and Crenner, eds., *Technological Change in Modern Surgery*. For orthopedic instrumentation, see Schlich, *Surgery, Science and Industry*. For joints, see Anderson, Neary, and Pickstone, *Surgeons, Manufacturers, and Patients*. For cardiac bypass, see, among others, Miller, *King of Hearts*. For the importance of immunosuppression to transplant surgery, see Hamilton, *A History of Organ Transplantation*. For artificial hearts, see McKellar,

Artificial Hearts. On laparoscopy, see Whitfield, "A Revolution through the Keyhole"; and Tang and Schlich, "Surgical Innovation and the Multiple Meanings of Randomized Controlled Trials."

10. M. L. Gross, *Bioethics and Armed Conflict.*

11. Lerner, *The Breast Cancer Wars*; Haiken, *Venus Envy*, 6, and chapter 3; Tang and Schlich, "Surgical Innovation and the Multiple Meanings of Randomized Controlled Trials."

12. David Jones articulates how surgeons' interest helped promote coronary artery bypass grafts in *Broken Hearts*, chapter 4.

13. Proving the equivalence of the modified radical mastectomy to the radical mastectomy was a major hurdle for the acceptance of the former. See Lerner, *Breast Cancer Wars*. Historians have analyzed the challenges of proving the efficacy and superiority of surgical interventions: Crenner, "Placebos and the Progress of Surgery," 156–84; and D. S. Jones, "Surgical Practice and the Reconstruction of the Therapeutic Niche."

14. Greene, *Prescribing by Numbers*; Morino, "The Impact of Technology on Surgery," 709–11.

15. This argument contradicts Christopher Lawrence's claim of the opposite in "Democratic, Divine, and Heroic" and may reflect some differences between nineteenth- and twentieth-century surgery.

16. While women certainly practiced surgery between 1880 and 1960, they remained few and far between. Based on both published and unpublished sources, women did not play a role in the development of arterial repair. For more on women surgeons in this era, see Brock, "Women in Surgery"; Dally, *Women under the Knife*; Morantz-Sanchez, *Conduct Unbecoming a Woman*; Drachman, *Hospital with a Heart*.

17. Barr, "The Education of American Surgeons and the Rise of Surgical Residencies."

18. Ludmerer, *Let Me Heal.*

19. Barr, "The Education of American Surgeons and the Rise of Surgical Residencies"; and Ludmerer, *Let Me Heal.*

20. For a review, see van Bergen's essay "Surgery and War," which itself concedes in the first paragraph that it examines war and medicine broadly, not surgery specifically.

21. Cooter, *Surgery and Society in Peace and War.*

22. Books focused on the medical aspects of the Korean War are limited to two official publications from the army and navy that mostly detail logistics and unit involvement, a collection of oral histories, and one history on the experience of nurses. Cowdrey, *The Medics' War: The History of the Medical Department of the United States Navy*; Herman, *Frozen in Memory*; Omori, *Quiet Heroes.*

23. Fulton, "Medicine, Warfare, and History." Roger Cooter has long argued for caution in assuming the medical benefits of war, as seen in "War and Modern Medicine" (1536–73). Some of his subsequent scholarship takes a more polemical tone. See, for example, Cooter, "Of War and Epidemics."

24. For two recent explorations of this topic focusing on the American Civil War, see Devine, *Learning from the Wounded*; and Humphreys, *Marrow of Tragedy*.

25. See, among many others, D. J. Kevles, *The Physicists*; T. P. Hughes, *American Genius*; Creager, "'What Blood Told Dr. Cohn'"; Creager, *Life Atomic*. The history of science literature has also largely ignored the Korean War; for an exception, see D. J. Kevles, "K1, S2."

26. Rhodes, *The Making of the Atomic Bomb*; and Buderi, *The Invention That Changed the World*.

27. Bud, *Penicillin*. This model applied to most medical interventions, like blood transfusions, antimalarial drugs, the insecticide DDT, and vaccines. Instructions on how and when to utilize these innovations did not necessarily lead to their appropriate use, but the physical nature of implementation remained markedly simpler than a surgical procedure.

28. Humphreys, *Marrow of Tragedy*, 80.

29. J. D. Howell, *Technology in the Hospital*, chapter 1.

30. Schlich, *Surgery, Science and Industry*; Wilde, "Practising Surgery"; Wilde and Hirst, "Learning from Mistakes."

31. Both Jones and Pickstone discuss how the World War II background of surgeons in heart and hip replacement surgery, respectively, proved crucial to pushing the operation through the early, experimental stages. D. S. Jones, *Broken Hearts*; Anderson, Neary, Pickstone, *Surgeons, Manufacturers, and Patients*, 1–4.

32. See Rosenberg, *The Care of Strangers*, chapter 6; Marks, *The Progress of Experiment*, 43. Devine explores this idea in *Learning from the Wounded*.

33. D. C. Smith, "Surgery."

34. Rogers, *Diffusion of Innovations*; Blume, *Insight and Industry*; Fennell and Warnecke, *The Diffusion of Medical Innovations*; Reiser and Anbar, *The Machine at the Bedside*; Stanton, *Innovations in Health and Medicine*; Riskin et al., "Innovation in Surgery."

35. J. D. Howell, *Technology in the Hospital*; Schlich, "Negotiating Technologies in Surgery." For CT scans, see Blume, *Insight and Industry*, chapter 5. Andrew Warwick has recently reevaluated the rapid adoption of X-rays by the German orthopedic surgeons in his article "X-Rays as Evidence in German Orthopedic Surgery," which demonstrates their importance in determining the efficacy of different procedures for congenital hip dislocation.

36. For crime, see Caplow, *The First Measured Century*, chapter 12. For automobiles, see Lewis, *Divided Highways*.

37. There were an estimated 51.4 million inpatient procedures in nonfederal hospitals and 53.3 million outpatient procedures. Procedures in VA, Public Health, and military hospitals are not accounted for and would drive the number millions higher. For outpatient data, see Cullen, Hall, and Golosinskiy, "Ambulatory Surgery in the United States." For inpatient, see Centers for Disease Control and Prevention, "National Hospital Discharge Survey."

Chapter One

1. Marvin Rynar to William Halsted, 4 April 1912, JHU Archives, Halsted Collection, Box 29/Folder 6. Marvin Rynar is a pseudonym to protect patient privacy. The operation took place in 1909, with the full chart, op note, and correspondence available in JHU Archives.

2. Thomas Schlich argues that for surgeons, many times the clinic, and more specifically the operating room, functioned as their laboratory. See his article "Surgery, Science and Modernity."

3. Majno, *The Healing Hand*; Albucasis, *On Surgery and Instruments*; Nicase, *The Major Surgery of Guy de Chauliac*.

4. De Moulin, "Aneurysms in Antiquity," 49–63.

5. Technically, pseudoaneurysms occurred following this trauma. Pseudoaneurysms differ from true aneurysms by the number of arterial layers involved. While the medical literature describes this distinction as early as ancient Rome, practically doctors did not treat the two pathologies differently during the years this book covers. As such, the term "aneurysm" will represent both.

6. For a description of this operation, see Billings, *The History and Literature of Surgery*, 21.

7. Stimson identified only a handful of attempts in his "An Inquiry into the Origin of the Use of the Ligature in the Treatment of Aneurysm," 13–25.

8. Pott, *Chirurgical Works*, 412–18. For a recent biography, see Payne, *The Best Surgeon in England*.

9. For biographies of Hunter, see Moore, *The Knife Man*; Kobler, *The Reluctant Surgeon*; and Home, "A Short Account of the Life of the Author." J. Hunter, "Observations on the Inflammation of the Internal Coats of Veins," 18–29; J. Hunter, *A Treatise on the Blood, Inflammation, and Gun-Shot Wounds*, chapter 2.

10. Unbeknownst to Hunter, Dominque Anel had performed a variant of this procedure almost fifty years earlier in France. Subsequently, Pierre Joseph Desault performed proximal ligation five months before Hunter, seemingly based on a scientific understanding of the disease. Despite the priority of these two Frenchmen, the operation remains closely associated with John Hunter in the English-language literature partly because of his contemporaneous fame as a surgeon. See de Moulin, "Dominique Anel and His Operation for Aneurysm," 498–507; and Stimson, "An Inquiry into the Origin of the Use of the Ligature in the Treatment of Aneurysm."

11. Hunter performed four of these operations, and only in the final case did he choose not to ligate the artery below the aneurysm. Despite Hunter never writing about the operations himself, they remain some of the most described procedures in surgical history. See Home, "An Account of Mr. Hunter's Methods of Performing the Operation for the Cure of the Popliteal Aneurysm," 143–45.

12. For critical analyses of how Hunter achieved the title of "father of scientific surgery," see Jacyna, "Physiological Principles in the Surgical Writings of John Hunter"; and Jacyna, "Images of John Hunter in the Nineteenth Century."

13. Woods, "From One Medicine to Two"; French, *Antivivisection and Medical Science in Victorian Society*, 15–23.

14. Collateral circulation refers to alternate pathways blood can travel to reach the same destination. You can think of the main artery as a highway and collateral circulation as the back roads; different regions of the body have varying degrees of collateral circulation. Collateral circulation is essential to maintaining the viability of an arm or leg if a surgeon (or trauma) severs the main artery. For a description of some of these experiments, see Home, "An Account of Mr. Hunter's Methods of Performing the Operation for the Cure of the Popliteal Aneurysm," 143–45. Despite numerous assertions otherwise, the reported stag experiments in Richmond Park demonstrating collateral circulation are unlikely ever to have occurred and, if so, certainly did not teach Hunter that collateral circulation existed—a conclusion he had previously reached through his dissections. Stevenson, "The Stag of Richmond Park"; and Stevenson, "A Further Note on John Hunter and Aneurism."

15. Wangensteen, *The Rise of Surgery*, 258. Most surgeons eschewed this division until the twentieth century.

16. Monti, *Antonia Scarpa in Scientific History and His Role in the Fortunes of the University of Pavia*.

17. Cooper, *The Lectures of Sir Astley Cooper on the Principles and Practice of Surgery*, 197–98. For a general biography, see Brock, *Life and Work of Astley Cooper*.

18. Cooper, "Case of Ligature on the Aorta," 111–41. See also Osler, "Sir Astley Cooper's Case of Ligature of the Abdominal Aorta," 277.

19. The patient died twenty-three days after the operation; Andrew Smyth performed the first successful innominate ligation in 1864 in New Orleans. See Mott, *Reflections on Securing in a Ligature the Arteria Innominata*; Post, *Eulogy on the Late Valentine Mott, M.D., LL.D.*; S. D. Gross, *Valentine Mott*, 49. By artery: innominate, 1; subclavian, 8; common carotid, 51; external carotid, 2; common iliac, 1; external iliac, 6; internal iliac, 2; femoral, 57; popliteal, 10.

20. Crowther and Dupree similarly illustrate the importance of students transferring surgical practice with regards to Listerism in their book *Medical Lives in the Age of Surgical Revolution*, chapters 8–10. Both their book and multiple other sources comment how surgeons who learned directly from Lister or one of his students enjoyed greater success in achieving antisepsis than those who tried to adopt the practice from reading alone.

21. Francis, *Biographical Sketches of Distinguished Living New York Surgeons*, cited in Brieger, "A Portrait of Surgery," 1181–216.

22. "Dorsey's Operation for Inguinal Aneurysm," *New England Journal of Medicine* 1 (1 January 1812): 106. Similarly, an article in the inaugural volume of *Annals of Surgery*, the first medical journal dedicated to surgery, also included an article on this topic: W. Thompson, "Simultaneous Double Distal Ligature of the Carotid and Subclavian Arteries for High Innominate Aneurysm," 582.

23. For a collection of these writings, see Erichsen, *Observations on Aneurism*.

24. Cooper, *A Dictionary of Practical Surgery*, 53–76.

25. Arnott, "The Hunterian Oration."

26. A Practitioner of Many Years Standing, "The Fellowship Examinations in Lincoln's-Inn-Fields," 16–17, cited in Cope, *The Royal College of Surgeons of England*, 142; see also p. 26.

27. Cutting for bladder stones was another. Stanley, *For Fear of Pain*.

28. Peterson, *The Medical Profession in Mid-Victorian London*; Loudon, *Medical Care and the General Practitioner*.

29. W. Hunter, "The History of an Aneurysm of the Aorta, with Some Remarks on Aneurysms in General," 354.

30. A vast literature exists on the history of anesthesia. For a start, see Pernick, *A Calculus of Suffering*. In the classic "first" operation under ether, John Collins Warren performed vascular ligation on Edward Abbot's neck.

31. Literature on anti/aseptic surgery is also vast. Lawrence and Dixey, "Practising on Principle," 153–214; Gariepy, "The Introduction and Acceptance of Listerian Antisepsis in the United States."

32. Schlich, "The Emergence of Modern Surgery"; Temkin, "The Role of Surgery in the Rise of Modern Medical Thought"; Kernahan, "Franklin Martin and the Standardization of American Surgery," chapter 2.

33. Rosenberg, *The Care of Strangers*, chapter 6. For the reciprocal relationship of how surgery led the construction and specific design of hospitals, see Atwater, "Of Grande Dames, Surgeons, and Hospitals"; and Kisacky, *Rise of the Modern Hospital*, especially chapter 3.

34. See, for example, the operating room at Cook Country Hospital in Chicago. Guinan et al., *A History of Surgery at Cook County Hospital*.

35. See, inter alia, Schlich and Hasegawa, "Order and Cleanliness," 106–21. For a broader overview, see Reverby, *Ordered to Care*.

36. Bonner, *Becoming a Physician*.

37. Walsh, "Post-graduate Medical School and Hospital," 573–93; Peitzman, "'Thoroughly Practical'"; Rutkow, "The Education, Training, and Specialization of Surgeons"; Warner, *Against the Spirit of System*; Bonner, *American Doctors and German Universities*.

38. Friederick Koenig produced the first practical steam-powered printing press in 1811. For more on the development of steam presses and its effects on journalism, see Musson, "Newspaper Printing in the Industrial Revolution"; R. White, *Railroaded*. Thanks to Ryan Shaw for suggesting this source. The professionalization of postal services also contributed to the rise and spread of periodicals. For the British context, see Daunton, *Royal Mail*, especially chapter 2. For the American context, see US Postal Service, *The United States Postal Service*, 11–26; Summerfield, *U.S. Mail*.

39. Bynum and Wilson, "Periodical Knowledge," 30; Loudon and Loudon, "Medicine, Politics and the Medical Periodical," 49–54; Kronick, *A History of Scientific and Technical Periodicals*, 24, 237, and passim.

40. Ziman, *Public Knowledge*, 102–6, 144. See also Ziman, "Information, Communication, and Knowledge," 318–24; Fye, "The Literature of Internal Medicine," 55–84.

41. Cope, *The Royal College of Surgeons of England*, 264.

42. The *Lancet* dramatically changed medical publishing. While not the first weekly medical periodical, it was certainly the most successful and the most widely read in England. Its flamboyant editor Thomas Wakley relished controversy and used the editorial space in the journal to raise passions—and readership—among British practitioners. Bostetter, "The Journalism of Thomas Wakley," 275–92; Richardson, *Vintage Papers from the Lancet*, see especially her introduction. For the *British Medical Journal*, see Bartrip, *Mirror of Medicine*; Brieger, "A Portrait of Surgery."

43. Cushing, "The Society of Clinical Surgery in Retrospect." For the history of Clinical Congresses, see Davis, *Fellowship of Surgeons*, chapter 2; Martin, *Fifty Years of Medicine and Surgery*, chapter 29; Stephenson, *American College of Surgeons at 75*, chapter 4.

44. Schlich, *Surgery, Science and Industry*; Wilde, "Practising Surgery"; Wilde and Hirst, "Learning from Mistakes"; Maulitz, *Morbid Appearances*, see especially chapter 6 and p. 226.

45. Schlich, "'One and the Same the World Over.'"

46. Fogelman and Reinmiller, "1880–1890," cited in Kernahan, "Franklin Martin and the Standardization of American Surgery," 43.

47. J. D. Howell, *Technology in the Hospital*, 57 and 62, cited in Kernahan, "Franklin Martin and the Standardization of American Surgery," 44. For similar numbers, see Halsted, "The Training of the Surgeon," 528–29; and Atwater, "Of Grande Dames, Surgeons, and Hospitals."

48. Schlich, "'The Days of Brilliancy Are Past,'" 379–403.

49. Brieger, "From Conservative to Radical Surgery in Late Nineteenth-Century America."

50. The best single-volume biography remains MacCallum, *William Stewart Halsted*. Also excellent is Crowe, *Halsted of Johns Hopkins*. George Heuer's monograph "Dr. Halsted" presents the fullest picture of the man. A 2010 account largely recapitulates the aforementioned sources: Imber, *Genius on the Edge*. Most recently, Markel has written a history that focuses on Halsted's work with and addiction to cocaine: *An Anatomy of Addiction*.

51. D. C. Smith, "Appendicitis, Appendectomy, and the Surgeon." Grob, "The Rise and Decline of the Tonsillectomy in Twentieth-Century America."

52. "Extract of a letter from Mr. Lambert," 360–64. The next successful vascular repair on a human did not appear in the literature until 1893 when Max Schede fixed a venous laceration. "Einige Bemerkungen über die Naht von Venenwunden."

53. Asman failed chiefly because of thrombi developing at the repair site. Others who tried, like Bensoul in 1833, met similarly grim results. Asman, "De aneurysmate." Horsley, *Surgery of the Blood Vessels*, 33; Watts, "The Suture of the Blood Vessels," 183; De Moulin, "Historical Notes on Vascular Surgery II," 321–30. For other

attempts and failures, see Gluck, "Über zwei Fälle von Aortenaneurysmen nebst Bemerkungen über die Naht der Blutgefässe"; Gluck, "Über Neuere Operationen an Blutgefäßen"; Van Horoch, "Die Gefässnaht."

54. Jassinowsky, "Die Arteriennhat." University of Dorpat in Estonia is now the University of Tartu. Jassinowsky, "Ein Beitrag zur Lehre von der Gefässnaht," 816–41; W. F. Barker, *Clio*, 44–45. Another important early innovator was Enrico Burci, who demonstrated that running sutures were equally effective as interrupted ones and also worked out some of the fundamental physiology of arteries. Burci, "Ricerche sperimentali sul processo di riparazione delle ferite longitudinali delle arterie."

55. Davis, *J. B. Murphy, Stormy Petrel of Surgery*.

56. Murphy, "Resection of Arteries and Veins Injured in Continuity," 73–88.

57. Murphy, "Resection of Arteries and Veins Injured in Continuity," 73–88.

58. See Watts, "The Suture of the Blood Vessels," 154–55, for a summary of these studies, most of which cite Murphy as their starting point.

59. F. Durante performed the first published suture of an artery in a human patient in 1892 when he closed a hole in the popliteal artery made accidentally when removing a tumor. For a complete listing, with references, see de Moulin, "Historical Notes on Vascular Surgery II"; and Watts, "The Suture of the Blood Vessels," 155.

60. Lesch, *Science and Medicine in France*.

61. For an overview of research in inflammation, see Rather, *Addison and the White Corpuscles*, especially the introduction.

62. Ackerknecht, *Rudolf Virchow*. Stephen Jacyna documents the uneven uptake of histopathology in his article "The Laboratory and the Clinic."

63. W. H. Welch, "Thrombosis," 110–92. This paper reviews the history of this research.

64. Dorrance, "An Experimental Study of Suture of Arteries with a Description of a New Suture"; Brewer, "Some Experiments with a New Method of Closing Wounds of the Larger Arteries."

65. Unless otherwise indicated, biographical information comes from Cohn with Deutsch, *Rudolph Matas*. The vascular exposure partly resulted from his surgery professor, Andrew Smyth, who performed the first successful innominate artery ligation in the world and thereafter treated aneurysms from all over that state. For Smyth's operation, see Duffy, *The Rudolph Matas History of Medicine in Louisiana*, 361–64.

66. Both the Society for Vascular Surgery and the Southern Association for Vascular Surgery honor him with awards in his name. Shumacker, *The Society for Vascular Surgery*, 17, 88, and chapter 10.

67. Matas, "Traumatic Aneurism of the Left Brachial Artery," 462–70.

68. Matas, "Traumatic Aneurism of the Left Brachial Artery"; Cohn, *Rudolph Matas*, 199–212.

69. Matas, "An Operation for the Radical Cure of Aneurism Based upon Arteriorrhaphy," 161–96.

70. Personal communication from George Crile to Rudolph Matas, 21 August and 8 October 1908, Tulane Archives, Matas Collection, Box 21, Folder 25.

71. Quoted in Isidore Cohn, "Rudolph Matas: His Influence on Vascular Surgery with Particular Reference to the Use of the Suture," Tulane Archives, Matas Collection, Box 2, Folder 31.

72. Bickham, "Arteriovenous Aneurisms." It offered an alternative to the then standard quadruple ligation.

73. Heringman, Rives, and Davis, "The Repair of Arteriovenous Fistulas."

74. Annual Reports of St. Mary's Hospital, 1903–1939, Mayo Clinic Archives.

75. "The Statistics of Endoaneurismorrhaphy," Tulane Archives, Matas Collection, Box 21, Folder 32. Of the 354, 333 recovered fully, 15 patients died, and the difference suffered from complications. Most (234) were of the obliterative type.

76. Lancisi, *De aneurysmatibus.*

77. Elkin, "Aneurysm of the Aorta."

78. Barr, "Battle of the Bulge."

79. Eck, "K voprosu o perevyazkie vorotnois veni." For an English translation of this article, see Child, "Eck's Fistula"; Ilia N. Kavarsky provided the translation.

80. Wangensteen and Wangensteen, *The Rise of Surgery*, 268.

81. Abbe, "The Surgery of the Hand," 33–40.

82. Abbe, "The Surgery of the Hand," 40.

83. Masini, "Ueber die Funktion der Leber"; Ehrenfried and Boothby, "The Technic of End-to-End Anastamosis"; Hoepfner, "Ueber Gefaessnaht, Gefaesstransplantationen und replantation von amputirten extremitaeten"; Ward, "Blood Vessel Anastamosis by Means of Rubber Tubing"; Winslow and Walker, "End-to-End Vascular Anastomosis."

84. Keen, *Surgery*, 5:131.

85. Murphy, "Resection of Arteries and Veins Injured in Continuity."

86. Cited in Brougham, "Arterial Anastamosis by Invagination," 410–12.

87. For references and examples, see Brougham, "Arterial Anastamosis by Invagination," 410–11; Watts, "The Suture of Blood Vessels," 380–81.

88. Keen, *Surgery*, 5:83.

89. Briau and Jaboulay, "Recherches expérimentales sur la suture et la greffe artérielles," 97–99. For an English translation of this article, see W. F. Barker, *Clio*, 61; Thomaselli, "Sutura circolare delle arterie coll'affrontamento dell'endoletio"; Thomaselli, "Esiti lontani della sutura col metocho dell'endothelio"; Salomoni, "Sutura circolare delle arterie con l'affrontamento dell'endotelio." See also Watts, "The Suture of Blood Vessels," 382; Guthrie, *Blood Vessel Surgery and Its Applications*, 6; and De Moulin, "Historical Notes of Vascular Surgery II."

90. Dörfler, "Ueber Arteriennaht," 781. For an English translation, see W. F. Barker, *Clio*, 49–59.

91. Guthrie, *Blood Vessel Surgery*, 1–8. See also Dale, "The Beginnings of Vascular Surgery," 849–66.

92. Hamilton, *The First Transplant Surgeon*, chapter 1; Malinin, *Surgery and Life*, chapter 1.

93. Carrel, *The Voyage to Lourdes*; Malinin, *Surgery and Life*, 13–17. See also accounts in Hamilton, *The First Transplant Surgeon*. Lourdes was, and is, a popular site in France for medical pilgrims to seek miraculous cures. Millions have visited the site since its opening in 1858, and thousands report magical cures, although no certified miracles have occurred since 1976. Its golden age occurred between 1890 and 1915, when Carrel visited. Lourdes has its own robust, thaumaturgic literature. For a critical analysis of "cures," see Francois, Sternberg, and Fee, "The Lourdes Medical Cures Revisited." For commentary on the article generally critiquing its presentist perspective, see Duffin, "Religion and Medicine, Again." For a more general history, see Harris, *Lourdes*.

94. Carl Beck, also a European immigrant, had established himself as a leading surgeon in Chicago. Having worked with both Hans Chiari and Theodor Billroth, Beck brought European surgical pathology to the United States, where he published the leading textbook on the subject in 1905. He cofounded the Chicago Surgical Society, over which he presided in 1917 and 1918, and was a founding member of the American College of Surgeons. See Baader and Nyhus, "The Life of Carl Beck and an Important Interval with Alexis Carrel."

95. Beck and Carrel, "A Demonstration of Specimens Illustrating a Method of Formation of a Prethoracic Esophagus," 463–64.

96. Harbinson, introduction to Guthrie, *Blood Vessel Surgery*, vi. The book includes a full bibliography of articles cowritten by Carrel and Guthrie.

97. Harbinson, "Origins of Vascular Surgery," 406; H. Stephenson, "A Brief Biography of Charles Claude Guthrie."

98. For Carrel's relationship with the media and self-promotion, see Hamilton, *The First Transplant Surgeon*.

99. Carrel, "La technique opératoire des anastomeses vasculaires et la transplantation des viscères."

100. Guthrie, "On Misleading Statements."

101. Harvey Cushing to Alexis Carrel, 7 November 1905, Carrel Collection, Georgetown Archives, Box 39, Folder 45.

102. See Carrel Collection, Georgetown Archives, Box 44, Folder 1907 for a trove of letters from surgeons around the world both complimenting Carrel and seeking additional details on his procedures so that they may replicate them.

103. Franklin Martin to Alexis Carrel, 1905, Carrel Collection, Georgetown Archives, Box 44, Folder 1905.

104. George Crile to Alexis Carrel, 7 February 1907, Carrel Collection, Georgetown Archives, Box 39, Folder 44. Cushing to Carrel, 7 November 1905.

105. Israel Brown to Alexis Carrel, 1 April 1909, Carrel Collection, Georgetown Archives, Box 45, Folder 1909.

106. Harvey Cushing to Alexis Carrel, 24 October 1905, Carrel Collection, Georgetown Archives, Box 41, Folder 45.

107. William Halsted to Alexis Carrel, 19 February 1907, JHU Archives, Halsted Collection, Box 4, Folder 18.

108. Akerman, "Award Ceremony Speech."

109. Lederer, *Flesh and Blood*, 20–22; "Our New Nobel Prize," *Literary Digest* 45, no. 21 (23 November 1912): 233–34. All the major newspapers covered the event.

110. Carrel, "The Transplantation of Organs"; Albert Fischer, "Alexis Carrel—as I Knew Him," Carrel Collection, Georgetown Archives, Box 39, Folder 67B, p. 21; Edward Pendray, "Twelve Men Who Changed the World," Carrel Collection, Georgetown Archives, Box 44, p. 6.

111. Schlich, *The Origins of Organ Transplantation*. Schlich argues that earlier efforts at tissue transplant (e.g., John Hunter's teeth transplants, skin grafts, etc.) had a fundamentally different philosophical and medical orientation. For more on this argument, see Schlich, "How Gods and Saints Became Transplant Surgeons." For a history of these early efforts of tissue transplantation, see Tilney, *Transplant*; Hamilton, *A History of Organ Transplantation*. For a history of skin transplants and particularly how American society saw and accepted them, see Lederer, *Flesh and Blood*.

112. Floresco, "Conditions anatomique et technique de la transplantation du rein."

113. Carrel and Guthrie, "Functions of a Transplanted Kidney," 473. They chose the neck because of the easy vascular access there and because dogs could not lick that region.

114. Druml, "The Beginning of Organ Transplant"; Hamilton, *A History of Organ Transplantation*. Carrel and Guthrie reported being unaware of Ullmann's work when they proceeded with their experiments, although they later gave him due credit in the literature. See Carrel, "The Transplantation of Organs"; and Carrel, "The Results of Transplantation of Blood Vessels, Organs, and Limbs." The first kidney transplants were performed in 1898 by Alfred Exner, but he did not publish his work. Carl Beck repeated Ullmann's kidney transplant in 1903 using the Murphy invagination technique; it failed but perhaps provided motivation for Carrel and Guthrie. See Schlich, *The Origins of Organ Transplantation*, 123–26.

115. Carrel and Guthrie, "Extirpation and Replantation of the Thyroid Gland with Reversal of the Circulation"; Carrel and Guthrie, "A New Method for the Homoplastic Transplantation of the Ovary." For a general summary, see Carrel, "The Transplantation of Organs," 1645–46; and Carrel and Guthrie, "Anastomosis of Blood Vessels by the Patching Method and Transplantation of the Kidney." They ultimately authored fifteen articles together on organ transplantation.

116. Carrel and Guthrie, "Results of a Replantation of the Thigh." For laboratory notes on this operation, see Carrel Collection, Georgetown Archives, Box 10, Folder 7.

117. Guthrie, *Blood Vessel Surgery*, 127, 250–52.

118. Mathieu Jaboulay, of U-stitch and everted suture lines, performed the first kidney transplant in humans, implanting a pig kidney into a young girl dying from Bright's disease. It failed. See Schlich, *The Origins of Organ Transplantation*, chapter 13.

119. Carrel, "The Transplantation of Organs"; Guthrie, *Blood Vessel Surgery*, 233–35; Carrel and Guthrie, "The Transplantation of Vein and Other Organs."

120. Pendray, *Twelve Men Who Changed the World*, 37. See also Alexis Carrel to M. D. Bloomfield, 7 October 1912, Carrel Collection, Georgetown Archives, Box 45, Folder 18. Hamilton, *The First Transplant Surgeon.*

121. Schlich, *The Origins of Organ Transplantation*, chapter 17. Various efforts at organ transplantation continued, but as Schlich demonstrated, by 1915 or so, all serious medical authorities had acknowledged the impossibility of allografts succeeding; Carrel's experiments provided essential convincing evidence.

122. Turney, *Frankenstein's Footsteps*, chapter 4, especially pp. 72–82. See also Lederer, *Frankenstein.*

123. Both Lederer and Hansen single out Carrel for the public attention he received from his organ transplantation experiments. See Lederer, *Flesh and Blood*, 20–22; Hansen, *Picturing Medical Progress from Pasteur to Polio*, 115–16.

124. "The Wizard Surgeon, by One Who Knew Him," Carrel Collection, Georgetown Archives, Box 39, Folder 65.

125. The Carrel Collection at Georgetown has literally hundreds of news clippings featuring Carrel and his work. See, for example, "Tissues of the Dead Live, Used to Replace Diseased Parts of the Human Body," *Washington Post*, 8 June 1912; "Elemental Death Is Banished, Dr. Carrel Tells Physicians," *New York Herald*, 6 June 1912; "Transferred Organs from One Animal to Another," *Toronto Globe*, 28 May 1912; "Surgeon Transplants Various Living Organs from One Animal to Another," *St. Louis Post Dispatch*, 19 June 1913; Lederer, *Flesh and Blood*, 20–22.

126. See Carrel Collection, Georgetown Archives, Box 45, Folder 18 for a variety of letters.

127. Z.L. to Alexis Carrel, 12 January 1912, Carrel Collection, Georgetown Archives, Box 45, Folder 13.

128. H.R.P. to Alexis Carrel, 11 February 1909, Carrel Collection, Georgetown Archives, Box 45, Folder 9. See also H.S. to Alexis Carrel, 11 March 1912, Carrel Collection, Georgetown Archives, Box 45, Folder 12; Hamilton, *The First Transplant Surgeon*, 115–16.

129. C.C.M. to Alexis Carrel, 14 March 1909, Carrel Collection, Georgetown Archives, Box 45, Folder 9. The issue of race that C.C.M. addressed so explicitly resounded throughout the popular and scientific discussions on organ transplant. See Lederer, *Flesh and Blood.*

130. Carrel never attempted organ transplants on humans, presumably because he recognized the rejection that occurred in animals would be equally parlous in human. Carrel performed little clinical surgery at all during his stay in the United States, preferring to focus his attention on research. A notable exception was a 1908 blood transfusion operation to save the life of the daughter of a prominent New York surgeon. Carrel used his anastomosis techniques, similar to George Crile's pioneering work on blood transfusion.

131. Harbinson, "Origins of Vascular Surgery," 408; H. Stephenson, "A Brief Biography of Charles Claude Guthrie."

132. Malinin, *Surgery and Life*, chapters 12 and 13; Hamilton, *The First Transplant Surgeon*, chapters 4–6; Corner, *History of the Rockefeller Institute*.

133. For a history of tissue cultures, see Landecker, "Technologies of Living Substance," with chapter 2 focusing on Carrel. For a history of tissue banks in America, see Swanson, *Banking on the Body*.

134. D. M. Friedman, *The Immortalists*. See *Time* 21, no. 24 (13 June 1938).

135. Carrel, *Man, the Unknown*. For a detailed, if hagiographic, discussion of this book, see Durkin, *Hope for Our Time*.

136. Reggiani, "Alexis Carrel, the Unknown," 331–56.

137. Bernheim, *Surgery of the Vascular System*. See also Yao, "First Textbook in Vascular Surgery," 269–72. For more on Bernheim see Williams, "Bertram M. Bernheim."

138. For a list of the studies, see Goodman, "A Histological Study of the Circular Suture of the Blood-Vessels."

139. Horsley, *Surgery of the Blood Vessels*; Jeger, "Die Chirurgie der Blutgefäße und des Herzens."

140. Grade, "Vascular Anastomosis and Transplantation of Organs."

141. Diamond, "A History of Blood Transfusion."

142. Lederer, *Flesh and Blood*, 48.

143. English, *Shock, Physiological Surgery, and George Washington Crile*; Crile and Crile, *George Crile*.

144. Crile, "Direct Transfusion of Blood in the Treatment of Hemorrhage."

145. Crile, *Hemorrhage and Transfusion*.

146. See, for example, Watts, "The Suture of Blood Vessels and Direct Transfusion of Blood by Vascular Anastomoses."

147. Rudolph Matas, "Vascular Surgery in War," read at AMA Surgical Section, Atlantic City, 1943, Tulane Archives, Matas Collections, Box 2, Folder 28, emphasis original.

148. Goyanes, "Nuevos trabajos de chirugia vascular"; Harrison, "Historical Aspects in the Development of Venous Autografts."

149. Lexer, "Die Ideale Operation des Arteriellen und des Arteriellvenösen Aneurysma."

150. Pringle, "Two Cases of Vein-Grafting for the Maintenance of a Direct Arterial Circulation."

151. Bernheim, "The Ideal Operation for Aneurysm of the Extremity." For a discussion of the failed 1909 attempt, see Halsted, "Partial Occlusion of Large Arteries by Aluminum Bands," 49–52.

152. Also known as the First and Second Balkan Wars, respectively. See Hall, *The Balkan Wars*.

153. Soubbotitch, "Military Experiences of Traumatic Aneurysms."

154. Rich et al., "The Matas/Soubbotitch Connection"; Rich and Rhee, "An Historical Tour of Vascular Injury Management."

155. Bernheim, "The Ideal Operation for Aneurisms of the Extremity," 94.

156. Bernheim, "The Ideal Operation for Aneurisms of the Extremity," 94–95, especially n9.

157. Rudolph Matas, "Commentaries on the Surgery of the Blood Vessels by Dr. Matas," Tulane Archives, Matas Collection, Box 22, Folder 2. For similar sentiments, see also Rudolph Matas, "The Technic of the Suture Applied to Vascular Surgery as Modified by the Experience of the World War," Tulane Archives, Matas Collection, Box 21, Folder 3; Rudolph Matas, "Discussion of Dr. Horsely's Paper," Tulane Archives, Matas Collections, Box 22, Folder 8; Rudolph Matas, "The Fallacies of Direct Arterial Suture," Tulane Archives, Matas Collection, Box 26, Folder 17.

Chapter Two

1. For an account of specialization, see Weisz, *Divide and Conquer*.

2. Terraine, *White Heat*.

3. Joy, "Historical Aspects of Medical Defense against Chemical Warfare."

4. Gillet, *The Army Medical Department*, see especially chapter 3; Whitehead, *Doctors in the Great War*, see chapters 2, 3, 4, and 7; Van Bergen, *Before My Helpless Sight*, 24; Schafer, "Fighting for Business."

5. Van Bergen, *Before My Helpless Sight*; Byerly, *Fever of War*; Bresalier, "Fighting Flu"; Linton, "'War Dysentery' and the Limitations of German Military Hygiene during World War I"; B. Shepherd, *A War of Nerves*; Jones and Wessely, *Shell Shock to PTSD*; Leese, *Shell Shock*.

6. M. Harrison, *The Medical War*; Jaffin, "Medical Support for the American Expeditionary Forces in France during the First World War"; Scotland, "Evacuation Pathway for the Wounded"; Marble, "Forward Surgery and Combat Hospitals," 73–80.

7. Makins, *Surgical Experiences in South Africa*, chapter 3, especially pp. 108–11; Barr, "Military Medicine of the Russo-Japanese War and its Influence on the Modernization of the US Army Medical Department."

8. Power, *Wounds in War*, 7–8.

9. Janeway, "War and Medicine," 222; M. Harrison, *The Medical War*, 27–28; Van Bergan, *Before My Helpless Sight*, 334.

10. Haller, "Treatment of Infected Wounds during the Great War," 303–15; Hamilton, *The First Transplant Surgeon*, chapter 8; Power, *Wounds in War*, 34–36; Crowther and Dupree, *Medical Lives in the Age of Surgical Revolution*, 346–49.

11. Wright, "Memorandum on the Treatment of Infected Wounds by Physiological Methods," 793–97; Haller, "Treatment of Infected Wounds during the Great War," 310–11; Whitehead, *Doctors in the Great War*, 207, 216.

12. Carrel, "Traitement abortif de l'infection des plaies," 361–68. For a detailed explanation of the method, see Carrel and Dehelly, *Le traitment des plaies infectées*. The book appeared in English that same year under the title *Treatment of Infected Wounds*.

13. An abundance of articles in the medical press touted its success. See, for example, Halsted, "Carrel-Dakin Method of the Treatment of Infected Wounds"; Rowe, "A Note on the Carrel-Dakin-Daufresne Treatment"; Sherman, "The Abortive Treatment of Wound Infection"; Gould, "Report to the Director-General Medical Services on Our Recent Visit to France to Study the Carrel-Dakin Treatment of Wounds"; Gibson, "The Carrel Method of Treating Wounds"; Janeway, "War and Medicine," 223–24; Loewy, "Carrel's Method of Treatment of Infected Wounds." Military medical textbooks also lauded the Carrel-Dakin solution; see Hughes and Banks, *War Surgery*, vi and 284–324.

14. See, for example, Bevan, "The Carrel-Dakin Treatment."

15. M. Harrison, *The Medical War*, 29–30; Helling and Daon, "In Flanders Fields."

16. For more on anesthesia, see Courington and Calverley, "Anesthesia on the Western Front"; and Robertson, "Anesthesia, Shock, and Resuscitation." For shock, see English, *Shock, Physiological Surgery, and George Washington Crile*, chapter 9; and Pelis, "Taking Credit."

17. Seaman, "Observations in the Russo-Japanese War," 6–7; Nimier, "The War in Manchuria and the Wounded by Small Arms Bullets."

18. Marble, *King of Battle*.

19. For American numbers, see *Report of the U.S. Surgeon General's Office, 1920*, 62–64. For British, see Scotland, "Evacuation Pathway for the Wounded."

20. MacPherson, *Medical Services*, 1:582–83.

21. These numbers refer only to soldiers and exclude marines. Again, they represent only those soldiers who survived to reach medical facilities. As 224,089 American soldiers were wounded, these numbers included the 42,023 second wounds some soldiers received. Wounds to the lower extremity were the most common battle injury; wounds to the thorax second, and wounds to the upper extremity third. See *Report of the U.S. Surgeon General's Office, 1920*, 65–66.

22. *Report of the U.S. Surgeon General's Office, 1920*, 84–85. A revised government document published in 1927 identified 1019 vascular injuries, for an incidence of 0.005 percent. See Ireland, *Medical Department of the United States in World War I*, 110.

23. Ireland, *Medical Department of the United States in World War I*, 110. *A History of United States Army Base Hospital No. 36*, 62.

24. "Evacuation Hospital No. 10," NARA 112/290/61/7/00/27/28. Out of 3,343 wounds, they recorded eight injuries to the femoral arteries, twelve to the brachial arteries, six to the popliteal arteries, three to the brachial veins, and seven to the femoral veins.

25. "Surgical Operations, 22 October–15 November 1918," NARA 120/270/64/15-21/00/1318/16.

26. DeBakey and Simeone, "Battle Injuries of the Arteries in World War II," 535.

27. Eccles, "A Clinical Lecture on Aneurysms of War Wounds."

28. Ireland, *Medical Department of the United States in World War I*, 302.

29. Makins, *On Gunshot Injuries to the Blood-Vessels*, 106–10, 175, 204–5, 225, 242–43. For Tuffier, see the quotation in Brooks, "Surgical Application of Therapeutic Venous Obstruction," 2–3; Shumacker, "Ramuald Weglowski."

30. *General Principles Guiding the Treatment of Wounds of War*, 29. It also recommended treating arteriovenous fistulae by restoring vessel continuity (31).

31. *Principles of War Surgery, Based on the Conclusions Adopted at the Various Interallied Surgical Conferences*, 4, 26–27.

32. Moure, "Etude des greffes vasculaires et particulièrement de leurs applications chirurgicales au rétablissement de la continuité des vaisseaux et des conduits musculo-membraneux."

33. Rudolph Matas, "The Technic of the Suture Applied to Vascular Surgery as Modified by the Experience of the World War," Tulane Archives, Matas Collection, Box 21, Folder 3; Makins, *On Gunshot Injuries to the Blood-Vessels*, 108; MacPherson, *Medical Services*, 2:201.

34. Rudolph Matas, "Discussion of Dr. Horsely's Paper," Tulane Archives, Matas Collection, Box 22, Folder 8, p. 1; Makins, *On Gunshot Injuries to the Blood-Vessels*, 108.

35. A 1917 German dissertation identified twenty-six Teutonic surgeons performing venous grafting, a negligible percentage of the twenty-six thousand German physicians in uniform; other armies cite rare individual examples, many of whom like Goodman and Jeger had researched vascular surgery before the war. Warthmüller, "Über die bisherigen Erfolge der Gefässtransplantation am Menschen"; Goodman, "A Histological Study of the Circular Suture of the Blood-Vessels"; Jeger, "Die Chirurgie der Blutgefäße und des Herzens."

36. Goodman, "Suture of Blood-Vessel Injuries from Projectiles of War."

37. Kuttner, "Gefässplastiken." Kuttner, "Kriegschirurgie der Grossen Gefässstämme." 741. Thanks to Robin Schmitz for his help with the German. Bier is most remembered today for his pioneering work on spinal anesthesia and the regional Bier block. He also invented the helmet German soldiers wore in World War I. See Reis, "Eulogy to August Karl Gustav Bier on the 100th Anniversary of Intravenous Regional Block and the 110th Anniversary of the Spinal Block."

38. Four died from unspecified complications (all in 1914). Shumacker, "Ramuald Weglowski," 95–96.

39. Macpherson, *Medical Services*, 2: chapter 6.

40. Nunn, Bunzendahl, and Handy, "Ernst Jeger."

41. Makins, *On Gunshot Injuries to the Blood-Vessels*, 217–26, 241–42.

42. Ireland, *Medical Department of the United States in World War I*, 159.

43. Coppard, *With a Machinegun to Cambrai*, 126–30.

44. Ireland, *Medical Department of the United States in World War I*, 302; Bourne, "Traumatic Aneurysm," 276–83.

45. *Report of the U.S. Surgeon General's Office, 1920,* 1819.

46. *Report of the U.S. Surgeon General's Office, 1920,* 1790. Similarly, if a ward officer at the 21st Evacuation Hospital "saw a bleeding vessel, [he] applied artery forceps and ligated" it. "Evacuation Hospital No. 21 History," NARA 112/290/61/7/00/30/27, p. 18.

47. MacPherson, *Medical Services,* 2: chapter 6.

48. A September 1918 report listed Dorrance as performing seventy-four operations, including four ligations and two primary amputations for avascular limbs that had already developed gangrene. See "Monthly Report of Operating Teams, September 1918," NARA 120/270/64/15-21/00/1324/2.

49. "Surgical Operations, 22 October–15 November 1918." See also "Surgical Operations, Sept 29, 1918 to Oct 15, 1918," NARA 120/270/64/15-21/00/1318/16.

50. "Memorandum No. 5," 2 October 1918, NARA 120/270/64/15-21/00/1318/21, p. 1. For a short biography of Harvey, see Taffel, "Samuel Clark Harvey."

51. "Surgical Operations, 22 October–15 November 1918," 42–43.

52. "Surgical Operations, 22 October–15 November 1918," 34.

53. For accounts of their reoperations, see "Surgical Operations, 22 October–15 November 1918," 46 (Griffen) and 47 (Boss).

54. *Report of the U.S. Surgeon General's Office, 1920,* 1818. For a similar British quote, see Eccles, "A Clinical Lecture on Aneurysms of War Wounds." See also Wallace, "Gas Gangrene as Seen at the Casualty Clearing Stations."

55. *Report of the U.S. Surgeon General's Office, 1920,* 1790.

56. "Surgical Operations, 22 October–15 November 1918," 42–43.

57. Mayhew, *Wounded,* 67. See also Macpherson, *Medical Services,* 3:11–53.

58. "A Yale Unit at the Front," *Yale Alumni Weekly* 37 (1918): 133–34. For similar numbers, see "Evacuation Hospital No. 10," 1–6.

59. "History of Evacuation Hospital No. 6," NARA 112/290/61/7/00/26/11; Gillet, *The Army Medical Department,* 82–83; Whitehead, *Doctors in the Great War,* 35, 40, 80.

60. Van Bergan, *Before My Helpless Sight,* 316–30.

61. *Report of the U.S. Surgeon General's Office, 1920,* 1291.

62. Van Bergan, *Before My Helpless Sight,* 92, 296–97.

63. For example, casualties waited an average of 6.25 hours for surgery after arriving at Mobile Hospital #1 in November, 1918. Joseph Flint, "Injury List," NARA 120/270/64/15/00/1325/8.

64. "History of Evacuation Hospital #9," NARA 112/290/61/7/00/27/10, p. 27. For a more complete breakdown, 2.5 percent of casualties received an operation within six hours of wounding; 21 percent within twelve hours; 48.5 percent within eighteen hours; 75 percent within twenty-four hours; 85 percent within thirty hours; 91 percent within thirty-six hours. Mobile Hospital No. 1, NARA 120/270/64/15/00/1313/9. The shortest recorded time from wounding to operating table was eight hours.

65. "Surgical Operations," 33–34, 42–43, and passim, for similar delays in other, nonvascular cases.

66. *Report of the U.S. Surgeon General's Office, 1920*, 1921.

67. A. A. Martin, *A Surgeon in Khaki*, 258.

68. Bernheim, "Blood-Vessel Surgery in the War." For similar sentiments regarding the difficulties of suture repair of vessels in an infected field, see Neff and O'Malley, "Some Observations on Military Surgery during One Year's Service in the 23rd General Hospital, B.E.F., France."

69. Bamberger, "The Adoption of Laparotomy for the Treatment of Penetrating Abdominal Wounds in War"; Heys, "Abdominal Wounds," 178–211; "Surgical Treatment of War Wounds of the Abdomen," *Review of War Surgery and Medicine* 1, no. 2 (April 1918): 20–26.

70. Brooks, "Surgical Application of Therapeutic Venous Obstruction." See also DeBakey and Simeone, "Battle Injuries of the Arteries in World War II," especially 551–55.

71. Rudolph Matas, "A Review of the Progress of Vascular Surgery during the World War, 1914–1918, with Commentaries," Tulane Archives, Matas Collection, Box 21, Folder 36.

72. *Principles of War Surgery, Based on the Conclusions Adopted at the Various Inter-allied Surgical Conferences*, 36.

73. See, for example, Cowell, "Simultaneous Ligation of Arterial and Venous Trunks in War Surgery," 577–78; Goodman, "Suture of Blood-Vessel Injuries from Projectiles of War"; Mitchiner, "Injuries of Blood Vessels and Their Treatment," 92–96. The debate continued to feature prominently in the vascular surgery literature after the war, with most surgeons, including the likes of Barney Brooks and Emile Holman, favoring its practice. Brooks et al., "Simultaneous Vein Ligation," 496–500; Holman, "Observations on the Surgery of the Large Arteries, with Report of Case of Ligation of the Innominate Artery for Varicose Aneurism of the Subclavian Vessels," 173–84.

74. MacPherson, *Medical Services*, vol. 1.

75. Gillet, *The Army Medical Department*, chapter 3 and especially 90–93; "History of Evacuation Hospital No. 9," NARA 112/290/61/7/0027/10, pp. 23–24.

76. *Report of the U.S. Surgeon General's Office, 1920*, 1087.

77. *Review of War Surgery and Medicine* 1, no. 1 (March 1918): 60–62. The issue also recommended repairs of pseudoaneurysms and arteriovenous fistulae that might result from arterial trauma. The September issue provided a particularly comprehensive review of vascular trauma and its proper management based on the French experience and similarly concluded suture repair to be ideal although recommended ligation for the vast majority of infected, disfigured wounds. "Vascular Injuries in War," *Review of War Surgery and Medicine* 1, no. 7 (September 1918): 1–26.

78. Munson, "The Needs of Medial Education as Revealed by War," 1050–55.

79. *Report of the U.S. Surgeon General's Office, 1920*, 444, 1135.

80. D. C. Smith, "Appendicitis, Appendectomy, and the Surgeon," see 416–17.

81. Finney, *A Surgeon's Life*, chapters 9 and 10; English, *Shock, Physiological Surgery, and George Washington Crile*, chapter 9. Other examples include Evarts Graham, Franklin Martin, Paul Magnuson, Alexis Carrel, the Mayo brothers, Harvey Cushing, et al.

82. Barr, "The Education of American Surgeons and the Rise of Surgical Residencies."

83. MacCallum, *William Stewart Halsted*.

84. Halsted, "The Training of the Surgeon"; Chesney, *The Johns Hopkins Hospital and the Johns Hopkins University School of Medicine*, 1:161–62; Ludmerer, *Let Me Heal*, chapter 2.

85. Halsted, "The Training of the Surgeon," 527.

86. Carter, "The Fruition of Halsted's Concept of Surgical Training," 518–27.

87. Harvey, "The Influence of William Stewart Halsted's Concepts of Surgical Training," 215–36.

88. Ludmerer, *Let Me Heal*, 56–57.

89. He also enabled residents to spend one to two years free from clinical duties to perform research, a model that quickly expanded to other academic programs and endures today. Mueller, *Evarts A. Graham*, 204–9.

90. Gillet, *The Army Medical Department*, 79.

91. Ludmerer, *Learning to Heal*.

92. *Graduate Medical Education*, 31. The first state to require internships was Pennsylvania, in 1914. American Medical Association, *A History of the Council on Medical Education and Hospitals of the American Medical Association*, 21.

93. For a list of common surgical procedures performed in the 1880s, see Bevan, "The Study and Teaching and the Practice of Surgery," 481–94, list p. 482.

94. Archibald, "Higher Degrees in the Profession of Surgery," 481–96, quote p. 481; Bevan, "The Study and Teaching and the Practice of Surgery." For the history of the association, see Ravitch, *A Century of Surgery*.

95. English, *Shock, Physiological Surgery, and George Washington Crile*; Brieger, "From Conservative to Radical Surgery in Late Nineteenth-Century America," 216–31; Schlich, "'The Days of Brilliancy Are Past,'" 379–403.

96. Whipple, "Opportunities for Graduate Teaching of Surgery in Larger Qualified Hospitals," 516–30; Heuer, "Graduate Teaching of Surgery," 729–32.

97. See Pool's comments in Whipple, "Opportunities for Graduate Teaching of Surgery in Larger Qualified Hospitals," 527. See also Heuer, "Graduate Teaching of Surgery in University Clinics," 507–15.

98. Ludmerer, *Let Me Heal*.

99. For an examination of how sociology often views medicine, and its efforts at self-regulation, as the prototypical profession, see Friedson, *Profession of Medicine*.

100. Olch, "Evarts A. Graham, the American College of Surgeons, and the American Board of Surgery," 247–61; Mueller, *Evarts A. Graham*, chapter 12; Kernahan, "Franklin Martin and the Standardization of American Surgery, 1890–1940," chapter 7.

101. For concerns of surgery splintering into multiple boards, see R. Stevens, *American Medicine and the Public Interest*, 235–42. The Board of Surgery was the fifteenth board formed in the United States.

102. Rodman, *History of the American Board of Surgery*; Ward O. Griffin, "The American Board of Surgery in the 20th Century."

103. Barr and Pappas, "The Role of the American Board of Surgery on the Development of Surgical Residences in Post–World War II America."

104. "Conference on the Teaching of Surgery and Surgical Specialties," ACS Archives, Graduate Education Committee, RG5/SG2/S8/Box 1/Folder 3, p. 1; George Crile, "Graduate Training for Surgery," June 1939, ACS Archives, Graduate Education Committee, RG5/SG2/S8/Box 1/Folder 3, p. 2. The hospital inspection process resulted from an effort to ensure patients received surgery in safe, modern facilities. Inspection continues today as part of the Joint Commission. See Nahrwold and Kernahan, *A Century of Surgeons and Surgery*, chapters 2–3 and 12; Davis, *Fellowship of Surgeons*, 172–85, 205–22, 272, 327, 379–88, 346–47; Kernahan, "Franklin Martin and the Standardization of American Surgery," chapter 4.

105. Crile, "Graduate Training for Surgery," 1.

106. The ACS had previously formed a variety of committees to assess and make recommendations on graduate medical education that served as forerunners to the Committee on Graduate Training in Surgery. For a description of those efforts, see G. W. Stephenson, *American College of Surgeons at 75*, chapter 4; G. W. Stephenson, "American College of Surgeons and Graduate Education in Surgery," 1–57, see pp. 12–31. See "Abstract of Minutes, Meeting of the Committee on Graduate Training in Surgery," 28 November 1937, ACS Archives, Graduate Medical Education, RG5/SG2/S8/Box 1/Folder 1. A list of initial requirements appears in "Report of Sub-committee of the Committee Graduate Training in Surgery," 11 February 1938, ACS Archives, Graduate Medical Education, RG5/SG2/S8/Box 1/Folder 1.

107. Joint Conference Committees of the American College of Surgeons and the American College of Physicians, 16 October 1938. ACS Archives, Conference Committee on Graduate Training in Surgery, RG5/SG2/S8/SS03/Box 1/Folder 7, p. 2.

108. See "Exhibit A to Abstract of Minutes, Committee on Graduate Training for Surgery," 28 December 1938, ACS Archives, Graduate Education Committee, RG5/SG2/S8/Box 1/Folder 1, pp. 6–7.

109. For opposition to uniformity of surgical GME, see Heuer, "Graduate Teaching in Surgery," 515. Whipple, "Opportunities for Graduate Teaching of Surgery in Larger Qualified Hospitals," 516, 520–21; G. W. Stephenson, "American College of Surgeons and Graduate Education in Surgery," 18.

110. Quoted in Ludmerer, *Let Me Heal*, 127.

111. In 1938, it cost roughly $22,500 ($388,000 in 2017 USD). Commission on Graduate Medical Education Tentative Budget 1938, ACS Archives, Graduate Education Committee, RG5/SG2/S8/Box 1/Folder 3. (All financial conversions completed through the US Bureau of Labor Statistics online inflation calculator, http://www.bls.gov/data/inflation_calculator.htm.)

112. Dallas B. Phemister, "Graduate Training for Surgery: Report of Survey," 16 October 1938, ACS Archives, Graduate Training for Surgery Survey of Hospitals, RG5/SG2/S8/SS07/Box 2/Folder 2, p. 13. They had intended to survey 436 hospitals, only reached 374, and only fully evaluated 270.

113. Melville H. Manson, "Report of Survey Graduate Training for Surgery," 1938?, ACS Archives, Graduate Education Committee, RG5/SG2/S8/Box 1/Folder 1, p. 20.

114. Of the 297 surgical residents surveyed in 1937, 118 were in one-year programs, 69 were in two-year programs, 71 were in three-year programs, 22 in four-year programs, and eight in programs lasting five or more years. These lengths reflect years after internship. Programs associated with medical schools tended to be longer. Manson, "Report of Survey," 7.

115. Manson, "Report of Survey," 9–10.

116. Hospitals associated with medical schools (26 percent of those inspected) produced 38 percent of graduating residents, who generally received superior training. Manson, "Report of Survey," 20, 24.

117. G. W. Stephenson, "American College of Surgeons and Graduate Education in Surgery," 28–30.

118. "Commission on Graduate Medical Education Tentative Budget, 1938," ACS Archives, Graduate Education Committee, RG5/SG2/S8/Box 1/Folder 3.

119. "Administrative Board," 23 April 1939, ACS Archives, Graduate Training for Surgery, RG5/SG2/S8/SS07/Box 2.

120. "Administrative Board."

121. Phemister, "Graduate Training for Surgery," 12, 32.

122. "Meeting Minutes," 15 October 1939, ACS Archives, Graduate Education Committee RG5/SG2/S8/Box 1/Folder 3, p. 11.

123. See, for example, the efforts of Methodist Hospital in Houston to ally with neighboring Baylor College of Medicine and the local county hospital explicitly to meet ACS requirements and gain approval. "Annual Reports of the Department of Surgery, Baylor University College of Medicine, 1949–1950," NLM Archives, DeBakey Collection, Box 9/Folder 43, p. 22.

124. The board used the ACS list with the exception that it insisted on three years of residency, rather than the two required by the college. Minutes, 7 May 1939, ABS Archives, p. 14. In comparison to the eleven-page 1941 specifications, the requirements for 1938 occupied a single page. "Minimum Standards Recommended by the Committee on Graduate Training in Surgery," *Manual of Graduate Training in Surgery*, 1 October 1941, ACS Archives, pp. 395–406.

125. "Minimum Standards" (1941), 395.

126. The shift in attention from pathology in the 1930s to physiology in the 1940s as the central basic science for surgeons is striking. See "Minimum Standards" (1941), 402.

127. Ludmerer, *Let Me Heal*, chapters 4, 6.

128. Grillo, "Edward D. Churchill and the 'Rectangular' Surgical Residency," 947–52, quote p. 951.

129. Edward D. Churchill, "A Pattern for Graduate Training in Surgery at the Massachusetts General Hospital," Report to the Trustees from the General Executive Committee, 1939, Countway Archives, Churchill Collection, Box 17, Folder 45; Churchill, "Graduate Training in Surgery at the Massachusetts General Hospital," 28–36; Edward D. Churchill, "Report to the General Executive Committee," 20 December 1961, Countway Archives, Churchill Collection, Box 17, Folder 50.

130. Mayo Clinic, for example, pioneered a rectangular model in the 1920s. Fye, *Caring for the Heart*, chapters 3–4. The American College of Surgeons had been debating the promotion of rectangular programs for years: "Joint Conference Committees of the American College of Surgeons and the American College of Physicians." Melville H. Manson, "Report of Survey of Graduate Training for Surgery," 1938, ACS Archives, Graduate Education Committee, RG5/SG2/S8/Box 1/Folder 1, p. 21; Minutes Committee on Graduate Training for Surgery, 28 December 1938, Graduate Education Committee, RG5/SG2/S8/Box 1/Folder 3, p. 27. Advocates for pyramidal programs remained, arguing that the competition it fostered drove students to achieve more and that the closer relationship between a chair and his picked chief produced the best academic surgeons. See Ravitch, "The Surgical Residency," 14; and Whipple, "Opportunities for Graduate Teaching of Surgery in Larger Qualified Hospitals," 518.

131. Churchill, "Report to the General Executive Committee." See also Ludmerer, *Let Me Heal*, 174.

132. Harold Earnheart, "Trends in the Graduate Training for General Surgery and the Surgical Specialties as Related to Hospitals," ACS Archives, Graduate Education Committee, RG5/SG2/S8/Box 1/Folder 3, p. 1. For the 2.5 million estimate, see "Executive Committee Meeting, 14 May 1938," ACS Archives, Graduate Training for Surgery Survey of Hospitals, 1938, RG5/SG2/S8/SS07/Box 2/Folder 2, p. 16.

133. Kirk, *Machine in Our Hearts*.

134. Lesch, *The First Miracle Drugs*; Bliss, *The Discovery of Insulin*; Apple, *Vitamania*.

135. Packard, *The Making of a Tropical Disease*; Pierce and Writer, *Yellow Jack*.

136. Mueller, *Evarts A. Graham*, chapter 7.

137. In 1912, Doyon published a paper that identified a natural anticoagulant that, in retrospect, may have contained heparin. Doyon could not follow up on this study, and it did not in any way lead to the development of the drug heparin. Doyon, "Rapport de foie avec la coagulation de sang," 229–40. On the controversy of heparin's discovery, see Marcum, "The Origins of the Dispute over the Discovery of Heparin," 37–66.

138. McLean, "The Thromboplastic Action of Cephalin," 250–57. For his account, see McLean, "The Discovery of Heparin," 75–78; and the letter quoted in Best, "Preparation of Heparin and Its Use in the First Clinical Cases," 79–86.

139. Fye, "Heparin," 1198–203; Howell and Holt, "Two New Factors in Blood Coagulation," 328–41.

140. Mason, "A Note on the Use of Heparin in Blood Transfusion," 203–6; W. H. Howell, "The Purification of Heparin and its Chemical and Physiological Reactions," 199; W. H. Howell, "The Purification of Heparin and Its Presence in the Blood," 553–62.

141. Marcum, "The Development of Heparin in Toronto," 310–37.

142. For more on Charles Best and the discovery of insulin, see Bliss, *The Discovery of Insulin*. For Best's role in heparin, see Best, "Preparation of Heparin and Its Use in the First Clinical Cases"; and Marcum, "Development of Heparin in Toronto."

143. Charles and Scott, "Studies on Heparin I," 425–29; Charles and Scott, "Studies on Heparin II," 431–35. Charles and Scott, "Studies on Heparin III," 437–48. Dog and beef liver proved too expensive and were replaced by beef lung. The beef lung smelled so pungent that purification operations had to move out of the lab to a farm outside of town. Eventually porcine intestine replaced bovine lung; it required forty thousand pounds of intestines to produce five pounds of heparin.

144. Charles and Scott, "Studies on Heparin IV," 1927–33.

145. McKellar, *Surgical Limits*.

146. Murray, "Embolism in the Peripheral Arteries," 61–66.

147. Crafoord, "Preliminary Report on Post-operative Treatment with Heparin as a Preventive of Thrombosis," 407–26. In Sweden, Erik Jorpes's lab was simultaneously working to extract and purify heparin. The Swedish and Canadian groups competitively collaborated during these years. For more details, see Marcum, "Development of Heparin in Toronto."

148. Murray et al., "Heparin and Vascular Occlusion," 621–22; Murray, "Heparin in Thrombosis and Embolism," 567–98.

149. Murray, "Heparin in Surgical Treatment of Blood Vessels," 307–25.

150. DeBakey, "The Development of Vascular Surgery," 697–738, see especially 698. For the German citation, see Haschek and Lindenthal, "Ein Beitrag zur Praktischen Verwerthung der Photographie nach Röntgen," 63–64. The pair—a physician and physicist—used a calcium carbonate emulsion as their contrast agent. The first visceral arteriogram—of a kidney—appeared in the literature a month later. Like the image of the arm, it occurred on a dead body and served a conceptual rather than clinical purpose. See Rowland, "Report on the Application of the New Photography to Medicine and Surgery," 492–96. The history of X-rays and radiology generally has received substantial attention in both the historical and medical literature. For an excellent place to start, see B. H. Kevles, *Naked to the Bone*.

151. Some exceptions occur, like when calcified plaque accumulates along the walls of blood vessels and outlines their course. The first identified X-ray image of an aortic aneurysm did not involve contrast. See Davy and Gates, "A Case of Dissecting Aneurysm of the Aorta," 4712.

152. Osbourne et al., "Roentgenography of Urinary Tract During Excretion of Sodium Iodid," 368–73. *JAMA* subsequently classified this contribution as a

"landmark paper in medicine" for establishing and validating a new technique. Graham was similarly working with iodine to image the gallbladder. See Mueller, *Evarts A. Graham*, chapter 6.

153. Sicard and Forestier, "L'huile idoée en clinique," 309–17; Bull and Fischgold, *A Short History of Neuroradiology*, 33–34.

154. Berberish and Hirsch, "Die Röntgenographische Darstellung der Arterien und Venen am Lebenden Menschen," 2226–28; Brooks, "Intra-arterial Injection of Sodium Iodid," 1016–19.

155. Rudolph Matas, "Arteriography with Radioopaque Solution," Tulane Archives, Matas Collection, Box 23, Folder 25. See also Rudolph Matas, "Radio-Vasography; Arteriography; Phlebography," 1932, Tulane Archives, Matas Collection, Box 23, Folder 28.

156. Moniz received his Nobel Prize for his work developing the frontal lobotomy to treat psychiatric conditions. See Pressman, *Last Resort*.

157. Bull and Fischgold, *A Short History of Neuroradiology*, 34–38.

158. Moniz, "Arterial Encephalography," 72–90.

159. Grainger, "Development of Intravascular Contrast Agents," 91; B. H. Kevles, *Naked to the Bone*, 105; Allen and Camp, "Roentgenography of the Arteries of the Extremities with Thorotrast," 61–63. Ongoing research into various contrast agents continued, with Uroselectan being another popular alternative in the 1930s and 1940s. Grainger, "Development of Intravascular Contrast Agents," 91–92. See also DeBakey, "The Development of Vascular Surgery," 698. For Swick's publication, which discusses the history of the molecule he used, see Swick, "Intravenous Urography by Means of Uroselectan," 405–14.

160. Brooks, "Intra-arterial Injection of Sodium Iodid."

161. Dale, with Johnson and DeWeese, *Band of Brothers*, 161.

162. Warwick has discussed the importance of radiological imaging to determining the efficacy of surgical intervention in his article "X-Rays as Evidence in German Orthopedic Surgery," 1–24.

163. For the delayed adoption of X-rays and other medical technologies, see J. D. Howell, *Technology in the Hospital*, chapter 4. Warwick presented a contrasting narrative highlighting their early use in Germany in "X-Rays as Evidence in German Orthopedic Surgery."

164. Nelson Barker, "The History of the Medical Vascular Section of the Mayo Clinic," Mayo Clinic Archives, MHU 0670—Staff Memoirs Collection, Box 1, Folder 16; H. Bjarnason and R. D. McBane, "A Brief History of Vascular Radiology at Mayo Clinic," Mayo Clinic Archives, MHU 0676 Subject Files Collection, Folder Section of Vascular Diseases.

165. For an article exploring doctors' disregard for scientific developments lacking therapeutic benefits, see D. C. Smith, "Austin Flint and Auscultation in America," 129–49.

166. Winslow, *An Anatomical Exposition of the Structure of the Human Body*, 60–72; Blair, "Winslow and the Sympathetic System," 1200; Olry, "Winslow's

Contribution to Our Understanding of the Cervical Portion of the Sympathetic Nervous System," 190–96.

167. W. J. Mayo, "Observations on the Sympathetic Nervous System," 627–28. For more on Bernard and French physiology, see Holmes, *Claude Bernard and Animal Chemistry*.

168. Jaboulay, *Chirurgie du grand sympathique et du corps thyroïde*. Jaboulay appeared in chapter 1 for his contribution of a new technique of vessel repair and kidney transplantation.

169. Leriche, "De l'elongation et de la section des nerfs périvasculaires dans certains syndromes douloureux d'origine artérielle et dans quelques troubles trophiques," 378–82. See also Leriche, "De la sympathectomie perí-artérielle et de ses résaltats," 513–15, which William S. Halsted translated in "A Striking Elevation of the Temperature of the Hand and Forearm Following the Excision of a Subclavian Aneurism and Ligations of the Left Subclavian and Axillary Arteries," 219–24.

170. Because sympathetic impulses are segmental, disrupting the sympathetic nervous plexi around the artery affects only that section of the artery and not anything more distal. Leriche later admitted his method made no anatomic sense but continued to advocate for it anyway. Davis and Kanavel, "Sympathectomy in Raynaud's Disease, Erythromelalgia, and other Vascular Diseases of the Extremities," 729–42; Leriche, "Experimental and Clinical Contribution to the Question of the Innervation of the Vessels," 631–43; Leriche, "Surgery of the Sympathetic System," 449–69; Barnes, "Discarded Operations," 109–23.

171. Royale, "A New Operative Procedure in the Treatment of Spastic Paralysis and its Experimental Basis," 77–86; J. I. Hunter, "The Postural Influence of the Sympathetic Innervation of Voluntary Muscle," 86–89; J. I. Hunter, "The Significance of the Double Innervation of Voluntary Muscle Illustrated by Reference to the Maintenance of the Posture of the Wing," 581–87; Royale, "The Operations of Sympathetic Ramisection," 587–91.

172. William Mayo to Normal Royale, 16 July 1924, Mayo Clinic Archives, MHU-0620, William J. Mayo Papers, Box 102, Folder 16.

173. "Australian Doctor Discovers Treatment for Three Diseases Deemed to Be Incurable," *New York Times*, 4 May 1924, A1; "Knife Relieves Victims of Paralysis," *San Antonio Texas Light*, 5 October 1924.

174. L. M. Roberts to William Mayo, 3 April 1925; and H. Davis to William Mayo, 23 January 1925, MHU-0620, William J. Mayo Papers, Box 102, Folder 16.

175. Royale, "The Treatment of Spastic Paralysis by Sympathetic Ramisection," 701–20.

176. C. H. Mayo, "Surgery of the Sympathetic Nervous System," 481–87.

177. Davis and Kanavel, "Sympathectomy in Raynaud's Disease, Erythromelalgia, and other Vascular Diseases of the Extremities," 729–42; Davis and Kanavel, "The Effect of Sympathectomy on Spastic Paralysis of the Extremities," 1890–93.

178. Brown and Adson, "Calorimetric Studies of the Extremities Following Lumbar Sympathetic Ramisection and Ganglionectomy," 232–40; Brown and Adson,

"Physiological Effects of Thoracic and of Lumber Sympathetic Ganglionectomy or Section of Trunk," 322–57; Barker, "The History of the Medical Vascular Section of the Mayo Clinic." The patient, who in retrospect probably had livedo reticularis (a diagnosis that did not exist in 1925), remained symptom-free when examined twenty years later.

179. Winchell McK. Craig, "History of the Development of the Section of Neurological Surgery at the Mayo Clinic," August 1958, Mayo Archives, MHU 0670 Staff Memoirs Collection, Box 4, Folder 78, p. 7.

180. Barker, "The History of the Medical Vascular Section of the Mayo Clinic," 5–6. Other posterior approaches were developed elsewhere; by the 1930s, the anterior, transabdominal approach effectively disappeared.

181. He actually injected procaine, a close cousin of Novocain. White, "Diagnostic Blocking of the Sympathetic Nerves to the Extremities with Procaine," 1382–88. George Brown had previously used the typhoid fever vaccine as a determinant of whether sympathectomies would be effective.

182. Flothow, "Surgery of the Sympathetic Nervous System," 8–18; Flothow, "Sympathetic Alcoholic Injection for Relief of Arteriosclerotic Pain and Gangrene," 408–12; Flothow, "Diagnostic and Therapeutic Injections of the Sympathetic Nerves," 591–604, 625.

183. C. H. Mayo, "Surgery of the Sympathetic Nervous System"; Ross, "Sympathectomy as an Experiment in Human Physiology," 5–19.

184. Review of Annual Reports of St. Mary's Hospitals from 1925 to 1939, Mayo Clinic Archives.

185. Review of Annual Reports of St. Mary's Hospitals from 1925 to 1939; Barnes, "Discarded Operations"; Leriche, "Surgery of the Sympathetic System."

186. For early enthusiasm for the operation, see, for example, Rowntree, "Result of Bilateral Lumbar Sympathetic Ganglionectomy and Ramisectomy for Polyarthritis of the Lower Extremities," 333–34.

187. Mulvihill and Harvey, "Studies on Collateral Circulation: I," 423–29; Theirs, "Effect of Neurectomy on the Collateral Arteriole Circulation of the Extremities," 737–44; Horton and Craig, "Evidence Shown in Roentgenograms of Changes in the Vascular Tree Following Experimental Sympathetic Ganglionectomy," 698–701; Moore, Williams, and Singleton, "Vasoconstrictor Fibers," 308–22; "Operative Schedule for Wednesday March 10th, 1937," Washington University Archives, RG 009, Box 1, Folder 2.

188. Ellis, "James Learmonth," 529.

189. Gage, "Mycotic Aneurysm of the Common Iliac Artery," 667–710; "Dr. Mims Gage," *Bulletin of the Tulane Medical Faculty* 11, no. 3 (1952): 172–74.

190. Bird, "Sympathectomy as a Preliminary to the Obliteration of Popliteal Aneurisms," 926–29.

191. See, for example, the future founder of the Society for Vascular Surgery, J. Ross Veal, "The Value of Sympathetic Interruption Following the Surgical Repair of Peripheral Aneurysms," 227–30.

192. The idea of traumatically induced vasospasm was a hotly debated topic in the 1930s. See Montgomery and Ireland, "Traumatic Segmentary Arterial Spasm," 1741–46; Jung, "Review of the Forty-Sixth French Congress of Surgery," 306–16. See especially the work of Hamiovici and Reynaldo dos Santos. For work promoting the use of sympathectomy in vascular trauma, see Gage, "Editorial," 792–95; Gage and Ochsner, "The Prevention of Ischemic Gangrene Following Surgical Operations upon the Major Peripheral Arteries by Chemical Section of the Cervicodorsal and Lumbar Sympathetics," 938–59; White, "Progress in Surgery of the Autonomic Nervous System," 491–517.

193. These schedules would not include emergent trauma cases. OR schedules, Washington University Archives, Barnes Hospital Records, RG 009, Box 1, Folders 2–3.

194. Review of annual reports of St. Mary's Hospitals from 1893 to 1939, Mayo Clinic Archives.

Chapter Three

1. For American military medicine in World War II, see a general overview in Cowdrey, *Fighting for Life*. For theater-specific experiences, see Cosmas and Cowdrey, *Medical Service in the European Theater of Operations*; Wiltse, *Medical Service in the Mediterranean and Minor Theaters*; Condon-Rall and Cowdrey, *Medical Service in the War against Japan*. For British military medicine in World War II, see M. Harrison, *Medicine and Victory*.

2. For the development of sulfas, see Lesch, *The First Miracle Drugs*.

3. Not a single US service member contracted yellow fever during the war. However, impurities in the human serum used to produce the yellow fever vaccine led to at least fifty thousand cases of serum hepatitis among US service members. See Pierce and Writer, *Yellow Jack*, chapter 16.

4. For more on the development of DDT and its use in World War II, see Russell, *War and Nature*, chapters 6–8. See also Soper, *Ventures in World Health*, chapters 15–17.

5. Malaria remained *the* disease problem in the Pacific theaters despite improved efforts at control. The literature on malaria in World War II is vast. For more on the development and use of atabrine, see Slater, *War and Disease*, chapters 3–5; and Bruce-Chwatt, "Changing Tides of Chemotherapy of Malaria," 581. For one of many articles on malaria in the Pacific, see Joy, "Malaria in American Troops in the South and Southwest Pacific in World War II," 192–207. Malaria posed less of a problem to forces in the western hemisphere, although it did complicate operations in Italy. See Snowden, *The Conquest of Malaria*, chapters 7 and 8.

6. Klasen, *History of Burns*.

7. Beebe and DeBakey, *Battle Casualties*.

8. Pelis, "Taking Credit," 238–77.

9. See chapter 2 of Kendrick, *Blood Program in World War II*. Kendrick's "Prevention and Treatment of Shock in the Combat Zone" provides a thorough review of the interwar literature, where theories of intravascular depletion slowly supplanted those of toxic etiologies of shock. In another important interwar advance, Karl Landsteiner et al. discovered the Rh factors (what makes blood "positive" or "negative") in 1940, making the transfusions safer and more effective. Most wartime transfusions were not typed so specifically given the priority of expediency and logistical simplicity. Moreover, Rh factor matching is less important in male patients, who predominated in war. Lederer, *Flesh and Blood*, 150.

10. M. Harrison, *Medicine and Victory*, 35, 55–56, 116–17.

11. Hedley-White and Milamed, "Our Blood, Your Money," 114–20.

12. Kendrick, "Prevention and Treatment of Shock in the Combat Zone," 106.

13. See, for example, Newhauser and Kendrick, "Blood Substitutes," 1–13; Elliot, Tatum, and Busby, "Blood Plasma," 118–28.

14. Kendrick, "Prevention and Treatment of Shock in the Combat Zone," 107.

15. Cowdrey, *Fighting for Life*, 171.

16. Creager, "'What Blood Told Dr. Cohn,'" 377–405, see especially 383.

17. Creager, "Biotechnology and Blood," 39–62; Creager, "Producing Molecular Therapeutics from Human Blood," 107–38.

18. Kendrick, *Blood Program in World War II*, chapter 3.

19. LTC Samuel A. Hanser, interview with the Office of the Surgeon General, 9 September 1944, NARA 112/390/17/8/1-2/2/2, p. 13.

20. See Crewes, "Colonel Edward Churchill's Transformation of Wound Care in the Mediterranean Theater of the Second World War," 20–39; Churchill, *Surgeon to Soldiers*, chapter 4.

21. "'Live Blood' Banks Save Soldiers' Lives in Sicily when Plasma Proves Inadequate," *New York Times*, 27 August 1943, 4.

22. Major Rafe N. Hatt, interview with the Office of the Surgeon General, 29 July 1944, NARA 112/390/16/33-34/7-1/1/5, p. 3. Hanser, interview with the Office of the Surgeon General, 13. Hospitals also collected blood from French civilians—some more eager to donate than others.

23. MAJ Samuel W. Windham, interview with the Office of the Surgeon General, 21 July 1944, NARA 112/390/17/8/1-2/2/2, pp. 6–7. Major Windham served as a physician in the 8th Evacuation Hospital, which was associated with the University of Virginia Hospital. For more on the 8th Evac, see Leavell, *The 8th Evac*.

24. "6703rd Blood Transfusion Unit Historical Report to 1 February 1945," NARA 112/390/17/27/1/459/22.

25. "Memo from the Office of the Chief Surgeon to Transfusion Services HQ," 30 October 1943, NARA 112/390/16/33-34/7-1/3/1.

26. "Essential Technical Medical Data from Overseas Forces," 5 May 1944, NARA 112/390/17/13/6/242/1, p. 9; Brigadier General Isidor Ravdin, interview with the Office of the Surgeon General, 23 January 1945, NARA 112/390/18/25/2/221, pp. 9–10. LTC Richard Shackelford, interview with the Office of the Surgeon General,

10 May 1944, NARA 112/390/18/25/2/219, pp. 5–6; "Technical Memorandum No. 13: Blood Bank, 21 Sept 1944," NARA 112/390/17/13/6242/6, p. 1. Helling, *Desperate Surgery in the Pacific War*, chapters 2, 4, and especially 9.

27. Edwards, "A System for an Efficient Transfusion Service," 481–85. For more on the establishment of blood banking in the United States, see Swanson, *Banking on the Body*.

28. Cowdrey, *Fighting for Life*, 165–73; Kendrick, *Blood Program in World War II*, chapters 4, 5, 8, 15–17; "Shipment of Whole Blood to Pacific Theaters of Operation," *Bulletin of the US Army Medical Department* no. 87 (April 1945): 45. Blood from the United States supplemented, not supplanted, in-theater supply. From May 1944 to May 1945, the European Theater of Operations used 385,231 pints of blood; 194,712 came from the United States. See Elliott C. Cutler, "Surgery—the US Forces," *Inter-Allied Conferences on War Medicine*, July 1945, NARA 112/390/17/7/6/428/1, p. 499; "The Wounded from Alamein: Observations on Wound Shock and Its Treatment," *Army Medical Department Bulletin* no. 7 (September 1943): 11–19.

29. Lesch, *The First Miracle Drugs*. See especially part 3 for their role in the American military effort in World War II.

30. For one of the most recent accounts of that history, see Bud, *Penicillin*. See also Parascandola, "The Introduction of Antibiotics into Therapeutics," 102–12.

31. Bud, *Penicillin*, 53. Parascandola, "Introduction of Antibiotics into Therapeutics," 107. In all of 1943, there were 21 billion units of penicillin produced; in 1945, 1,663 billion units. The drug became generally available to American civilians in 1945.

32. "Annual Report of the Surgery Division for Fiscal Year 1944," 20 June 1944, NARA 112/390/18/35/2/1/8 pp. 37–39. Training programs occurred at Bushnell Hospital in Utah and Halloran Hospital in New York City. Additionally, they distributed multiple circulars to deployed physicians discussing the drug and appropriate usage.

33. "Technical Memorandum No. 5: Penicillin," 26 February 1944, NARA 112/390/17/13/6/242/6.

34. *Burns, Shock, Wound Healing, and Vascular Injuries*.

35. See, for example, Holman, "War Injuries to Arteries and Their Treatment," 183–92; de Takáts, "Vascular Surgery in the War," 291–96.

36. See the curriculum at Tulane, for example: "Fundamental Surgery for Medical Officers, United States Army, August 16 through August 26, 1943," Matas Collection, Tulane Archives, Box 23, Folder 56. The Mayo Clinic also provided substantial continuing medical education to army medical officers. Later in the war, the Office of the Surgeon General came to question the value of these courses, suggesting that they covered material too superficially and too briefly to be of much benefit to the war surgeon. See "Annual Report of the Surgery Division for Fiscal Year 1944," 22; "Annual Report of the Surgery Consultants Division for Fiscal Year 1945," NARA 112/390/18/35/2/2/4-6, p. 20.

37. Specifically, they insisted on ligation with division of the artery and warned that ligation in continuity presented a serious risk of secondary hemorrhage and distal arteriospasm. *Burns, Shock, Wound Healing, and Vascular Injuries,* 199–206; Holman, "War Injuries to Arteries and Their Treatment," 184, 191, 211–26.

38. Circular letter No. 178, Office of the Surgeon General of the Army, 23 October 1943. http://history.amedd.army.mil/booksdocs/wwii/StandarizedCare/CL178. htm (accessed 26 April 2018); War Department Technical Bulletin 147: Notes on Care of Battle Casualties, Washington DC: War Department, March 1945, http://history.amedd.army.mil/booksdocs/wwii/StandarizedCare/TBMED147.pdf (accessed 26 April 2018).

39. "Circular Letter No. 8: Notes on Care of Battle Casualties," HQ MTO Office of the Surgeon, March 1945, NARA 112/390/17/9/2/5/5, p. 14; "Circular Letter No. 5: Gas Gangrene," NATOUSA, 5 August 1943, NARA 112/390/17/8/1/4/17, p. 1; "Medical Circular No. 4 Gas Gangrene," Office of the Surgeon, 5th Army, 20 October 1943, NARA 112/390/17/8/1/4/18, p. 2; "Circular Letter No. 2: Surgery," HQ 7th Army, 18 July 1944, NARA 112/390/17/8/1/4/1/18, p. 5; Holman, "War Injuries to Arteries and Their Treatment," 186–87.

40. "Medical Circular No. 4 Gas Gangrene," 2; "Circular Letter No. 2: Surgery," 5; *Burns, Shock, Wound Healing, and Vascular Injuries,* 199–206.

41. *Burns, Shock, Wound Healing, and Vascular Injuries,* 204–5; Holman, "War Injuries to Arteries and Their Treatment," 185; De Takáts, "Vascular Surgery in the War," 293–94; John Homans, A. W. Allen, Géza de Takáts, and W. G. Maddock, "Wounds of the Large Blood Vessels," in *Technical Manual 8–210: Guide to Therapy for Medical Officers,* War Department, Government Printing Office, 1942, in Washington University Archives, General Hospital 21 Collection, Series 7, Box 15, Folder 23, pp. 34–50; DeBakey, "Traumatic Vasospasm," 23–28.

42. War Department Technical Bulletin 147; J. J. Mason Brown, "A Plea for Conservatism in the Primary Surgery of Wounds of the Main Arteries of the Limbs," and Ruscoe Clark, "Forward Surgery of Injuries to Major Blood Vessels," both in "Proceedings of the Congress of CMF Army Surgeons," Rome, 12–19 February 1945, NLM Archives, DeBakey Collection, Box 27, Folder 21, pp. 103–6 and 107–11, respectively.

43. For an explication of this system, see *Activities of Surgical Consultants.*

44. DeBakey and Simeone, "Battle Injuries of the Arteries in World War II," 534–79, especially 537; DeBakey and Simeone, "Acute Battle-Incurred Arterial Injuries," 60–148, see especially 64–66 and chart 2. The Medical Statistics Division of the Office of the Surgeon General reviewed the latter article and suggested that vascular injuries comprised 1.7 percent of all war wounds, although it readily admitted that this number was a rough guestimate. See "Corrections" in NARA 112/390/16/11/6/481/1. As in World War I, doctors were not required to document or catalog vascular injuries; moreover, many patients suffering from these wounds bled to death before reaching a physician. A review of one thousand autopsies from the Italian campaign clearly indicates that vascular trauma caused far more than 1

percent of battlefield deaths. William W. Tribby, "Examination of One Thousand Americans Killed in Action in Italy," NARA 112/390/16/4/4-5/1408-1409.

45. The 2nd Auxiliary Surgery Group documented seventy-five injuries to major blood vessels in 3,154 abdominal and abdominal-thoracic cases; 55 (73 percent) of these patients died. "Forward Surgery of the Severely Wounded: A History of the Activities of the 2nd Auxiliary Surgery Group, 1942–1945," NARA 112/390/16/11/6/358/3 pp. 385–95.

46. Data from DeBakey and Simeone, "Acute Battle-Incurred Arterial Injuries," table 3.

47. "Injuries and Diseases Common to War," Medical Department, Enlisted Technicians School, NARA 112/390/16/4/4-5/1402, pp. 27–32. Minimal literature on enlisted combat medics in World War II exists, paradoxical to their prominence in popular culture. See Engle, *Medic*; Greenwood and Berry, *Medics at War*; Shilcutt, "First Link in the Chain."

48. Cutler, "Military Surgery, United States Army, European Theater of Operations," 262.

49. The Pacific theaters presented unique strategic, logistical, and geographic considerations that influenced the practice of vascular surgery. See Barr, Cherry, and Rich, "Vascular Surgery in the Pacific Theaters of World War II."

50. C. B. Odom, "Vascular Injuries, Report to Anglo-American Consultants Conference, 10 December 1944," NARA 331/290/7/34/4/3/2.

51. DeBakey and Simeone, "Acute Battle-Incurred Arterial Injuries," 109–15.

52. Barr, Cherry, and Rich, "Vascular Surgery in the Pacific Theaters of World War II."

53. "Forward Surgery of the Severely Wounded," 734–40; Rose, Hess, and Welch, "Vascular Injuries of the Extremities in Battle Casualties," 866–72; Bradford and Moore, "Vascular Injuries in War," 667.

54. New research also recommended ligating just distal to a branch point to avoid leaving blind sacs that attenuated flow into the collaterals; it is unclear how closely front-line surgeons followed this specific recommendation. Holman, "Further Observations on Surgery of the Large Arteries," 275–87.

55. Odom, "Causes of Amputations in Battle Casualties with Emphasis on Vascular Injuries." Grantley W. Taylor, "Report of the Surgical Section," in "Historical Records and Annual Report, 95th Evacuation Hospital," by Paul K. Sauer, 1944, NARA 331/290/8/25/1/31/25, p. 3; Rose, Hess, and Welch, "Vascular Injuries of the Extremities in Battle Casualties," 161.

56. Odom, "Causes of Amputations in Battle Casualties with Emphasis on Vascular Injuries," 562–69.

57. Taylor, "Report of the Surgical Section," 3; Carl P. Schlicke, "Arterial Injuries," 247th General Hospital, 7 December 1944, NARA 112/390/17/13/6/235/1, p. 1; Fiorindo Simeone, "Wounds of the Arteries of the Extremities," August 1945, NARA 112/390/16/11/6/359/3, p. 5; Rose, Hess, and Welch, "Vascular Injuries of

the Extremities in Battle Casualties," 166; Kirtley, "Arterial Injuries in a Theater of Operations," 223–24.

58. Ogilivie, "War Surgery in Africa," 321; Bradford, "Vascular Injuries in Battle Casualties," 106.

59. See tables 5, 7, 19, 27, and 47 and the text on page 5 in Simeone, "Wounds of the Arteries of the Extremities." These statistics do not reveal any deleterious effect, but nor do they evidence any advantage.

60. "Annual Report of the Surgery Consultants Division for Fiscal Year 1945," 97c.

61. "Anglo-American Consultants Conference," 10 December 1944, NARA 331/290/7/34/4/3/2, p. 6. Some sources continued to recommend concomitant venous ligation. See, for example, Elkin, "Vascular Injuries of Warfare," 284–306, especially page 289.

62. In addition to the Inter-Allied Medical Conference, see also "Proceedings of the Congress of CMF Army Surgeons," Rome, 12–19 Feb 1945, NLM Archives, DeBakey Collection, Box 27, Folder 21.

63. Simeone, "Wounds of the Arteries of the Extremities," 29; Taylor, "Report of the Surgical Section," 3. See also Snyder, "Vascular Wounds," 77–85.

64. Taylor, "Report of the Surgical Section," 3. See also Snyder, "Vascular Wounds."

65. "3rd Auxiliary Surgery Group Annual Report, 1945," NARA 112/390/17/17/5/393/3, pp. 23–34.

66. "Anglo-American Consultants Conference," 5.

67. LTC Donald Glover, interview with the Office of the Surgeon General, 14 August 1944, NARA 112/390/18/25/2/219, p. 5. For analogous results, see Bradford and Moore, "Vascular Injuries in War," 668; Odom, "Causes of Amputations in Battle Casualties with Emphasis on Vascular Injuries," 567–68; MacFee, "Arterial Anastomosis in War Wounds of the Extremities," 381–83.

68. "Annual Report 9th Evacuation Hospital, 1944," NARA 112/390/17/25/6/400/3, p. 20; "Semi-annual Report of the 9th Evacuation Hospital, 1 January–30 June 1945," NARA 112/390/17/25/6/400/3, pp. 16–17. For similar sentiment, see M. K. Smith, "Arterial Injuries," 871; and Warren, "War Wounds of Arteries," 86–99, especially 97.

69. "Arterial Injuries in War Wounds," from the 2nd Auxiliary Surgical Group, NARA 112/390/16/11/6/358/2, Tables 6C, 7D, 9F, 10D, 11D, 11E, 14, 15A and 15B; DeBakey and Simeone, "Acute Battle-Incurred Arterial Injuries," 135–39 and chart 17; DeBakey and Simeone, "Battle Injuries of the in World War II," 564–66.

70. DeBakey and Simeone particularly praised it; DeBakey's role in developing the technique prior to the war possibly clouded his objectivity. DeBakey and Simeone, "Acute Battle-Incurred Arterial Injuries," 135–39 and chart 17; DeBakey and Simeone, "Battle Injuries of the Arteries in World War II," 564–66. See also Elkin, "Vascular Injuries of Warfare," 285–89; Harbinson, "Experiences with Aneurysms

in an Overseas General Hospital," 128–37; Kirtley, "Arterial Injuries in a Theater of Operations," 223–24; Snyder, "Vascular Wounds," 77–85.

71. Albright and Van Hale, "Traumatic Aneurysms," 459. See also Harbinson, "Experiences with Aneurysms in an Overseas General Hospital," 131–32.

72. *Burns, Shock, Wound Healing, and Vascular Injuries*, 204–5; Holman, "War Injuries to Arteries and Their Treatment," 185; De Takáts, "Vascular Surgery in the War," 293–94. See also Langely, "Repair of Ruptured Popliteal Artery," 161–65.

73. "Report of the Surgical Consultant, 6th Army, 1945," NARA 112/390/ 17/13/6/232/22, p. 8; Snyder, "Vascular Wounds," 77–85; Thomas J. Kelly, "Major Vessel Injury of the Upper and Lower Extremities: A Report and Analysis of 58 Cases," 28 March 1946, MHI Archives, Medical Historical Unit Collection, Box 64, Folder 6, p. 1; "27th Evacuation Hospital Semi-annual Report, 1 January 1945 thru 30 June 1945," NARA 112/390/17/25/6/403/2, p. 3.

74. "Report of the Surgical Consultant, 6th Army, 1945," 8; "Annual Report 9th Evacuation Hospital, 1944," 18.

75. DeBakey and Simeone, "Acute Battle-Incurred Arterial Injuries," 98–99; DeBakey and Simeone, "Battle Injuries of the Arteries in World War II," 563–64.

76. "Annual Report of the Surgery Division for Fiscal Year 1944," 97d. In contrast to the American experience, the Canadians employed heparin safely in the majority of their arterial repairs, partially explaining their greater success rates in arterial repair. See "Report of Consulting Surgeon Allied Force Headquarters to Cover the Period 1 March 1944–31 October 1944," to Director of Medical Services, Allied Force Headquarters, NARA 112/390/17/7/6/436/10, pp. 25–26. For more on Canadian efforts with vascular repair, see Mustard, "The Technic of Immediate Restoration of Vascular Continuity after Arterial Wounds," 46–59. Unfortunately, Mustard was only a major at time of publication; one hopes he received promotion to colonel.

77. Craig Miller is currently writing the definitive biography of Michael DeBakey and graciously shared some of his material. For available biographical sources, see both published sources and interview transcripts in the DeBakey Papers, NLM Archives, and a video interview through the Society for Vascular Surgery: "Interview with Dr. Michael DeBakey on the 50th anniversary of SVS," YouTube video, posted by SVS Vascular, 1 December, 2014, https://www.youtube.com/watch?v=hdQfrZo fAcc&list=PLdMQA5pt2x0JuwVQ-c-DO7LUPus4QB0yZ&index=5 (accessed 19 May 2018).

78. *Burns, Shock, Wound Healing, and Vascular Injuries*, 211.

79. DeBakey and Simeone, "Battle Injuries of the Arteries in World War II," 536; DeBakey and Simeone, "Acute Battle-Incurred Arterial Injuries," 69. Their numbers roughly correspond with other, smaller studies. See "Semi-annual Report of the 9th Evacuation Hospital," 1 January–30 June 1945, NARA 112/390/17/25/6/400/4, pp. 16–17. This number excluded so-called traumatic amputations—limbs so severely damaged that surgeons lopped them off without any effort to preserve them. Many of these traumatic amputations would have resulted from damage to blood

vessels that created avascular extremities, although precise numbers are unavailable. One study that included primary amputations suggested vascular injuries caused 60 percent of limbs lost. "Arterial Injuries in War Wounds," table 2B.

80. Meillier et al., "Arthur Hendley Blakemore's Life and Contributions to Vascular Surgery," 1094–97.

81. For more on the effects of disability in World War I, see Linker, *War's Waste*; and Bourke, *Dismembering the Male*.

82. Arthur H. Blakemore and Jere W. Lord Jr., "The Damaged Main Artery in Extremity Wounds of World War II: A Surgical Problem," Tulane Archives, Matas Collection, Box 22, Folder 25, p. 2.

83. "Dr. Jere Lord Jr., 88; Led Heart Association," *New York Times*, 3 May 1999, A26.

84. Blakemore, Lord, and Stefko, "The Severed Primary Artery in the War Wounded," 488–508.

85. In fact, Blakemore and Lord believed that because not even suture material extended into the lumen, their method would prove superior to traditional suture anastomosis à la Carrel. Blakemore and Lord, "The Damaged Main Artery in Extremity Wound of World War II," 5.

86. Blakemore, Lord, and Stefko, "Restoration of Blood Flow in Damaged Arteries," 481–97; Blakemore and Lord, "A Nonsuture Method of Blood Vessel Anastomosis: Review of Experimental Study, Report of Clinical Cases," 435–51; Blakemore and Lord, "A Nonsuture Method of Blood Vessel Anastomosis," 685–91 and 748–53.

87. Blakemore and Lord, "The Damaged Main Artery in Extremity Wounds," 5. They also asserted that, unlike in suture anastomosis, their method allowed for significant differences in the diameters of the artery and vein.

88. They grimly noted that one dead GI would produce twelve to fifteen prostheses. In theory, pathologists would harvest the veins aseptically in the base hospitals, prepare and freeze them, and then bank the veins in field hospitals. Problematically, the refrigerators used to store blood were not cold enough to preserve the vein grafts, thus requiring a separate, rare piece of equipment for that purpose. Arthur H. Blakemore and Jere W. Lord Jr., "A Non-suture Method of Blood Vessel Anastamosis: A Program for Handling War Wounded," Tulane Archives, Matas Collection, Box 22, Folder 25, p. 13; Arthur H. Blakemore and Jere W. Lord Jr., "Measures Contributing to the Success of a Non-suture Method of Anastomosing Blood Vessels in the War Wounded with Vitallium Tubes," Tulane Archives, Matas Collection, Box 24, Folder 34, p. 5; Blakemore and Lord, "A Nonsuture Method of Blood Vessel Anastamosis," 438–39.

89. Odom, "Causes of Amputations in Battle Casualties with Emphasis on Vascular Injuries," 564; Snyder, "Vascular Wounds," 77–85.

90. DeBakey and Simeone, "Battle Injuries of the Arteries in World War II," 559. See note in NARA 112/390/17/13/6/241/7.

91. "Anglo-American Consultants Conference," 10–11 December 1944, NARA 112/390/17/7/6/436/4, p. 5.

92. Simeone, "The Anastomosis of Severed Arteries by a Nonsuture Method," 1088–99; DeBakey and Simeone, "Battle Injuries of the Arteries in World War II," 559. They reported multiple instances of surgeons abandoning the procedure mid-operation because of technical difficulties. Other surgeons similarly report taking two to three hours per case: Rose, Hess, and Welch, "Vascular Injuries of the Extremities in Battle Casualties," 169; Odom, "Causes of Amputations in Battle Casualties with Emphasis on Vascular Injuries," 564–65.

93. Simeone, "The Anastomosis of Severed Arteries by a Nonsuture Method"; "Semi-annual Report of the 9th Evacuation Hospital," 17; C. B. Odom, "Vascular Injuries," in "Anglo-American Consultants Conference," p. 5; Steward, "War Experiences with Nonsuture Technic of Anastomosis in Primary Arterial Injuries," 157–70.

94. MacFee, "Arterial Anastomosis in War Wounds of the Extremities"; M. K. Smith, "Arterial Injuries"; Bradford and Moore, "Vascular Injuries in War," 667–68.

95. "Annual Report of the Surgery Division for Fiscal Year 1944," 97c–97d.

96. Odom, "Vascular Injuries." For a similar experience, see Taylor, "Historical Records and Annual Report, 95th Evacuation Hospital," 3.

97. DeBakey and Simeone, "Acute Battle-Incurred Arterial Injuries," 109–13; DeBakey and Simeone, "Battle Injuries of the Arteries in World War II," 555–58.

98. Toland, *Battle*.

99. Beebe and DeBakey, *Battle Casualties*, 55–57.

100. Barr, Cherry, and Rich, "Vascular Surgery in the Pacific Theaters of World War II."

101. Wilde, "Practising Surgery"; Wilde and Hirst, "Learning from Mistakes," 38–77.

102. Randomly selecting 1 May 1944 as a division point, Carter and DeBakey noticed the overall case fatality rate in the 2nd Auxiliary Surgical Group drop from 11.3 percent to 8.3 percent despite increasing severity of the casualties. Carter and DeBakey, "Special Reports and Statistical Data," 530–31.

103. Imes, "Suture of the Popliteal Artery," 644–46, quote p. 644. Imes had ligated eight popliteal artery injuries in the Italian campaign, and all resulted in amputation. When his unit transferred to Europe, he repaired three popliteal artery lesions; all three patients kept their limbs, although even Imes questioned the long-term patency of the repairs. For similar experiences (and similar quotes), see M. K. Smith, "Arterial Injuries," 866; Bradford and Moore, "Vascular Injuries in War," 667; Rose, Hess, and Welch, "Vascular Injuries of the Extremities in Battle Casualties," 161. For a similar experience among British surgeons, see Brown, "A Plea for Conservatism in the Primary Surgery of Wounds of the Main Arteries of the Limbs"; and Clark, "Forward Surgery of Injuries to Major Blood Vessels."

104. Simeone, "Wounds of the Arteries of the Extremities," 17–18. Simeone goes on to cite a series of eighteen cases of suture repair where seventeen limbs survived.

105. This percentage discounts wounds to the tibial arteries, which even today generally are ligated in trauma. Snyder, "Vascular Wounds," 77–85. Snyder's unit also performed a rare venous autograft on a German POW who suffered an injury to the common femoral artery. The hospital lacked heparin, and a thrombus formed at the site of repair which embolized to the posterior tibial artery and required amputation distal to that level, but the graft remained patent.

106. Odom, "Causes of Amputations in Battle Casualties with Emphasis on Vascular Injuries," 564. Prentice, *I Was Patton's Doctor*, 117.

107. "5th Evacuation Hospital Period Report to Surgeon General, 30 June 1945," NARA 112/390/17/25/6/400/2, p. 21.

108. For more on the development of these groups, see Marble, "Forward Surgery and Combat Hospitals," 68–100, especially pp. 80–92. For more on the 2nd Auxiliary Surgery Group, see L. A. Brewer, "The Contributions of the Second Auxiliary Surgical Group to Military Surgery During World War II," 318–26; and "Forward Surgery of the Severely Wounded," the introductory chapters of which provide a useful unit history. For more on the 3rd Auxiliary Surgery Group, see "3d Auxiliary Surgical Group Unit History," https://www.med-dept.com/unit-histories/3d-auxiliary-surgical-group/ (accessed 18 April 2019); Graves, *Front Line Surgeons*. The other three auxiliary surgical groups did not publish their history, although annual reports and operational histories are available in NARA at 112/390/17/7/2, Boxes 220–22. Unfortunately, they did not document their medical statistics and no information regarding their treatment of vascular patients survives.

109. Some teams logged upward of 1,200. Graves, *Front Line Surgeons*, 317–18.

110. "Forward Surgery of the Severely Wounded," data compiled from pp. 717–41.

111. "3rd Auxiliary Surgery Group Annual Report, 1945," 21–24. Members of the 3rd Group also cite the positive results obtained by Canadian surgeons performing arterial repairs as a motivating factor.

112. DeBakey and Simeone, "Acute Battle-Incurred Arterial Injuries," 112. The medical statistics division of the Office of the Surgeon General did find statistical significance in this difference, although with a sample size of eighty-one for suture repair and percentages that do not align with their earlier tables, broad conclusions are not justified.

113. "Forward Surgery of the Severely Wounded," data compiled from pp. 717–41. These data reflect a subset of 220 vascular cases for which the group recorded details of therapy. For the entire series of vascular wounds (463), patients suffered a 58 percent amputation rate (a number that included ligated and repaired arteries), making the decrease to 25 percent following arterial repair all the more significant.

114. Serlin, *Replaceable You.*

115. "Annual Report of the Surgery Division for Fiscal Year 1944," 103. See also Albright and Van Hale, "Traumatic Aneurysms"; Snyder, "Vascular Wounds," 78.

116. "Circular Letter No. 8," 14; "Delay Advised in Treatment of Aneurysm," *Bulletin of the U.S. Army Medical Department* 80 (September 1944): 3; War Department

Technical Bulletin 147; J. D. Martin, "Pulsating Hematoma," 219–24; John M. Willis, ed., "Data for Surgical History Pacific Ocean Areas and Middle Pacific," NARA 112/390/16/11/6/359/3, p. 3; Conway and Plain, "Pulsating Hematoma, False Aneurysm, and Arteriovenous Fistula Due to War Injuries," 383–406.

117. Harbinson, "Experiences with Aneurysms in an Overseas General Hospital," 131.

118. "Combined Diagnostic Analysis Report (1 January 1945 to 31 August 1945)," NARA 112/390/17/13/6/241/5; Elkin and Shumacker, "Arterial Aneurysms and Arteriovenous Fistulas," 149–80.

119. "Annual Report of the Surgery Division for Fiscal Year 1944," 18; "Annual Report of the Surgery Consultants Division for Fiscal Year 1945," 14–15; Michael E. DeBakey, "The Organization of Surgical Services in the Zone of the Interior, with a Consideration of Specialty Centers," 20 April 1951, NLM Archives, DeBakey Collection, Box 27, Folder 23.

120. "Ashford General Hospital," NARA 112/390/17/13/6/241/5, p. 3. See also Daniel C. Elkin to Michael E. DeBakey, 12 February 1944, NARA 112/390/17/13/6/241/5.

121. Link and Coleman, *Medical Support of the Army Air Forces in World War II*, 399.

122. For an overview of these centers, see Elkin, "Specialized Centers for the Management of Vascular Injuries and Diseases," 1–16; Michael E. DeBakey, "Report of Visit to Ashford General Hospital," 13 September 1944, NARA 112/390/17/13/6/241/5, p. 1; "Ashford General Hospital."

123. Ambrose H. Storck, "Designation, Organization, Development, and Function of the Vascular Center at De Witt General Hospital, Auburn, California," NARA 112/390/17/13/6/241/5, p. 1.

124. Harris B. Shumacker Jr., "History of the Vascular Center at Mayo General Hospital," NARA 112/390/17/13/6/241/5.

125. Storck, "Evaluation of the Vascular Status in Traumatic and Nontraumatic Lesions of the Blood Vessels," 17–59; Not every vascular unit had the full array of equipment available, and some had to rely on the personal stores of medical officers or borrowed from nearby universities. Nonetheless, their vascular testing capabilities far exceeded any other military medical facility and almost all civilian centers as well.

126. Shumacker, *The Society for Vascular Surgery*, 20; "Department of Surgery, Emory University School of Medicine, Atlanta, Georgia," *Archives of Surgery* 139 (2004): 359–61.

127. "Harris Shumacker," in Dale, with Johnson and DeWeese, *Band of Brothers*, 412–18. See also Harris B. Shumacker Jr., interview with the Society for Vascular Surgery, YouTube video, posted by SVS Vascular, December 1, 2014, https://www.youtube.com/watch?v=c31e1OSCFLs&feature=youtu.be&list=PLdMQA5pt2x0JuwVQ-c-DO7LUPus4QB0yZ (accessed 19 May 2019).

128. Shumacker, *The Society for Vascular Surgery*, 13; Dale, with Johnson and DeWeese, *Band of Brothers*, 64–66.

129. Daniel C. Elkin to Michael E. DeBakey, 12 February 1944, NARA 112/390/17/13/7/241/8. See also Elkin, "Vascular Injuries of Warfare," 305.

130. Elkin and Shumacker, "Arterial Aneurysms and Arteriovenous Fistulas," 162, table 9.

131. Elkin and Shumacker, "Arterial Aneurysms and Arteriovenous Fistulas," 161, table 8; Bigger, "Treatment of Traumatic Aneurysms and Arteriovenous Fistula," 170–79.

132. Freeman and Shumacker, "Arterial Aneurysms and Arteriovenous Fistulas," 287–88; Bigger, "Treatment of Traumatic Aneurysms and Arteriovenous Fistula," 178.

133. Freeman and Shumacker, "Arterial Aneurysms and Arteriovenous Fistulas," quote and data p. 267.

134. All cases are described in detail: Freeman and Shumacker, "Arterial Aneurysms and Arteriovenous Fistulas," 273–86.

135. Storck, "Evaluation of Vascular Status in Traumatic and Nontraumatic Lesions of the Blood Vessels," 50–54.

136. Shumacker, Abramson, and Lambert, "Arterial Aneurysms and Arteriovenous Fistulas," 310–17.

137. Storck, "Designation, Organization, Development, and Function of the Vascular Center at De Witt General Hospital," 10.

138. J. W. Kahn, "Survey of Sympathectomies," NARA 112/390/17/13/6/241/3; Shumacker, "Arterial Aneurysms and Arteriovenous Fistulas," 318–60; Daniel C. Elkin, "Memorandum to Brigadier General Fred W. Rankin," 7 February 1945, NARA 112/390/17/13/6/241/5.

139. Elkin, "Vascular Injuries of Warfare," 306; Shumacker, *Society for Vascular Surgery*, 29.

140. Nicholson, "The Effects of Local Context on the Development of Obstetric Ultrasound Scanning in Two Scottish Hospitals," 21–36.

141. Freeman and Shumacker, "Arterial Aneurysms and Arteriovenous Fistulas," for the lack of postoperative complications, see 287–88, 297–98, 300; for clinical improvement, see 287 and 299–300.

142. Odom, "Causes of Amputations in Battle Casualties with Emphasis on Vascular Injuries," quote p. 568; Province, *I Was Patton's Doctor*, 117–21.

143. DeBakey and Simeone, "Battle Injuries of Arteries in World War II," see chart 6, p. 541; De Takáts, "Vascular Surgery in War," 292.

144. Beebe and DeBakey, *Battle Casualties*, 99–101; DeBakey and Simeone, "Battle Injuries of Arteries in World War II," 542; "Forward Surgery of the Severely Wounded," 593 and table 9. "Essential Technical Medical Data," 13 July 1945, NARA 112/390/17/13/6/242/4, p. 14.

145. Snyder, "Vascular Wounds," 78. In comparison, the entire Mayo Hospital, with two thousand physicians on staff, performed only 5,800 operations a month in 2012. "Mayo Clinic," http://health.usnews.com/best-hospitals/area/mn/mayo-clinic-661MAYO (accessed 1 September 2013).

146. Steward, "War Experiences with Nonsuture Technic of Anastomosis in Primary Arterial Injuries," 160–65; "War Journal 94th Evacuation Hospital, April–July 1944," Countway Archives, Edward Churchill Papers, Box 35, Folder 2. In comparison, at the 94th Evac an average laparotomy required 117 minutes; thoracotomy, 148 minutes; and standard thigh debridement, 69 minutes.

147. Wolff, *Forward Surgeon*, 157–59. Thanks to Richard Mullins for directing me to this source.

148. "Memo: Staffing of Medical Units Destined for Movement to ETO," NARA 112/390/16/33/7/3/5, p. 1; Graham, "What Kind of Medical Officers do the Armed Services Want?," 217–19; Beebe and DeBakey, *Battle Casualties*, chapter 6.

149. Ludmerer, *Time to Heal*, chapter 7. For a history of the military medical training of these officers, see Parks, *Medical Training in World War II*, chapter 2.

150. Ludmerer, *Let Me Heal*, chapters 5–6.

151. The number of surgical residents in approved ACS programs peaked above 1,800 in 1941 and dropped to a nadir of 1,000 in 1945. Dallas B. Phemister, "Report on Graduate Training in Surgery," 12 December 1943, ACS Archives, Graduate Training Committee, Annual Reports to the Board of Regents, RG5/SG2/S8/SS09/Box 1/Folder 2, p.1; and Malcolm T. MacEachern, "The Expanded Program of the American College of Surgeons for Graduate Training in Surgery," 9.

152. Charles R. Reynolds, "Department of Graduate Training in Surgery," 1945, ACS Archives, Graduate Training Committee Annual Reports to the Board of Regents, RG5/SG2/S8/SS09/Box 1/Folder 2, p. 1.

153. "The 1945 Graduate Training in Surgery," *Special Bulletin of the American College of Surgeons* (September 1945): 38.

154. Graham, "What Kind of Medical Officers Do the Armed Services Want?," 217–19, quote 218–19. See also Graham, "Have the Armed Services Crippled Medical Education?," 34, 39, 41–42. Hundreds of physicians wrote to Graham expressing support for this position. See Becker Archives, Graham Collection, FC003/Box 118/Folder 1559.

155. Shackelford, interview with the Office of the Surgeon General, 3.

156. Kuite, interview with the Office of the Surgeon General, 8.

157. Ben Eiseman, interview with Justin Barr, 3 August 2011, Navy Bureau of Medicine and Surgery Office of Medical History, p. 7. See also Chandler et al., "Ben Eiseman, MD (1917–2012)," 529–35.

158. Helling, *Desperate Surgery in the Pacific War*, 221.

159. DeBakey and Simeone, "Battle Injuries of Arteries in World War II."

160. DeBakey and Simeone, "Battle Injuries of Arteries in World War II," 551.

161. Simeone, "Wounds of the Arteries of the Extremities." See also page proofs of the final article that explicitly note its reliance on Simeone's report: NARA 112/390/16/11/6/482/2.

162. Those hospitals were 94th Evacuation Hospital, 8th Evacuation Hospital, 171st Evacuation Hospital, and statistics from the 7th Army.

163. The field of memory studies is vast; for classic historical examples, see Blight, *Race and Reunion*; and Fussel, *The Great War and Modern Memory*.

Chapter Four

1. "Andrew Callow," in Dale, with Johnson and DeWeese, *Band of Brothers*, 34.

2. See, for example, Callow and Welch, "Arterial Anastomosis in Experimental Arterial Injury," 77–85; Swan, "Arterial Grafts," 115–17; Schloss and Shumacker, "Studies in Vascular Repair: IV," 273–90; Johnson et al., "The Experimental and Clinical Use of Vein Grafts to Replace Defects of Large Arteries," 945–56. For new methods, see, for example, Blakemore, "Restorative Endoaneurysmorrhaphy by Vein Graft Inlay," 461–69; LeVeen, "Nonsuture Method for Vascular Anastomosis Utilizing the Murphy Button Principle," 504–10.

3. Hufnagel, "The Use of Rigid and Flexible Plastic Prostheses for Arterial Replacement," 165–74; Donovan, "The Uses of Plastic Tubes in the Reparative Surgery of Battle Injuries to Arteries with and without Intra-arterial Heparin Administration," 1024–43.

4. For advocates of vein grafts, see Johnson et al., "The Experimental and Clinical Use of Vein Grafts to Replace Defects of Large Arteries"; Shumacker et al., "Studies in Vascular Repair: V," 81–93; Cooke et al., "Homologous Arterial Grafts and Autogenous Vein Grafts Used to Bridge Large Arterial Defects in Man," 183–89. For advocates of arterial grafts, see Mille et al., "The Fate of Arterial Grafts in Small Arteries," 581–88; Swan, "Arterial Grafts"; Klotz, Permar, and Guthrie, "End Results of Arterial Transplants," 305–20.

5. Heringman, Rives, and Davis, "The Repair of Arteriovenous Fistulas," 663–68; Johnson et al., "The Experimental and Clinical Use of Vein Grafts to Replace Defects of Large Arteries."

6. List of operations, DeBakey Collection, NLM Archives, Box 44, Folder 3. He created an Eck fistula and repaired a brachial aneurysm; the list does not describe how the aneurysm was repaired.

7. C. E. Welch, *A Twentieth Century Surgeon*, 161.

8. Even in their study of fifty-three arteriovenous fistulae that recognized the dangers inherent to ligation and specifically sought opportunities to repair the pathology, Herngman's team ligated over 80 percent of their patients' vessels. Heringman, Rives, and Davis, "The Repair of Arteriovenous Fistulas."

9. Aortic coarctation is a congenital condition that involves a severe narrowing of the aorta just distal to its cardiac origin so that little blood can pass through the vessel. The repair operation involved extirpating that constriction and reuniting the two ends. Kvitting and Olin, "Clarence Crafoord," 342–46.

10. Tetralogy of Fallot is a complex congenital cardiac condition with multiple pathologies that condemns its sufferers to an early death without treatment. Blalock's initial operation was palliative, not curative, but it nonetheless sparked hope and

attention. While numerous articles in the surgical literature address it, the historical literature unfortunately ignores this seminal surgery except for Stefan Timmermans's social history exploring the role and importance of Blalock's African American laboratory assistant: "A Black Technician and Blue Babies," 197–228. Thanks to Todd Olszewski for this reference.

11. William Glenn, interview with William S. Stoney, 15 September 2000, Vanderbilt University Oral History Collection. In the adult cardiac world, Dwight Harken and others were simultaneously inventing surgical procedures to treat mitral valve stenosis. While not involving arterial anastomosis, the operations further demonstrate changes in and attention to cardiac surgery in these years. Wertenbaker, *To Mend the Heart*. Miller, *King of Hearts*.

12. Johnson et al., "The Experimental and Clinical Use of Vein Grafts to Replace Defects of Large Arteries"; Schmitz et al., "The Influence of Diameter Disproportion and of Length on the Incidence of Complications in Autogenous Venous Grafts in the Abdominal Aorta," 190–206.

13. Gross, Bill, and Pierce, "Methods for Preservation and Transplantation of Arterial Grafts," 689–701.

14. Carrel, "The Preservation of Tissues and Its Application in Surgery," 523–27, quote p. 523. For more on the development of tissue banks in America, see Swanson, *Banking on the Body*.

15. Carrel, "Heterotransplantation of Blood Vessels Preserved in Cold Storage," 226–28; Guthrie, "Transplantation of Formaldehyde-Fixed Blood Vessels," 473; Guthrie, "End Results of Arterial Restoration with Devitalized Tissue," 186–87.

16. Landecker, "Technologies of Living Substance."

17. Radin, *Life on Ice*.

18. Carrel, "Results of Transplantation of Blood Vessels, Organs, and Limbs," 1662–67. See also Carrel, "The Preservation of Tissues and Its Application in Surgery"; Carrel, "Latent Life of Arteries," 460–90. Guthrie was also involved in this work: Klotz et al., "End Results of Arterial Transplants."

19. Pierce et al., "Tissue-Culture Evaluation of Viability of Blood Vessels Stored by Refrigeration," 333–48; Gross et al., "Methods for Preservation and Transplantation of Arterial Grafts."

20. Gross et al., "Preliminary Observations on the Use of Human Arterial Grafts in the Treatment of Certain Cardiovascular Defects," 578–79; Gross et al., "Methods for Preservation and Transplantation of Arterial Grafts"; Miller, *King of Hearts*.

21. Keefer et al., "The Blood Vessel Bank," 888–93.

22. Deterling, Coleman, and Parshley, "Experimental Studies of the Frozen Homologous Aortic Graft," 419–40; Hufnagel and Eastcott, "The Preservation of Arterial Grafts by Freezing," 531–37; Deterling, Parshley, and Blunt, "A Critical Study of Present Criteria Governing Selection and Use of Blood Vessel Grafts," 213–32.

23. Interviews with leaders in vascular surgery reveal the nearly simultaneous founding of artery banks across the country in the early 1950s, with almost all based

on frozen specimens. See Dale, with Johnson and DeWeese, *Band of Brothers*, 36, 158–59, 173, 190, 209, 362, 466, for banks established in Boston (Allan Callow), New York (Ralph Deterling), Chicago (Géza de Takáts), Rochester, NY (James DeWeese), Birmingham (Sterling Edwards), Baltimore (Mark Ravitch), and Houston (Jesse Thompson). For Chicago, see also Frank Milloy, interview with Michael Bullington, 8 March 1995, Rush Medical Archives, Accession No. RG052000 095-029.

24. See Kenneth Mattox's comments in *Michael DeBakey*, film produced by the Society for Vascular Surgery, 2018, due to be published.

25. Pernick, *A Calculus of Suffering*. Bollet, *Civil War Medicine*, 76–81.

26. In contrast, the British chiefly used chloroform, which was far more dangerous and complicated. As such, physicians took control of the anesthesia profession much earlier in Britain. D. Shephard, *From Craft to Specialty*, 67–70.

27. Lundy, "Factors That Influenced the Development of Anesthesiology," 38–43, quote p. 41. Thanks to Doug Bacon for directing me toward this and other articles.

28. Ellis, Narr, and Bacon, "Developing a Specialty," 226–29.

29. D. Shephard, *From Craft to Specialty*, chapter 5.

30. For the history of professional organizations in anesthesia, see Betcher et al., "The Jubilee Year of Organized Anesthesia," 226–64.

31. Betcher et al., "The Jubilee Year of Organized Anesthesia," 243–45. In 1938, the anesthesiology board was affiliated with the board of surgery; in 1941, it became its own independent board.

32. Graves, *Front Line Surgeons*, 53; and "Forward Surgery of the Severely Wounded," 55–57, 169.

33. Martin et al., "The Mayo Clinic World War II Short Course and Its Effect on Anesthesiology," 209–13.

34. "Annual Report of the Surgery Consultants Division for Fiscal Year 1945," 20.

35. Grantley W. Taylor, "Report of the Surgical Section," in Paul K. Sauer, "Historical Records and Annual Report, 95th Evacuation Hospital," 1944, NARA 331/290/8/25/1/31/25, p. 2.

36. Romanelli and Bacon, "The Origins of Modern Anesthesia throughout the American Experience Spanning the World Wars," 1, 4–7; statistics on p. 5. Thanks to Matthew Edwards for pointing me to this and similar articles.

37. Waisel, "Norman's War," 995–1003, see table 1.

38. Waisel, "The Role of World War II and the European Theater of Operations in the Development of Anesthesiology as a Physician Specialty in the USA," 907–14.

39. Martin, "The Mayo Clinic World War II Short Course and Its Effect on Anesthesiology," 211–12.

40. Waisel, "The Role of World War II and the European Theater of Operations in the Development of Anesthesiology as a Physician Specialty in the USA," 908; Romanelli and Baker, "The Origins of Modern Anesthesia throughout the American

Experience Spanning the World Wars," 7; Beecher et al., "The Anesthetist as a Physician," 49–55; Betcher et al., "The Jubilee Year of Organized Anesthesia," left figure p. 246, 260.

41. Ravitch, *A Century of Surgery*; Nahrwold and Kernahan, *A Century of Surgeons and Surgery*. This emergence and formalization of surgical organizations occurred internationally. For Germany's Deutsche Gesellschaft für Chirurgie, see Trendelenburg, *Die ersten 25 Jahre der Deutschen Gesellschaft für Chirurgie*. For England, see Cope, *The Royal College of Surgeons of England*.

42. Weisz, *Divide and Conquer*.

43. For surgery, see Gavrus, "Men of Strong Opinion"; and Rosen, *The Specialization of Medicine, with Particular Reference to Ophthalmology*, chapter 4. For medicine, see Fye, *American Cardiology*, chapters 2 and 4. Again, this theme extended beyond the borders of the United States: Nancy M. Frieden explicitly links the development of a profession to the formation of an association in *Russian Physicians in an Era of Reform and Revolution*, 107. For more on professionalization, see Freidson, *Profession of Medicine*.

44. The history of the SVS is well documented. See Shumacker, *The Society for Vascular Surgery*; Lilly, "The First Ten Years of the Society for Vascular Surgery," 1–5; J. E. Thompson, "The Founding Fathers," 801–8. See the special issue, fiftieth anniversary edition of the *Journal of Vascular Surgery* 23 (June 1996) for a series of articles documenting the history of the organization. Yao, "Society for Vascular Surgery (SVS)," 776–79.

45. Shumacker, *The Society for Vascular Surgery*, 11.

46. Shumacker, *The Society for Vascular Surgery*, 11; Lilly, "The First Ten Years of the Society for Vascular Surgery"; Yao, "Society for Vascular Surgery (SVS)."

47. Interview with Harris B. Shumacker Jr., Society for Vascular Surgery Archives, available online: https://vascular.org/about-svs/history (accessed 17 July 2018).

48. Shumacker, *The Society for Vascular Surgery*, appendix K for a list of all early programs.

49. Barr, "The Education of American Surgeons and the Rise of Surgical Residencies," 274–302; R. Stevens, *American Medicine and the Public Interest*, chapter 14, especially pp. 278–79 and 297–300; Ludmerer, *Let Me Heal*, chapters 7–8.

50. Irvin Abell, "Medicine in the National Defense Program," October 1940, ACS Archives, Eleanor Grimm Scrapbook, XXIV-A; "Minutes of the Business Meetings of the Council on Medical Education and Hospitals," 29 November 1948, AMA Archives, pp. 11–12; Edward Churchill to J. Stewart Rodman, 4 January 1946, Countway Archives, Churchill Collection, Box 1, Folder 38; R. Stevens, *American Medicine and the Public Interest*, 78, 278–79. The board actively campaigned for this distinction, recognizing the value of federal imprimatur in establishing the relevancy of the boards: "Chairman's Annual Report," ABS Archives, ABS Minutes, 31 March 1942, pp. 3–4. ABS Minutes 13–14 December 1946, p. 1. Fellows of the college were upset that fellowship did not count as certification, a transition that poignantly emphasized the rising importance of the specialty boards. They

confronted the government in 1946 to no avail. "ACS, ABS, and Surgical Specialties, Summary from the Minutes of Board of Regents Meeting," 17 December 1946, ACS Archives, Board of Regents Statements on Education and Specialization, RG5/SG2/S8/SS11/Box 2/Folder 1; "Report of the Washington Conference on October 25, 1946," Becker Archives, Graham Collection, FC003/Box 130/Folder 50.

51. Section 8 of Public Law 293 of the Seventy-Ninth Congress gave specialists a 25 percent pay bonus and defined specialist based solely on their board status.

52. "Meeting of the Committee on Postwar Medical Service," 28 October 1944, in ACS Archives, Department of Graduate Training Collections, RG5/SG2/S8/SS10 Box: Correspondence and Reports, Folder 4, p. 1; "Report of the Committee on Postwar Medical Service," 23 June 1945, ACS Archives, Eleanor Grimm Scrapbook vol. XXIV-A, pp. 68–69; Bowman C. Crowell, "Program of the Graduate Training in Surgery," 1945, ACS Archives, Department of Graduate Training, Correspondence, and Reports, 1944–1946, RG5/SG2/S8/SS10/Box 1/Folder 3, pp. 1–6.

53. Senior residents in Churchill's program earned $500/year; the secretary earned $1,500. Churchill, "Graduate Training in Surgery at the Massachusetts General Hospital," 30–32. See also Ludmerer, Let Me Heal, chapter 5.

54. "Post War Planning: Graduate Education of Physician Veterans Under GI Bill," AMA Archives, CMEH Series 2.1 Graduate Medical Education, Box 27–14, Folder 1412, pp. 2–4; "Minutes of the Business Meetings of the Council on Medical Education and Hospitals," 2 December 1945, AMA Archives, p. 8; "The Program of Graduate Training in Surgery of the American College of Surgeons," Becker Archives, Blair Papers, FC025/Box 10/Folder 62, p. 5. For more on the effect of the GI Bill in post–World War II America, see Altschuler and Blumin, The GI Bill.

55. John, "Practicing Physicians," chapter 1, for salary increases in the 1960s; Ludmerer, Let Me Heal.

56. Stevens, A Time of Scandal; Adler, Burdens of War.

57. Administration for Veterans Affairs Annual Report Fiscal Year 1946, Washington, DC: Government Printing Office, 1946, https://www.va.gov/vetdata/docs/FY1946.pdf (accessed 11 August 2017).

58. John Paul North, "Annual Report of the Surgical Residency and Training Programs and the Surgical Services Veterans Administration Hospitals, Dallas and McKinney Texas, 1956–1957," ACS Archives, Board of Regents Statements on Education and Specialization, RG5/SG2/S8/SS11/Box 1/Folder 4, p. 3; Bricker, Gerbode, and Habif, "The Effect of Health Insurance Programs on Residency Training in Surgery," 333–40.

59. Adkins, Medical Care of Veterans, chapter 10; Magnuson, Ring the Night Bell, chapters 18, 19, 21; Paul B. Magnuson to Deans of Medical Schools, Becker Archives, Barnes Hospital Records, RG009/Box 19/Folder 14; Paul B. Magnuson and William T. Doran, "Plans of Future Medical Cooperation between Teaching Institutions and Veterans Hospitals in Proximity," Becker Archives, Barnes Hospital Records, RG 009/Box 19/Folder 14; George H. Miller, "Report on the Development of Graduate Training Programs through the Collaboration of Medical Schools

with Civilian Hospitals and Government Hospitals," 15 December 1946, ACS Archives, Graduate Training Committee Annual Reports to the Board of Regents, RG5/SG2/S8/SS09/Box 1/Folder 2, p. 1.

60. See, for example, the challenges of Ashburn's Veterans Hospital in McKinney, Texas, highlighted in "The Surgical Service and its Residency Training Program Second Annual Report: July 1, 1947 to June 30, 1948," Countway Archives, Churchill Collection, Box 17, Folder 49; Malcolm T. MacEachern, "Report on Graduate Training Activities During 1944," 17 September 1944, ACS Archives, Graduate Training Committee Annual Reports to the Board of Regents, RG5/SG2/S8/SS09/Box 1/Folder 2, p. 1; "Complete Minutes of the Meetings of the Committee on Graduate Training in Surgery," 6–7 February 1944, ACS Archives, Graduate Education Committee, RG5/SG2/S8/Box 2/Folder 4, p. 4.

61. Paul S. Ferguson and Charles R. Reynolds, "Progress Report on Graduate Training in Surgery," ACS Archives, Graduate Training Committee Annual Reports to Board of Regents, RG5/SG2/S8/SS09/Box 1/Folder 2, p. 5.

62. "Report of the Department of Graduate Training in Surgery to the Annual Meeting of Fellows of the ACS," 11 September 1947, ACS Archives, Graduate Education Committee, RG5/SG2/S8/Box 2/Folder 5, pp. 2–3; Charles Reynolds, "General Statement of Activities of the Department," 15 December 1946, ACS Archives, Graduate Training Committee, Annual Reports to Board of Regents, RG5/SG2/S8/SS09/Box 1/Folder 2, p. 6; Paul S. Ferguson, "Report of Hospital Surveys in Graduate Training in Surgery," 1946, ACS Archives, Graduate Training Committee Annual Reports to Board of Regents, RG5/SG2/S8/SS09/Box 1/Folder 2, p. 2.

63. "Minutes of the Business Meetings of the Council on Medical Education and Hospitals," 3–4 June 1949, AMA Archives, p. 12; Charles R. Reynolds, "Report of the Department of Graduate Training in Surgery, 1 January 1947–1 August 1947," 7 September 1947, ACS Archives, Graduate Training Committee Annual Reports to Board of Regents, RG5/SG2/S8/SS09/Box 1/Folder 2, pp. 3–4.

64. "Meeting of the Committee on Graduate Training in Surgery," 2 November 1941, ACS Archives, Graduate Education Committee, RG5/SG2/S8/Box 1/Folder 4, p. 2.

65. "Graduate Training Army General Hospitals and to a Limited Extent in AAF and ASF, 1945," ACS Archives, Department of Graduate Training, Correspondence and Reports, 1944–1946, RG5/SG2/S8/SS10/Box 1/Folder 3, p. 1.

66. MacEachern, "Report on Graduate Training Activities During 1944," 1–2; Charles R. Reynolds, "The Training Program," in "Complete Minutes of the Meeting of the Committee on Graduate Training in Surgery," 30 November 1945, ACS Archives, Graduate Education Committee Collection, RG5/SG2/S8/Box 2/Folder 5, p. 11; "Meeting at ACS, Abstract of Discussion of 13 February 1945," ACS Archives, Graduate Training Committee for Surgery, RG5/SG2/S8/SS14/Box 1/Folder 1, p. 2.

67. The ACS also approved twenty-nine orthopedic and two thoracic programs at naval hospitals for a combined 285 positions and two orthopedic programs at

Public Health Service hospitals. Ferguson and Reynolds, "Progress Report on Graduate Training in Surgery," 4–7.

68. COL Paul I. Robinson, MC, USA, "Presentation before the Council on Education and Hospitals," 7 February 1948, appendix H to "Minutes of the Business Meetings of the Council on Medical Education and Hospitals," 6–7 February 1948, AMA Archives, p. 46. The exact number of physicians electing to remain is barely legible on the document but appears to read 822.

69. Cowdrey, *The Medics' War*, chapter 1. The army, for example, had to shrink from providing a ratio of 6 physicians per 1,000 soldiers during World War II to 3.8:1,000 in 1949. See p. 32. For the shortage in the navy, see *The History of the Medical Department of the United States Navy*, chapters 2–5.

70. Robinson, "Presentation before the Council on Education and Hospitals." See especially his six-point plan (47–49) detailing the various measures the Army was taking to recruit doctors. See also Cowdrey, *Medics' War*, 15–16; "Appendix E: Conference with Representatives of the Government Agencies, Minutes of the Business Meetings of the Council on Medical Education and Hospitals," 7–10 June 1951, AMA Archives, p. 5. For naval efforts, see *History of the Medical Department of the United States Navy*, chapter 5.

71. "Graduate Training Army General Hospitals and to a Limited Extent in AAF and ASF," 1; "Minutes of the Board of Regents," 1 April 1946, ACS Archives, Graduate Training Committee Annual Reports to the Board of Regents, RG5/SG2/S8/SS09/Box 1/Folder 2, p. 76.

72. "Meeting at ACS, Abstract of Discussion of 13 February 1945," ACS Archives, "Graduate Training Committee for Surgery, RG5/SG2/S8/SS14/Box 1/Folder 1, pp. 1–4.

73. "Meeting at ACS, Abstract of Discussion of 13 February 1945," p. 2; "Complete Minutes of the Meeting on Graduate Training in Surgery," 30 November 1945, ACS Archives, Graduate Education Committee, RG5/SG2/S8/Box 2/Folder 5, p. 17; Charles R. Reynolds, "General Statement of Activities of the Department," 15 December 1946; ACS Archives, Graduate Training Committee, Annual Reports to Board of Regents, RG5/SG2/S8/SS09/Box 1/Folder 2, p. 3; Paul S. Ferguson, "Report to the Board of Regents on the Graduate Training in Surgery," 1 October 1948, ACS Archives, Graduate Training Committee, Annual Reports to the Board of Regents, RG5/SG2/S8/SS09/Box 1/Folder 1, p. 3.

74. See documents in Department of Graduate Training: Correspondence and Reports, ACS Archives, RG5/SG2/S8/SS10; Floyd E. Wergeland, "Progress Report," 19 June 1950, Appendix F, "Minutes of the Business Meetings of the Council on Medical Education and Hospitals," 23–24 June 1950, AMA Archives, p. 5. In 1946, there were 70 regular army board-certified physicians; this had increased to 187 by 1950.

75. The navy dropped from 430 positions to 300; the army eliminated 167 slots. Wergeland, "Progress Report," 2; "Minutes of the Business Meetings of the Council on Medical Education and Hospitals," 23–24 June 1950, AMA Archives, p. 25;

"Minutes of the Business Meetings of the Council on Medical Education and Hospitals," 8–9 February 1949, AMA Archives, p. 6.

76. R. Stevens, *In Sickness and in Wealth*, 216–30. It funded 4,678 projects.

77. Ludmerer, *Let Me Heal*.

78. George H. Miller, "Report on Surveys of Hospitals and Visits to Medical Schools for Consultations on Graduate Training to the Board of Regents," 1 April 1946, ACS Archives, Board of Regents, Board of Governors, Fellows, and Committees Collection, RG4/SG04/S02/Box 28/Folder 1, p. 2228.

79. "Fundamental Requirements for Graduate Training in Surgery," *Special Bulletin of the American College of Surgeons* (September 1945): 26–36.

80. "Abstract of the Minutes, Board of Regents Meeting," 5 May 1944, ACS Archives, Department of Graduate Training, Correspondence and Reports, 1944–1946, RG5/SG2/S8/SS10/Box 1/Folder 1, p. 2. For a similar, public declaration, see *Special Bulletin of the American College of Surgeons* 30 (1945): 5.

81. "Program of Graduate Training in Surgery," 6; "Complete Minutes of the Meeting on the Committee on Graduate Training in Surgery, 30 November 1945," Becker Archives, Blair Papers, FC025/Box 10/Folder 62, exhibit C. Exhibit F is a nine-page, single-spaced list of programs to evaluate.

82. "Joint Meeting of Committee of American College of Surgeons with Executive Committee of Board of Trustees of the American Medical Association for Discussion of Problems of Mutual Interest," 21 February 1948, ACS Archives, Conference Committee on Graduate Training in Surgery, RG5/SG2/S8/SS03/Box 1/Folder 6, p. 7.

83. "Hospitals Surveyed for Graduate Training in Surgery and Not Approved, January 1 1945 to December 31 1947," ACS Archives, Conference Committee on Graduate Training in Surgery, RG5/SG2/S8/SS03/Box 1/Folder 4.

84. "Minutes of the Business Meetings of the Council on Medical Education and Hospitals, Appendix A: Memo to the Board of Trustees of the American Medical Association, 8 July 1945," 18–20 June 1948, AMA Archives, pp. 1–3; "Minutes of the Business Meetings of the Council on Medical Education and Hospitals," 4–5 October 1947, AMA Archives, p. 13.

85. Firor, "Residency Training in Surgery," 154; "Graduate Training Committee Meeting," 17 October 1948, ACS Archives, Graduate Education Committee, RG5/SG2/S8/Box 2/Folder 5, p. 4; Guy A. Caldwell, "Suggestions for the Improvement of Resident Training in the Surgical Specialties and for Better Cooperation of Agencies Concerned in Approval of Training, 18 February 1948, in Joint Meeting of Committee of American College of Surgeons with Executive Committee of Board of Trustees of the American Medical Association for Discussion of Problems of Mutual Interest," 21 February 1948, ACS Archives, Conference Committee on Graduate Training in Surgery, RG5/SG2/S8/SS03/Box 1/Folder 6, pp. 15–17.

86. Quoted in Caldwell, "Suggestions for the Improvement of Resident Training," 21.

87. Barr and Pappas, "The Role of the American Board of Surgery on the Development of Surgical Residencies in Post–World War II America."

88. Barr, "The Education of American Surgeons and the Rise of Surgical Residencies," 296–302.

89. *Surgery in the United States.*

90. Minutes of the Seventy-Fourth Meeting of the American Surgical Association, April 1954, NLM Archives, American Surgical Association Collection, Box 1, Folder 1; Barr, "The Education of American Surgeons and the Rise of Surgical Residencies."

91. Minutes of the Seventy-Eighth Meeting of the American Surgical Association, April 1958. NLM Archives, American Surgical Association Collection, box 5, folder 9, p. 16; Green v. City of St. Petersburg, 154 Fla 339, 17 So 2d 517, 518.

92. Study relied on BCBS data from Michigan and Massachusetts and was collated by Frederick Coller. Coller presented data that showed these cases represented about 50 percent of the total operations in each state. Massachusetts consistently had a higher percentage of cases performed by residency-trained surgeons than did Michigan (which was higher than Oklahoma). Minutes of the Seventy-Seventh Meeting of the American Surgical Association, May 1957, NLM Archives, American Surgical Association Collection, Box 1, Folder 8, pp. 11–14.

Chapter Five

1. Millett, *The War for Korea, 1945–1950.*

2. Appleman, *South to the Naktong, North to the Yalu*; Millett, *The War for Korea, 1950–1951*; Halberstam, *The Coldest Winter*; Fehrenbach, *This Kind of War.* For a broader view of how the Korean War fit into geostrategic Cold War considerations, see Stueck, *Rethinking the Korean War.*

3. Hoyt, *The Pusan Perimeter.* See also Appleman, *South to the Naktong, North to the Yalu*; Millett, *War for Korea, 1950–1951*; and Fehrenbach, *This Kind of War.*

4. Futrell, *The United States Air Force in Korea.*

5. Mossman, *Ebb and Flow.* Fehrenbach and Millett also cover these months well; Halberstam focuses more on political-strategic issues (including the failure/denial at McArthur's headquarters) than events on the ground in Korea.

6. Hermes, *Truce Tent and Fighting Front.*

7. Fehrenbach, *This Kind of War.*

8. The shortage of military medical personnel is well covered for the army in Cowdrey, *The Medics' War*, chapters 1 and 2; and for the navy in *The History of the Medical Department of the United States Navy*, chapters 2, 4, 5, and especially 8.

9. Department of the Army, *History of the Korean Conflict (25 June 1950–8 September 1951)*, MHI Archives, see pp. 1–3 under heading "Personnel Division."

10. Tribble, *Doctor Draft Justified?*

11. For army casualty data in Korea, see Reister, *Battle Casualties and Medical Statistics*; the army suffered 78,000 wounded (total hospital admissions were 443,000, with disease and non-battle injury making up the remainder). The navy suffered 1,500 wounded and the marines 24,000. See "Casualties: U.S. Navy and Marine Corps Personnel Killed and Wounded in Wars, Conflicts, Terrorist Acts, and Other Hostile Incidents," https://www.history.navy.mil/research/library/online-reading-room/title-list-alphabetically/c/casualties1.html (accessed 18 April 2019).

12. Engle, *Medic*. From the point of view of a casualty, see W. L. White, *Back Down the Ridge*.

13. Jensen, *Bloody Snow*; Phelps, *Battalion Surgeon*, self-published, MHI Archives, DS921.25.P54 A3 2000. Buerger, "Medical Support for Mountain Fighting in Korea," 694–700.

14. Ginn and Ziperman, "Surgery in Division Clearing Stations," 443–47; "SOP for Surgery in Eighth Army Hospitals and Division Clearing Companies," 18 November 1952, NARA 112/631/19/6/6, see procedure 3.b; "Transmittal of Draft Monograph *The Surgical Hospital in Korea*," NARA 112/390/16/9/3/241, p. 6.

15. The navy instituted medical units at the division level (often within five miles of the front line) that performed forward surgery. Twenty-one percent of army soldiers hit by enemy fire died; only 14 percent of marines so struck did. Howard E. Snyder et al., "Report to the Surgeon General of the Ad Hoc Committee on the Emergency Care of Casualties," 9 April 1955, NARA 112/390/17/34/05/342/3, p. 4 in the appendix; Hermes Grillo, interview with Jan K. Herman, 1 July 1999, BUMED Library and Archives; Howard Sirak, interview with Jan K. Herman, 17 January 2001, BUMED Library and Archives; Herman, *Frozen in Memory*, 151; see interviews with Henry Litvin and Donald Kent for information on the battalion aid stations and interview with Chester Lessenden Jr., for information on the regimental aid stations.

16. Marble, "Forward Surgery and Combat Hospitals," 68–100; Marble, "The Evolution and Demise of the MASH," 22–39. For histories of the television show, see Diffrient, *M*A*S*H*; Wittebols, *Watching "M*A*S*H," Watching America*. For a comparison of the real MASH with the TV show, see Cowdrey, "MASH vs. *M*A*S*H*," 4–11. The MASH units were also well known at the time in lay society, covered in newspaper articles and Hollywood movies: e.g., *Battle Circus*, directed by Richard Brooks.

17. "Eighth United States Army Annual Report, 1951: Army Medical Services Activities," NARA 112/390/17/34/5/196/2, p. 25. Cowdrey, *Medics' War*, 172–73.

18. For the best single history of the MASH in Korea, see *The Surgical Hospital in Korea*, prepared by the Military History Department, 8086th AU, NARA 112/390/16/9/3/241. A. W. Schulz, "Historical Narrative Report, 31 January 1949–31 December 1949," 1st Mobile Army Surgical Hospital, NARA 407/270/68/20/04/4717/3; "Narrative Report, 1 January 1949—31 December 1949," 5th Mobile Army Surgical Hospital, NARA 407/270/68/20/04/4717/4; Woodard, "The Story of the Mobile Army Surgical Hospital," 506–13. Cowdrey,

Medics' War also addresses it frequently. For an excellent account of a surgeon who served in a MASH in Korea, see Apel and Apel, *MASH*.

19. Berman, "The X-Ray Service in an Army Area Surgical Hospital," 135–44. The 1951 annual report of the 8164th MASH reviewed all films taken—a total of 7,526 for 2,435 inpatients and 4,487 outpatients; while it performed eighty-five intravenous pyelograms, it does not record any arteriograms (nor do any other similar reports). "Annual Report of 1951 for the Department Radiology, 8164 Army Unit," NARA 338/290/73/6/1/4797/1.

20. There was no army policy on anesthesia methodology—practitioners used the drugs with which they were most comfortable, reflecting the autonomy of medical practitioners. At times, MASHs did lack sufficient anesthesiology support; there were just not enough fully trained anesthesiologists in the army. This shortage probably explains the move to nurse anesthetists in July 1950 and the reversal to two MD anesthesiologists in January 1951. While the switch to more modern drugs like nitrous oxide had obvious benefits to the patient, it also required more technical support than older methods did, resulting in a variety of different models of anesthesia machines deploying to Korea. "Combat Operations Command Report 46th Surgical Hospital: May 1953," NARA 319/270/69/17/7/6211/20, p. 1; "Combat Operations Command Report for May 1953, 47th Surgical Hospital," NARA 319/270/69/17/7/6211/20, p. 2; *The Surgical Hospital in Korea*, 11–15; Dripps, "Anesthesia for Combat Casualties on the Basis of Experience in Korea," 241–55.

21. Neither evacuation nor field hospitals had significant roles in Korea. The increase in bed numbers did not include a proportional increase in physicians and nurses: the army added only four more of each. See Westover, *Combat Support in Korea*, 116.

22. *The Surgical Hospital in Korea*, 40; Apel, *MASH*, 80; Woodward, "The Story of the Mobile Army Surgical Hospital," 510.

23. Edgcomb et al., "Primaquine, SN 13272, a New Curative Agent in vivax Malaria," 285–92; Alving, Arnold, and Robinson, "Status of Primaquine," 1558–62; Alving et al., "Korean vivax Malaria," 970–76; Smadel, "Epidemic Hemorrhagic Fever," 1327–30. See Ricketts, "Report of the Clinical and Physiological Research at Hemorrhagic Fever Center, Korea, Fall of 1953," 29–31; Katz, "Hemorrhagic Fever of the Far Eastern Type," 109–17.

24. Peitzman, *Dropsy, Dialysis, Transplant*, 87–88; Peitzman, "Science, Inventors, and the Introduction of the Artificial Kidney in the United States," 276–81; Meroney, introduction to *Post-traumatic Renal Insufficiency*, 2.

25. Meroney and Herndon, "The Management of Acute Renal Insufficiency," 52; Balch, Meroney, and Sako, "Observations on the Surgical Care of Patients with Post-traumatic Renal Insufficiency," 94.

26. Kendrick, *Blood Program in World War II*, chapter 20; Steer, Hullinghorst, and Mason, "The Blood Program in the Korean War," 150–65; Kendrick, "Operation of Blood Bank Systems," 148; Link, "Development of the Armed Services Blood, Blood Derivatives, and Plasma Expanders Program," 1221–25.

27. Artz, "Massive Transfusions, Blood Derivatives, and Plasma Expanders," 202–9; Artz, Sako, and Brownwell, "Massive Transfusion in the Severely Wounded," 66–71.

28. Paul W. Sanger, "Report to Surgeon General, U.S. Army, on Tour of Medical Installations of the Far East Command," 20 May 1953, Countway Library, Beecher Collection, Box 51, Folder 27, p. 2.

29. Podolsky, *The Antibiotic Era.*

30. Herman, *Frozen in Memory*, 159. This widespread empirical dosing of antibiotics did lead to resistant organisms: whereas 94 percent of *Clostridia* strains were sensitive to penicillin in 1952, only 84 percent were in 1953. See Lindberg, "The Bacterial Flora of Wounds in the Korean War," 319.

31. Howard and Inui, "Clostridial Myositis—Gas Gangrene," 196.

32. Altemeir and Pulaski, "The Occurrence of Wound Infection in Korean War Battle Casualties during May–June 1953," 334–63.

33. "The Value of a Field Research Project," NARA 319/270/69/17/07/6211/20, p. 3.

34. Howard, "Introduction—Historical Background and Development"; Howard, "The Value of a Field Research Project," NARA 319/270/69/17/07/6211/20, p. 1.

35. Several postwar conferences, resulting in published collections of papers, also ensued. See *Recent Advances in Medicine and Surgery*; C. W. Hughes, *The Systemic Response to Injury*; Crosby, *Tools for Resuscitation*; Artz, *The Battle Wound*; Meroney, *Post-traumatic Renal Insufficiency.* For the challenges of medical research in combat, see Barr, "A Short History of Dapsone," 425–67.

36. Postwar reports frequently cited improvements in vascular care as justification for intra-war military medical research efforts. See Howard and Mason, "The Value of a Field Research Project," 1–2, 16–17; Howard, "Introduction—Historical Background and Development," 4, 9.

37. Seeley, "Vascular Surgery at Walter Reed Army Hospital," 8–9. For a history of Walter Reed Hospital, see Standlee, *Borden's Dream.*

38. Howard, "Dedication," 1009; Elmer K. Miller, "A Chronological History of the 100th General Hospital from June 25 1943 to November 8 1945," US Army Medical Department Center of History and Heritage Historical Research Collection, Fort Sam Houston, TX.

39. Seeley et al., "Traumatic Arteriovenous Fistulas and Aneurysms in War Wounds," 471–79; C. W. Hughes, "Vascular Surgery in the Armed Forces," 30–46.

40. "Walter Reed Army Hospital Annual Report, 1952," NARA 112/390/17/34/05/131/6, p. 169. The first 101 patients suffered from seventy-three arteriovenous fistulae and thirty-three false aneurysms (some patients had both).

41. For Elkin's conservatism, see Elkin, "Vascular Injuries of Warfare," 284–306.

42. Seeley et al., "Traumatic Arteriovenous Fistulas and Aneurysms in War Wounds," 471–72.

43. Seeley et al., "Traumatic Arteriovenous Fistulas and Aneurysms in War Wounds," 478. For a similar transition, see also Seeley, Hughes, and Jahnke, "Surgery of the Popliteal Artery," 712–17.

44. Seeley et al., "Surgery of the Popliteal Artery," 714–16. They used two guy sutures instead of three, preferred anastomosis when such an operation would not place undue tension on joining, reverted to venous grafts when the defect was too large for primary anastomosis, and declined to use any anticoagulation. They did not report any failures related to operative technique.

45. Initially, the team did not repair veins, but increasing evidence of venous insufficiency led to the initiation of reparative venous operations. Seeley et al., "Surgery of the Popliteal Artery," 715; C. W. Hughes, "Vascular Surgery in the Armed Forces," 37.

46. Seeley et al., "Traumatic Arteriovenous Fistulas and Aneurysms in War Wounds," 479. For raw numbers, there were twenty-nine ligations and thirty-five arterial repairs (twenty-three suture repairs, seven vein grafts, and five arterial grafts). While the absolute numbers are relatively small, the true statistical significance matters less than how the participants interpreted the significance of the data, which they believed clearly favored arterial repair. Similar statistics, with a smaller subset of data, appear in Seeley et al., "Surgery of the Popliteal Artery," 716.

47. Seeley et al., "Traumatic Arteriovenous Fistulas and Aneurysms in War Wounds," 479. At the time, this policy affected cases only at Walter Reed under their care—it was not yet army-wide.

48. For the 1950 numbers, see Seeley et al., "Traumatic Arteriovenous Fistulas and Aneurysms in War Wounds," 479. For the 1951 numbers, see "Walter Reed Army Hospital Annual Report, 1951," NARA 112/390/17/34/05/131/4, p. 157. The 87 percent refers only to "successful" operations, a category the report does not define.

49. Dickinson, Ashley, and Gerbode, "The Definitive Treatment of Injuries to Major Blood Vessels Incurred in the Korean War," 625–34.

50. "Walter Reed Army Hospital Annual Report, 1952," 169. See also Dickinson, Ashley, and Gerbode, "The Definitive Treatment of Injuries to Major Blood Vessels Incurred in the Korean War," 625.

51. C. W. Hughes, "Vascular Surgery in the Armed Forces," 38; "Walter Reed Army Hospital Annual Report, 1951," 159; "Walter Reed Army Hospital Annual Report, 1952," 167–69.

52. Armistice talks began 10 July 1951; Communist forces broke off talks on 23 August, and fighting recommenced.

53. Information from this section comes mostly from two oral histories, Grillo, interview with Herman; Herman, *Frozen in Memory*, 164–72; and Hermes C. Grillo, interview with G. Kurt Piehler and Crystal Dover as part of the University of Tennessee's Veteran's Oral History Project, 8 July 2002, http://csws.utk.edu/oral-history-project/read-an-interview/korea/ (accessed 18 April 2019). Additional

biographical information may be found in Austen et al., "Hermes C. Grillo." See also Negri, "Hermes C. Grillo, 83, Thoracic Surgeon at MGH."

54. Grillo, interview with Herman, 14.

55. Grillo, interview with Herman, 11. Grillo related the same story in his interview with Piehler and Dover. Grillo apparently worked with vascular expert Fiorindo Simeone at Harvard as well. See DeBakey and Amspacher, "Acute Arterial Injuries," n49, which lists the two as collaborators on an unpublished study examining the effects of vein occlusion on muscles.

56. See Apel, *MASH*, and especially chapter 7, for information in the following paragraphs.

57. Apel, *MASH*, 169–77.

58. Apel, *MASH*, 157.

59. Apel, *MASH*, xi–xiii.

60. For information on his early life in Texas, see Kolsti, "Beat of a Different Drummer."

61. Frank C. Spencer, interview with C. Rollins Hanlon, 4 May 2004, ACS Archives, p. 13.

62. For the best description of Spencer's activities in Korea, see Frank C. Spencer, interview with Justin Barr, 1 December 2011, Navy Bureau of Medicine and Surgery Office of Medical History; and Spencer, "Historical Vignette," 906–9.

63. "Daily Intelligence and Operations Report, 1–2 August 1952," 1st Medical Battalion, 1st Marine Division, NARA 127/470/902/9/7/219/4, p. 1. A note dated a week before Spencer's arrival in Korea states that a Dr. Marecki had attended a postgraduate course in vascular surgery in Korea. See "Daily Intelligence and Operations Report, 22–23 July 1952," 1st Medical Battalion, 1st Marine Division, NARA 127/470/902/9/7/219/4, p. 1. Other daily intelligence and operations reports from around the time discuss navy physicians participating in a variety of army-sponsored postgraduate courses, including those on orthopedic and abdominal surgery.

64. Spencer, interview with Barr, 4–5.

65. In addition to informal, ad hoc teaching, records indicate that Spencer also delivered formal seminars on arterial repair to fellow naval medical officers. See "Historical Diary for April 1953, 1st Medical Battalion, 1st Marine Division," NARA 127/170/61/18/7/38/45, p. 6.

66. Spencer, interview with Barr, 15.

67. Grewe later became a neurosurgeon in Portland, Oregon.

68. Spencer and Grewe, "The Management of Arterial Injuries in Battle Casualties," 304–13.

69. The authors conceded that ligation might have prevented the deaths of two of the patients who underwent repair. Spencer and Grewe, "The Management of Arterial Injuries in Battle Casualties," 310–11.

70. Given the severity of the marines' other injuries, Spencer and Grewe, like the other Korean War surgeons, elected not to heparinize the patient systemically. Spencer and Grewe, "Management of Arterial Injuries in Battle Casualties," 305–6.

71. S. G. Friedman, "Korea, M*A*S*H, and the Accidental Pioneers of Vascular Surgery," 666–70.

72. "Eighth United States Army Annual Report, 1951," 29.

73. Frank E. Hagman, "Surgery in the Orient," *Surgeon's Circular Letter* 7, no. 1 (1 January 1952), in NARA 112/390/17/34/05/27/2.

74. Calvin H. Goddard, "Summary of Medical Service Activities, 25 June 1950–8 September 1951," NARA 112/390/17/34/05/34/2. See also *Surgeon's Circular Letter* 6, no. 1 (1 January 1951), NARA 112/390/17/34/05/27/2, p. 1.

75. Upon arriving in Korea, members of the team did visit Apel and observe his work; the significance of this encounter is unclear. Apel, *MASH*, 163.

76. Beger, "John M. Howard, MD,"140. Howard, "Historical Vignettes of Arterial Repair," 716–18; Fernández-Zapico, "'Keep at It!' Accept the Challenge of Your Critics," 551–53.

77. Correspondence demonstrates that Howard and DeBakey remained in touch about vascular surgery during the former's tour in Korea. See "Annual Report of the Department of Surgery, Baylor University College of Medicine, 1949–1950," Countway Archives, Edward D. Churchill Papers, Box 3, Folder 19, p. 31; Michael E. DeBakey to Edward C. Churchill, 23 December 1952, Countway Archives, Edward D. Churchill Collection, Box 3, Folder 17.

78. Howard, "Historical Vignettes of Arterial Repair." It is challenging to verify the precise accuracy of that statement, but certainly very few board-certified surgeons deployed to Korea. In March 1951, only six board-certified surgeons had deployed to the Far East Command, which included hospitals in Japan. See John D. Stewart, "Report to the Surgeon General U.S. Army on Tour of Medical Installation of Far East Command, March 1951," Countway Archives, Edward D. Churchill Collection, Box 51, Folder 20, p. 2.

79. Norman Rich, "Carl W. Hughes: In Memoriam," personal communication, 2008.

80. Howard engaged in some preliminary studies at the 46th MASH starting in December 1951, but the bulk of the research took place at the 43rd the following spring and summer. "Combat Operations Report—46th Surgical Hospital," 2.

81. Howard, "Introduction—Historical Background and Development," 9; Notes of interview with Edward J. Jahnke by Sam Milner, 1 September 1966, US Army Medical Department Center of History and Heritage Historical Research Collection, Fort Sam Houston, TX.

82. Journal articles in chronological order: Jahnke and Howard, "Primary Repair of Major Arterial Injuries," 646–49; Jahnke, "The Surgery of Acute Vascular Injuries," 249–51; Jahnke and Seeley, "Acute Vascular Injuries in the Korean War"; C. W. Hughes, "Acute Vascular Trauma in Korean War Casualties," 91–100; Jahnke, Hughes, and Howard, "The Rationale of Arterial Repair on the Battlefield," 396–401; C. W. Hughes, "The Primary Repair of Wounds of Major Arteries," 297–303; Hughes and Bowers, "Blood Vessel Surgery," 174–78; Inui, Shannon, and Howard, "Arterial Injuries in the Korean Conflict," 850–57; C. W. Hughes, "Arterial

Repair in the Korean War"; C. W. Hughes, "Vascular Surgery in the Armed Forces." For national meetings, see, for example, program, 1951 Clinical Congress, ACS Archives, Clinical Congresses of Surgeons of North America, RG0/SG2/S1/Box 3.

83. Ziperman, "Acute Arterial Injuries in the Korean War," 1–8.

84. C. W. Hughes, "Acute Vascular Trauma in Korean War Casualties," 91; Jahnke and Seeley, "Acute Vascular Injuries in the Korean War," 163; C. W. Hughes, "The Primary Repair of Wounds of Major Arteries," 298. The percentage for vascular wounds is higher than for wounds in general, where fragmentary explosions caused only 65.5 percent of nonfatal wounds, 61.9 percent of died of wounds, and 63.4 percent of killed in action. Reister, *Battle Casualties and Medical Statistics*, table 40, p. 36.

85. In the first fifty-eight cases, there were two exceptions for patients whom the team deemed too unstable to tolerate a lengthy repair operation. The ensuing primary ligations resulted in an above-the-knee amputation and symptoms of arterial insufficiency in an arm. Jahnke and Howard, "Primary Repair of Major Arterial Injuries," 646.

86. Spencer and Hughes both reported repairing venous injuries after several of their arterial repairs failed because of venous thrombosis secondary to trauma. Spencer and Grewe, "The Management of Arterial Injuries in Battle Casualties," 312; C. W. Hughes, "Acute Vascular Trauma in Korean War Casualties," 98. Spencer repaired seven and Hughes thirteen, relatively small numbers given the incidence of venous trauma. Routine repair of venous injuries awaited the Vietnam War. Rich and Rhee, "An Historical Tour of Vascular Injury Management," 1199–1215; Rich, Baugh, and Hughes, "Acute Arterial Injuries in Vietnam," 359–69.

87. Jahnke and Seeley, "Acute Vascular Injuries in the Korean War," 162–67.

88. A study between the wars demonstrated the everted mattress technique had slightly fewer complications associated with it, but the difference was marginal and the technique more challenging to master. No difference between interrupted versus continuous suturing appeared. See Shumacker and Lowenberg, "Experimental Studies in Vascular Repair: I," 79–89.

89. One minor difference involved the tendency of Korean War–era surgeons to strip the adventitia off the segment of artery they sutured, a technique they claimed facilitated the suturing. It also provided a de facto periarterial sympathectomy and theoretically reduced the risk of arteriospasm over the anastomosis site, although no study specifically examined this possibility and what effect it might have had.

90. Jahnke and Howard, "Primary Repair of Major Arterial Injuries," 647, emphasis added.

91. Jahnke and Seeley, "Acute Vascular Injuries in the Korean War," 171.

92. Michael E. DeBakey to the National Research Council, 2 September 1950, reproduced in Churchill, *Surgeon to Soldiers*, 280–81. The army had established an artery bank at Walter Reed in 1949 with which at least Jahnke should have been familiar, given that he completed his residency there. However, the technology just

never achieved the same popularity in the army as in the navy. Cooke et al., "Blood Vessel Bank," 1779–85.

93. See the next chapter for a discussion on US naval involvement in artery bank creation. For more on naval artery grafts in the Korean War, see Grant, "Front Line Surgery in Korea," 268. N. E. Adamson Jr., "Treatment of Arterial Injuries," 19 November 1953, NARA 52/470/56/6/7/291/5.

94. Spencer and Grewe, "The Management of Arterial Injuries in Battle Casualties," 306.

95. Jahnke and Howard, "Primary Repair of Major Arterial Injuries," 647.

96. Spencer and Grewe, "The Management of Arterial Injuries in Battle Casualties," 306; Thomas, "Continuous Lumbar Sympathetic Block by the Catheter Technique," 47–48.

97. For evidence of its inefficacy, see "Organization of Medical Service, 11th Evacuation Hospital Semimobile," November 1951, NARA 338/290/73/5/6/4786/1, p. 2; Richard Warren, "Report to Surgeon General, U.S. Army, on Tour of Medical Installations of Far East Command, April 1952," Countway Archives, Edward D. Churchill Collection, Box 51, Folder 24, pp. 2 and 5.

98. C. W. Hughes, "Vascular Surgery in the Armed Forces," 37; Seeley, "Surgery of the Popliteal Artery," 717.

99. For a description of methods to control arteries without clamps, see Guthrie, *Blood Vessel Surgery and Its Applications*, 31–34.

100. Spencer, interview with Barr, 8; Spencer, "Historical Vignette," 908. Spencer had experience using the bulldog clamp in this capacity during his time at Hopkins. Apel, *MASH*, 162. A surgical consultant later observed a false aneurysm develop at the site where a defective Japanese copy of the Potts clamp had occluded the artery. See Frank Gerbode, "Report to Surgeon General, U.S. Army, on Tour of Medical Installations of Far East Command," Countway Archives, Edward D. Churchill Collection, Box 51, Folder 26, p. 7.

101. Howard, "Historical Vignettes of Arterial Repair," 717. Howard tried commissioning the army engineering department to produce an atraumatic vascular clamp, but the devices they produced similarly failed.

102. Potts, "A New Clamp for Surgical Division of the Patent Ductus Arteriosus," 321–24; Richter, "Surgical Forceps." Richter manufactured the clamp for Potts. Surgeons in the 1950s rarely filed patents on instruments they invented; the AMA Code of Ethics actually forbade the practice. See Edmonson, "Asepsis and the Transformation of Surgical Instruments," 75–91. The ductus arteriosus (also known as ductus Botalli) is an embryological structure that connects the pulmonary artery to the aorta. This connection allows fetal blood to bypass the lungs, which do not participate in oxygenation while in utero. Normally, the ductus arteriosus closes a few days after birth, but in some babies it remains open (patent). The high likelihood for medical complications with a patent ductus arteriosus mandates treatment, which in the mid-twentieth century meant surgery (either ligation or division).

103. Gross and Hubbard, "Surgical Ligation of a Patent Ductus Arteriosus," 729–31.

104. Gross also performed the first intentional division of a patent ductus arteriosus. See R. E. Gross, "Complete Surgical Division of the Patent Ductus Arteriosus," 36–43. For a brief historical review of the ligation vs. division discussion, see Conklin and Watkins, "Use of the Potts-Smith-Gibson Clamp for Division of Patent Ductus Arteriosus," 361–70.

105. Potts et al., "Diagnosis and Surgical Treatment of Patent Ductus Arteriosus," 612–22, quote p. 617; Potts, "A New Clamp for Surgical Division of the Patent Ductus Arteriosus," 321. Other thoracic surgeons had invented their own clamps, but none worked as well or gained the popularity of Potts's. See Gross and Hufnagel, "Coarctation of the Aorta," 286–93, especially pp. 288–89; and Deterling and Essex, "An Instrument Designed Primarily for Use in Surgical Procedures on the Aorta,"132.

106. Bush, "Doctor's Idea Leads to Firm and Success," F5. Potts initially approached a medical instrument company, which rejected the idea for fear of cost overruns during the research and development phase; Richter quit the firm and began manufacturing the device out of his garage. He eventually established quite a successful business and, working with other surgeons, produced a variety of vascular clamps. See, for example, Riker, Nielson, and Potts, "A Technic of Portacaval Anastomosis," 937–43. This partnership between Potts and Richter reflected longstanding collaboration between surgeons and instrument makers, characterized in C. L. Jones, *The Medical Trade Catalogue in Britain.*

107. Jahnke, "The Surgery of Acute Vascular Injuries," 249.

108. For copies of the correspondence between Stone and the company, see Howard, "Historical Vignettes of Arterial Repair," 717–18.

109. Adamson, "Treatment of Arterial Injuries," see appendix. See also Organization of Medical Services, 11th Evacuation Hospital Semimobile," July 1952, NARA 338/290/73/5/6/4786/1, p. 1.

110. Ghislaine Lawrence explores the role of surgical instrument innovation in the creation/expansion of surgical operations in her important historical and historiographical article, "The Ambiguous Artifact: Surgical Instruments and the Surgical Past," 295–311. As Lawrence notes, the scholarly literature on the history of surgical instruments, especially modern ones, is thin. For Americana, the standard starting point is Edmonson, *American Surgical Instruments.* See also Kirkup, *The Evolution of Surgical Instruments.*

111. C. W. Hughes, "Primary Surgery of Blood Vessels in Korea."

112. Lindsey, "Evacuation and Specialty Centers," 30.

113. Jahnke, Hughes, and Howard, "The Rationale of Arterial Repair on the Battlefield," 399. See also Melvin to Dorothy Horwitz, 22 March 1953, in Horowitz, *We Will Not Be Strangers,* 249.

114. "Daily Intelligence and Operations Report, 5–6 July 1952," 1st Medical Battalion, 1st Marine Division, NARA 127/470/902/9/7/219/4, p. 1; "Daily Intelligence and Operations Report, 1–2 August 1952," 1.

115. Howard and Mason, "The Value of a Field Research Project," 17; Gerbode, "Report to Surgeon General," 7. Apel noted that the average tour of duty for a medical officer at the 8076th MASH was 10.3 months. Apel, *MASH*, 98. Doctors would usually serve for a year overseas but, due to the intensity of MASH work, would rotate to a rear hospital after several months at the front.

116. Howard, "Introduction—Historical Background and Development," 9. According to head OR nurse Ruth Kegler, Jahnke could obtain only four dogs for the first seventeen surgeons who came to learn arterial repair, so the students used and reused the animals. Questionnaire of Ruth A. Kegler, AMEDD Archives.

117. Howard, "Historical Vignettes of Arterial Repair," 718; Edward J. Jahnke, interview with Sam Milner, 1 September 1966, US Army Medical Department Center of History and Heritage Historical Research Collection, Fort Sam Houston, TX, p. 3; Salyer, "Training of Medical Officers," 90.

118. Other historians have discussed the importance/necessity of hands-on education in surgery. See, for example, Schlich, *Surgery, Science and Industry*; Wilde, "Practising Surgery"; Wilde and Hirst, "Learning from Mistakes," 38–77.

119. Sanger, "Report to Surgeon General," 3.

120. Jahnke, interview with Milner, 4.

121. "Organization of Medical Service, 11th Evacuation Hospital Semimobile, June 1952," NARA 338/290/73/5/6/4786/1, p. 3; "Organization of Medical Service, 11th Evacuation Hospital Semimobile, July 1952," pp. 1–2. The course occurred from 18 to 21 July 1952.

122. See, for example, "Sample Training Course for 11th Evacuation Hospital," December 1951, NARA 338/290/73/5/6/4786/1. Salyer, "Training of Medical Officers," 90.

123. Francis D. Moore, "Report of Visit to Far East Command, July–August 1952," Countway Archives, Edward D. Churchill Collection, Box 51, Folder 24, p. 16. See also Francis D. Moore, "Report of the Surgeon-in-Chief," Archives of Peter Bent Brigham Hospital, 45.

124. Gerbode, "Report to Surgeon General," 7.

125. Sanger, "Report to Surgeon General," 2.

126. Hughes tentatively identifies seventy-one arterial repairs performed by non-members of the Surgical Research Team based on follow-up studies of patients evacuated to Japan but makes no claims for completeness. His analysis does not separate the results of these cases from the results of those performed by research team members. C. W. Hughes, "Arterial Repair in the Korean War," 556.

127. Howard, "Introduction—Historical Background and Development," 9.

128. Statistical data for this paragraph is drawn from C. W. Hughes, "Arterial Repair in the Korean War"; C. W. Hughes, "The Primary Repair of Wounds of Major Arteries"; and Spencer and Grewe, "Management of Arterial Injuries in Battle Casualties."

129. See, for example, Brooks, "Pathological Changes in Muscle as a Result of Disturbances of Circulation," 188–216, especially pp. 207–8, 214–15; Reichert,

"The Importance of Circulatory Balance in the Survival of Replanted Limbs," 86–93. Barnes and Trueta detail the microscopic findings in such edema but do not explore its etiology in their article "Arterial Spasm," 74–79.

130. Miller and Welch, "Quantitative Studies on the Time Factor in Arterial Injuries," 428–38.

131. Altemeir and Pulaski, "The Occurrence of Wound Infection in Korean War Battle Casualties during May–June 1953," 346–47. The idea that curing one disease effectively created another has received some attention in the literature. For the best explication of this concept, see Feudtner, *Bittersweet*.

132. Fasciotomy is the surgical opening of the fascial compartments. C. W. Hughes, "Primary Surgery of Blood Vessels in Korea," 448.

133. C. W. Hughes, *Debridement*. The MHI Archives houses this publication of a lecture Hughes delivered at the Management of Mass Casualties course at the Army Medical Service Graduate School.

134. Jahnke, "Late Structural and Functional Results of Arterial Injuries Primarily Repaired," 175–83.

135. Jahnke, "Late Structural and Functional Results of Arterial Injuries Primarily Repaired," 176. Five patients wounded in the upper extremity retained excellent circulation due to collateral vessels, but the rest suffered from some degree of vascular insufficiency. Other patients with apparently patent arteries nonetheless complained of symptoms of arterial deficiency during exercise tests. Some of these patients had constriction but not occlusion at the site of repair; Jahnke presumed others developed some element of arteriospasm.

136. Jahnke, "Late Structural and Functional Results of Arterial Injuries Primarily Repaired," 179. All these series have relatively small denominators, but the dramatic differences among the series impart statistical significance.

137. Jahnke, "Late Structural and Functional Results of Arterial Injuries Primarily Repaired," 175. Eight patients suffering from arterial insufficiency elected to receive a second operation to replace the thrombosed section of artery with another venous graft. At time of publication, all eight patients had recovered from the surgery and obtained relief from their symptoms of arterial insufficiency.

138. Jahnke, "Late Structural and Functional Results of Arterial Injuries Primarily Repaired," 175.

139. "Monthly Historical Report, 1 October–31 October 1950, 8055th Mobile Army Surgical Hospital," NARA 407/270/68/20/04/4714/1, p. 1, 5; "Unit History, 45th Surgical Hospital, 19 July 1950 to 19 July 1954," NARA 112/390/18/7/1/144/18, pp. 2–4; between 4 October 1950 and 31 January 1951, the hospital moved an average of once a week.

140. Lindsey, "Professional Considerations of Patient Evacuation," 71, emphasis original; Albert, "Air Evacuation from Korea," 256–59; A. D. Smith, "Medical Air Evacuation in Korea and Its Influence on the Future," 323–32.

141. "Unit History, 45th Surgical Hospital," p. 2. In defense of Pusan, the same hospital had admitted 5,674 patients in one month, with 608 admitted in a single twenty-four-hour span, with similar triage challenges.

142. Woodard, "The Story of the Mobile Army Surgical Hospital," 510.

143. "Unit History, 45th Surgical Hospital," p. 7; "Combat Operations Command Report for May 1953, 47th Surgical Hospital," pp. 1–2.

144. For the position of hospital units in North Africa to minimize the effects of German air raids, see Ogilvie, "War Surgery in Africa," 313–24; and Churchill, *Surgeon to Soldiers*, 124. For the Pacific theaters, Condon-Rall and Cowdrey, *Medical Service in the War against Japan*, 167–68, 239, 324, 389, and elsewhere.

145. "Annual Report 8164th Army Unit, 1951," NARA 338/290/73/ 6/1/4797/3, see chart on occupied beds indicating a dramatic and sustained decline after stemming the Chinese counterattack in the spring of 1951. See also "Health of Army Troops, FEC," *Surgeon General's Circular* 7, no. 1 (1952): 18.

146. Beyer, Enos, and Holmes, "Personnel Protective Armor," 663–73; Herget, Coe, and Beyer, "Wound Ballistics and Body Armor in Korea,"697–725; R. H. Holmes, "Wound Ballistics and Body Armor," 73–78; *The History of the Medical Department of the United States Navy*, 113–14; Cowdrey, *The Medics' War*, 210–11; "Semiannual Report, Medical Research and Development Boards, 1 January–30 June 1952," NARA 112/631/19/6/6/6/22, p. 5; Holmes et al., "Medical Aspects of Body Armor Used in Korea," 1477–78.

147. Reister, *Battle Casualties and Medical Statistics*, 49–51.

148. Spencer, interview with Barr, 16. See, among others, Cowdry, "MASH vs *M*A*S*H**"; Benjamin Eiseman, interview with Justin Barr, 3 August 2011, Navy Bureau of Medicine and Surgery Office of Medical History; Grant, "Front Line Surgery in Korea," 268; "Eighth United States Army Annual Report, 1952: Army Medical Services Activities, Section 2, Annex VI," NARA 112/390/18/11/2/197/1; D. M. Friedman, *A History of Vascular Surgery*.

149. Animal studies in the interwar era had clearly demonstrated this principle. See Miller and Welch, "Quantitative Studies on the Time Factor in Arterial Injuries," 428–38. That military surgeons were aware of these results is apparent through their discussion in Hughes and Bowers, "Blood Vessel Surgery."

150. Barr and Montgomery, "Helicopter Evacuation of Casualties in Korea—Did It Matter?"

151. "Command Report for June 1953," 2–3, "Command Report for August 1953, 1st Helicopter Ambulance Company," NARA 112/390/18/11/ 2/192/1, p. 2; Dorland and Nanney, *Dustoff*, 11, 14–15; Whitcomb, *Call Sign—Dustoff*, 16.

152. W. L. White, *Back Down the Ridge*, chapter 2; Cowdrey, *Medics' War*, 179; Lindsey, "Professional Considerations of Patient Evacuation," 93; Buerger, "Medical Support for Mountain Fighting in Korea," 695; Carle, "Medical Experiences in Korea," 1628.

153. Sako et al., "A Survey of Evacuation, Resuscitation, and Mortality in a Forward Surgical Hospital," 9–11; Reister, *Battle Casualties and Medical Statistics*, 80, see especially tables 72 and 73; C. W. Hughes, "Primary Surgery of Blood Vessels in Korea," 446. No conflict-wide statistics on time lag from wounding to surgery exist for World War II. In data collected by the 2nd Auxiliary Surgical Group, 26 percent of casualties reached the operating table within six hours and 65 percent within twelve hours. "Time Interval, Wounding to Operation," NARA 112/390/17/17/5/393/1. "Essential Technical Medical Data," 13 July 1945, NARA 112/390/17/13/6/242/4, p. 14.

154. Inui, Shannon, and Howard, "Arterial Injuries in the Korean Conflict," 854. See also Jahnke and Seeley, "Acute Vascular Injuries in the Korean War," 168; C. W. Hughes, "Primary Surgery of Blood Vessels in Korea"; and Jahnke and Howard, "Primary Repair of Major Arterial Injuries."

155. Readers should take this figure as a guestimate. The army suffered 443,163 casualties in the war; the navy and Marine Corps combined for 30,090. Army helicopters evacuated about 17,700 patients. US Air Force helicopters carried roughly 8,400 medevac patients. Numbers for the navy/marines are unavailable, although by the end of 1951 the tally was 8,500. Obviously, helicopters rarely transported servicemen classified as killed in action, but they did transport diseased patients (especially hemorrhagic fever and cerebral malaria cases), further complicating the accounting. These statistics register each trip a patient made by helicopter separately and included evacuations of ROK and other UN forces as well, making the percent evacuated by helicopter particularly difficult to quantify. See Reister, *Battle Casualties and Medical Statistics*, 5; Cowdrey, *Medics' War*, 341–42; Kirkland, *MASH Angels*, 268; Driscoll, "U.S. Army Medical Helicopters in the Korean War," 290; "Casualties: U.S. Navy and Marine Corps Personnel Killed and Wounded in Wars, Conflicts, Terrorist Acts, and Other Hostile Incidents"; Herman, *Frozen in Memory*, 113.

156. For a work specifically on nursing during the Korean War, see Omori, *Quiet Heroes*. See also Herman, *Frozen in Memory*, chapter 5 and *passim*.

157. Inui, Shannon, and Howard, "Arterial Injuries in the Korean Conflict," 851–52.

158. Warren was a prominent surgeon at Harvard who specialized in the vascular system. See Warren, "Report to Surgeon General," 4.

159. Pratt, "Vascular Wounds," 272–73.

160. Simeone, "Notes of the Treatment of Wounds of the Arteries," 72–73.

161. For an assessment of the intellectual flexibility of young medical officers in Korea, see Stewart, "Report to the Surgeon General," 8–9.

Chapter Six

1. Michel et al., "Quantitative Analysis of Culture Using Millions of Digitized Books," 176–82. Thanks to Sonal Singhal for directing me to this source. Search

conducted in English. https://books.google.com/ngrams/graph?content=vascular+s urgery&year_start=1900&year_end=1970&corpus=15&smoothing=3&share=&dir ect_url=t1%3B%2Cvascular%20surgery%3B%2Cc0 (accessed 28 April 2014).

2. Search conducted in English. https://books.google.com/ngrams/graph?conte nt=arterial+repair&year_start=1900&year_end=1970&corpus=15&smoothing=3 &share=&direct_url=t1%3B%2Carterial%20repair%3B%2Cc0 (accessed 28 April 2014).

3. Program, 1951 Clinical Congress, ACS Archives, Clinical Congresses of Surgeons of North America, RG0/SG2/S1/Box 3. They returned the following year, having definitively demonstrated the superiority of arterial repair over ligation, declaring it their "procedure of choice." Program, 1952 Clinical Congress, ACS Archives, Clinical Congresses of Surgeons of North America, RG0/SG2/S1/Box 3. The year with minimum attendance was 1951, with 4,084 surgeons; maximum was 1958, with 8,450 surgeons. The college did not track—or at least did not store— data on attendance at specific sessions. Data collated from Programs of Clinical Congresses, 1950–1960, ACS Archives, Clinical Congresses of Surgeons of North America, RG0/SG2/S1/Boxes 3–9.

4. Data collated from Programs of Clinical Congresses, 1950–1960, ACS Archives, Clinical Congresses of Surgeons of North America, RG0/SG2/S1/Boxes 3–9.

5. Program, 1953 Clinical Congress, ACS Archives, Clinical Congresses of Surgeons of North America, RG0/SG2/S1/Box 3.

6. Conley and Schroeder, "Session on Principles of Arterial Surgery."

7. Shumacker, *The Society for Vascular Surgery*. Appendix K lists all the programs from first through the thirty-sixth annual conference.

8. Coleman, Katz, and Menzel, *Medical Innovation*.

9. The four journals also represented the major surgical organizations of the era: *Annals of Surgery* (American Surgical Association), *Archives of Surgery* (Surgical Section of the American Medical Association), *Surgery* (official organ for the Society for Vascular Surgery in these years and the Society of University Surgeons), and *Surgery, Gynecology, and Obstetrics* (American College of Surgeons). Journals were manually reviewed every three years for a total of 6,489 articles individually inspected.

10. Fox, "The Politics of the NIH Extramural Program," 447–66.

11. National Institutes of Health, Office of Budget, "Appropriations History by Institute/Center (1938 to Present)," https://officeofbudget.od.nih.gov/approp_hist. html (accessed 1 November 2018).

12. See, for example, Crawford, DeBakey, and Cooley, "Clinical Use of Synthetic Substitutes in Three Hundred Seventeen Patients," 261–70; Hurwitt, "Cardiovascular Surgery at Montefiore Hospital in 1957 as Compared to 1952," 1516–20.

13. Morris, Creech, and DeBakey, "Acute Arterial Injuries in Civilian Practice," 565–72, quote p. 570.

14. See, for example, Seidenberg, Hurwitt, and Carton, "The Technique of Anastomosing Small Arteries," 743–46; W. P. Nelson, "Treatment of Acute Vascular Catastrophes," 3487–92.

15. Dickinson, Ashley, and Gerbode, "The Definitive Treatment of Injuries to Major Blood Vessels Incurred in the Korean War," 625–34.

16. See, for example, Tarizzo et al., "Atherosclerosis in Synthetic Vascular Grafts," 826–32.

17. For naval distribution and usage, see M. W. Arnold, CPT USN MC, Assistant Head, Training Branch, to Michael Mason, 26 February 1957. The letter and statistics on sales of the first edition through 17 February 1959 are available in ACS Archives, Committee on Trauma Administrative Records, RG5/SG3/S5/Box 21, Folder 5.

18. Shumacker, "Vascular Injuries" [1954], 148.

19. Shumacker, "Vascular Injuries" [1960], 88.

20. Christopher, A Textbook of Surgery by American Authors; "An American Textbook of Surgery," Review of A Textbook of Surgery by American Authors, ed. Frederick Christopher. British Medicine Journal 2 (4 July 1936): 16–17.

21. Holman, "Diseases of the Arteries," 147–64.

22. Holman and de Takáts, "The Vascular System," in A Textbook of Surgery by American Authors, 3rd ed., 187–230; Holman and de Takáts, "The Vascular System," in A Textbook of Surgery by American Authors, 5th ed., 620–65.

23. Shumacker, "The Arteries," 1298–315. The chapter in the 1960 edition is essentially unchanged.

24. Allen, Barker, and Hines, Peripheral Vascular Diseases; Allen, Barker, and Hines, Peripheral Vascular Diseases, 2nd ed.

25. Fye, "The Literature of Internal Medicine," 55–84.

26. "Questions for Consideration in Residency Programs in General Surgery, Jan 1956," ACS Archives, Board of Regents Statements on Education and Specialization, RG5/SG2/S8/SS11/Box 1/Folder 1.

27. Interviews with leaders in vascular surgery reveal nearly simultaneous founding of artery banks across the country in the early 1950s, with almost all based on frozen specimens. See Dale, with Johnson and DeWeese, Band of Brothers, 36, 158–59, 173, 190, 209, 362, 466 for banks established in Boston (Allan Callow), New York City (Ralph Deterling), Chicago (Géza de Takáts), Rochester, NY (James DeWeese), Birmingham (Sterling Edwards), Baltimore (Mark Ravitch and Henry Bahnson), and Houston (Jesse Thompson). For Chicago, see also Frank Milloy, interview with Michael Bullington, 8 March 1995, Rush Medical Archives, Accession No. RG052000 095-029. For Madison, see Phelan, Young, Botham, et al., "The Development of the Artery Bank at the University Hospitals," 232–34, 248. For the military vessel bank in DC, see Hurwitt, "A Blood Vessel Bank under Military Conditions," 19–27. MGH News 133 (April 1954), 2.

28. For naval funding supporting multiple projects investigating refrigeration technology, see Radin, Life on Ice, 136, 140, 142–43, 144–45. For studies relying on

naval funding, see Deterling, Parshley, and Blunt, "A Critical Study of Present Criteria Governing Selection and Use of Blood Vessel Grafts"; Shumacker et al., "Studies in Vascular Repair: V"; Schloss and Shumacker, "Studies in Vascular Repair: IV."

29. A. Stevens, "Spare Parts for People," 74–76. Other journalists repeated this trope in popular articles about vessel banks. Bundesen, "Artery Banks Now Aid Patients with Aneurysms," 4. Other historians have previously discussed this idea of the body being composed of replaceable, interchangeable parts. Lederer, *Flesh and Blood*; McKellar, *Artificial Hearts*; and especially Fox and Swazey, *Spare Parts*.

30. Strong, "The US Navy Tissue Bank," 9–16.

31. "Redesignation of Bone Bank Technicians, Recommendation Concerning," 10 June 1952, NARA 52/470/56/6/7/291/5, p. 1; and "Redesignation of Bone Bank Technicians, Advisory Board Action Concerning," 9 July 1952, NARA 52/470/56/6/7/291/5, p. 1.

32. "Augmentation of Supply of Tissue for the Tissue Bank, Information Concerning," 5 October 1953, NARA 52/470/56/4/2/303/5, p. 2.

33. "Tissue Homografts, Follow-up Studies Concerning," 15 March 1955, NARA 52/470/56/4/2/303/5, p. 2.

34. F. S. Hoffmeister to B. W. Hogan, 19 July 1955, NARA 52/470/56/6/7/291/5.

35. Keshishian and Prandoni, "The Surgical Management of Occlusive Vascular Disease," 1–12.

36. By 1955, the bank had only shipped four to nonfederal hospitals. See "Tissue Homografts, Follow-up Studies Concerning," 2; A. Stevens, "Spare Parts for People," 76; J. Maxwell Chamberlain to W. E. Kellum, 22 December 1954, NARA 52/470/56/6/7/291/5.

37. They paid the navy in kind: for every three arteries they sent, the navy kept one for research. See W. F. Moehlman and E. Converse Pierce to chief, BuMed, 12 November 1955, NARA 52/470/56/6/7/291/5 and J. R. V. Norman to East Tennessee Heart Association, 7 December 1955, NARA 52/470/56/6/7/291/5.

38. Spencer and Grewe, "The Management of Arterial Injuries in Battle Casualties," 304–13.

39. Seeley, "Vascular Surgery at Walter Reed Army Hospital," 8–9; Seeley et al., "Traumatic Arteriovenous Fistulas and Aneurysms in War Wounds," 471–79; C. W. Hughes, "Vascular Surgery in the Armed Forces," 30–46; Seeley, Hughes, and Jahnke, "Surgery of the Popliteal Artery," 712–17; Dickinson, Ashley, and Gerbode, "The Definitive Treatment of Injuries to Major Blood Vessels Incurred in the Korean War," 625–64; Spencer and Grewe, "The Management of Arterial Injuries in Battle Casualties"; Jahnke and Howard, "Primary Repair of Major Arterial Injuries," 646–49; Jahnke, "The Surgery of Acute Vascular Injuries," 249–51; C. W. Hughes, "Acute Vascular Trauma in Korean War Casualties," 91–100; Jahnke, Hughes, and Howard, "The Rationale of Arterial Repair on the Battlefield," 396–401; C. W. Hughes, "The Primary Repair of Wounds of Major Arteries," 297–303; Hughes and Bowers, "Blood Vessel Surgery," 174–78; Inui, Shannon, and Howard, "Arterial Injuries in the Korean Conflict," 850–57.

40. Holman, *New Concepts in Surgery of the Vascular System*, 9–10.

41. Holman, *New Concepts in Surgery of the Vascular System*, 44.

42. Morris, Creech, and DeBakey, "Acute Arterial Injuries in Civilian Practice," 565.

43. Their role was analogous to the one Joel Howell documented for returning World War I doctors and the subsequent rapid acceptance of X-rays in *Technology in the Hospital*.

44. Bowers performed the original work highlighting the importance of interpersonal channels in 1938, focusing on ham radios; subsequent studies in physicians have consistently revealed that scientific publications, regardless of the strength of their evidence, educate clinicians about an innovation, but that contact with peers and opinion leaders actually causes change in practice. For ham radios, see Bowers, "Differential Intensity of Intra-societal Diffusion," 21–31. For medical diffusion, see John Harley Warner's account of how American doctors studying in France in the nineteenth century brought back and disseminated empiricism in *Against the Spirit of System*, especially chapter 4. For the role of interpersonal connection in innovation diffusion generally, see Rogers, *Diffusion of Innovations*, 18–19, 205, 304.

45. Hermes C. Grillo, interview with Jan K. Herman, 1 July 1999, BUMED Library and Archives; Hermes C. Grillo, interview with G. Kurt Piehler and Crystal Dover as part of the University of Tennessee's Veteran's Oral History Project, 8 July 2002, http://csws.utk.edu/oral-history-project/read-an-interview/korea/ (accessed 18 April 2019). Additional biographical information may be found in Austen et al., "Hermes C. Grillo." See also Negri, "Hermes C. Grillo, 83, Thoracic Surgeon at MGH."

46. Mullins, "Albert Starr." Starr served as an intern on Blalock's service at Johns Hopkins before beginning a surgical residency at Presbyterian Hospital, associated with Columbia University. Both training locales would have likely exposed Starr to some vascular surgery. See D. K. Cooper, *Open Heart*, 261–69.

47. Frank C. Spencer, interview with Justin Barr, 1 December 2011, BUMED Library and Archives, 9–13.

48. DeAnda and Galloway, "Historical Perspectives of the American Association for Thoracic Surgery." Spencer helped pioneer the use of the internal mammary artery in coronary artery bypass grafts.

49. Rich and Spencer, *Vascular Trauma*. The diffusion studies literature would classify Spencer as a change agent; see Rogers, *Diffusion of Innovations*, chapter 9.

50. DeAnda and Balsam, "Historical Perspectives of The American Association for Thoracic Surgery," 762–64.

51. Condie, *Russell M. Nelson*; R. M. Nelson, *From Heart to Heart*, see 75–79 for Korean experience. For a similar example of a surgeon who went into private practice, see Melvin to Dorothy Horwitz, 22 March 1953, in Horwitz, *We Will Not Be Strangers*, 249.

52. Seeley, "Vascular Surgery at Walter Reed Army Hospital," 8–9; Rich, "Carl W. Hughes: In Memoriam," personal communication. Every army surgery resident at Walter Reed would come to rotate on the vascular surgery service.

53. Phelan, Young, and Gale, "The Effect of Suture Material on Small Artery Anastomoses," 79–83; Phelan et al., "The Effect of Suture Material in Determining the Patency of Small Artery Grafts," 969–73; Phelan, "A New Method of Artery Graft Anastomosis," 990–93.

54. Phelan, "Newer Aspects of Peripheral Vascular Surgery," 691–93. See also Phelan and Young, "The Recognition and Management of Disease of the Aorta and Great Vessels," 373–78.

55. Cooke et al., "Blood Vessel Bank," 1779–86; Seeley et al., "Traumatic Arteriovenous Fistulas and Aneurysms in War Wounds," 471–79; Cooke, Hughes, Jahnke, Seeley, "Homologous Arterial Grafts and Autogenous Vein Grafts Used to Bridge Large Arterial Defects in Man," 183–89.

56. Cooke, Kurzweg, and Starzl, "Blood Vessel Bank," 26–31.

57. Starzl, *The Puzzle People*, see p. 48 for his experience training under Cooke and learning vascular surgery.

58. Caplow, *The First Measured Century*, chapter 12 discusses crime. For murder rates, a stand-in for violent crime and more carefully tracked, see Eckberg, "Estimates of Early Twentieth Century U.S. Homicide Rates," 1–16, see the figure on p. 3; Eckberg, "Crimes Known to Urban Police, by Type of Offense," table Ec21–29.

59. For example, in a series of eighty-five instances of arterial damage from 1958 to 1966 in St. Louis, Missouri, knives, guns, and glass combined to cause 77 percent of the cases; blunt trauma, only 22 percent. Dillard, Nelson, and Norman, "Review of 85 Major Traumatic Arterial Injuries," 391–94. Other cases series evidenced similar rations. For a thorough review of civilian vascular trauma, see Rich, "Historical and Military Aspects of Vascular Trauma," 1–72, especially pp. 28–39.

60. Sinkler and Spencer, "The Importance of Early Exploration of Vascular Injuries," 228–34; Whitaker, Durden, and Ferguson, "Acute Arterial Injuries," 129–34; Ferguson, Byrd, McAfee, "Experience in the Management of Arterial Injuries," 980–86.

61. Jackson, *Crabgrass Frontier*.

62. Lewis, *Divided Highways*; Kay, *Asphalt Nation*.

63. "Motor Vehicle Traffic Fatalities and Fatality Rate, 1899–2016," https://cdan.nhtsa.gov/tsftables/Fatalities%20and%20Fatality%20Rates.pdf (accessed 23 April 2019).

64. Fink, *The Automobile Age*.

65. "Motor Vehicle Traffic Fatalities and Fatality Rate, 1899–2003."

66. *AMA News* 3, no. 23 (14 November 1960).

67. "Congress Opens Today with Trauma as Keynote," *Clinical Congress News* (15 November 1954): 1–5, in ACS Archives, Committee on Trauma Administrative Records, RG5/SG3/S5/Box 1/Folder 2.

68. J. F. TerHorst, "Auto Safety Devices Gain Public Favor," *Detroit Michigan News*, 18 March 1956, in ACS Archives, Committee on Trauma Administrative Records, RG5/SG3/S5/Box 22/Folder 1. See also *AMA News*, 14 November 1960. For a detailed description of the changes car companies made to their vehicles to improve safety, see Eastman, *Styling vs. Safety*.

69. Gangloff, "Medicalizing the Automobile"; Lerner, *One for the Road*; Simpson, "Transporting Lazarus," 163–97; Zink, *Anyone, Anything, Anytime*; Barr and Smith, "The History of Trauma Care." Of note, John Howard, who had led the surgical research team in Korea that promoted arterial repair, cowrote the seminal 1966 *Accidental Death and Disability Report*, and Sam Seeley, the army surgeon who published the first data on the superiority of reparative operations on Korean War casualties, played a prominent role on the first national Emergency Medical Services Committee.

70. Zollinger, "Traffic Injuries—a Surgical Problem," 694–700. For specific vascular concerns, see W. P. Nelson, "Treatment of Acute Vascular Catastrophes."

71. Dickinson et al., "The Definitive Treatment of Injuries to Major Blood Vessels Incurred in the Korean War," 634.

72. For the early scientific history of atherosclerosis, see Olszewski, "Cholesterol," chapter 1. Technically, atherosclerosis (coined 1904) is a cause of arteriosclerosis, but the two terms were often used interchangeably through the mid-twentieth century.

73. D. S. Jones, *Broken Hearts*.

74. Rosen, *A History of Public Health*, chapters 7 and 8.

75. Chris Feudtner commented on the chronic health problems newly identified in diabetics treated with insulin in his book *Bittersweet*, see especially chapter 8. For references in the vascular surgery literature, see Silbert, "Surgical Consideration in the Treatment of Infection and Gangrene in the Diabetic," 895–903; Cole, "Results of Sympathectomy in Diabetic Arteriosclerotic Peripheral Vascular Disease," 1607–8.

76. Starr, *The Social Transformation of American Medicine*, book 2, chapter 3.

77. Turow and Gans-Boriskin, "From Expert in Action to Existential Angst," 263–81; Hansen, *Picturing Medical Progress from Pasteur to Polio*, chapter 9. For a similar trend in science, see Lafollette, *Making Science Our Own*.

78. Oshinsky, *Polio*, 188–213.

79. R. Stevens, *In Sickness and in Wealth*, chapter 7. The war itself helped drive the expansion of health insurance as companies tried to recruit workers in an era of salary freezes by offering benefits.

80. Anderson, *Blue Cross Since 1929*, 45. The US population in 1950 was 151 million. Population data available from US Census, http://www.census.gov/history/www/through_the_decades/fast_facts/1950_fast_facts.html (accessed 29 April 2014). See also Steckel, "Persons with Hospital and Surgical Benefits, by Type of Private Health Insurance Plan," table Bd294–305.

81. Anderson, *Blue Cross Since 1929*, 45, 62.

82. By 1960, only about half of all health-care costs were paid out of pocket, down from 65 percent in 1950 and practically 100 percent in 1900. This increased the utilization of medical services. Anderson and Newman, "Societal and Individual Determinants of Medical Care Utilization in the United States," 95–124.

83. Brandt, *The Cigarette Century*.

84. Hogan, *Selling 'em by the Sack*.

85. See US Census data, https://hsus.cambridge.org/HSUSWeb/toc/tableToc.do?id=Aa125-144 (accessed 16 July 2018).

86. For the importance of postoperative care in modern surgery, see Fye, *Caring for the Heart*, especially chapter 13.

87. In 1986, JAMA included this article as one of the fifty-one landmark publications that most dramatically influenced the field of medicine. Enos, Holmes, and Beyer, "Coronary Disease among United States Soldiers Killed in Action in Korea," 1091–93. They published a follow-up study in 1953: Enos, Beyer, and Holmes, "Pathogenesis of Coronary Disease in American Soldiers Killed in Korea," 912–14.

88. Yater, "Coronary Artery Disease in Men Eighteen to Thirty-Nine Years of Age," 481–526. Olszewski, *Cholesterol*, 100.

89. List of applicants for charter membership in the American Society for the Study of Arteriosclerosis, Mayo Archives, MHU 0633, Nelson W. Barker Papers, Series 1, Folder 2.

90. N. W. Barker, "Diagnosis and Treatment of Chronic Occlusive Disease of the Peripheral Arteries," 470–74; Moore, "Endocrine Therapy of Arteriosclerosis," 26–30; Mufson et al., "An Evaluation of Priscoline by Artery in the Treatment of Peripheral Arterial Obliterative Disease," 2651–54.

91. Lowenberg, "Treatment of Peripheral Arterial Insufficiency," 809–14; Pratt, "Surgical Sympathectomy for Obliterative Vascular Disease," 3357–61.

92. Deterling, "Experience with Permanent By-pass Grafts in Treatment of Occlusive Arterial Disease," 247–60, quote p. 247.

93. Julian et al., "Direct Surgery of Arteriosclerosis," 459–73.

94. While national journals reflect leading research from academia, state medical journals more accurately capture the interests and practices of regular physicians. The following state medical journals were reviewed in totality from 1950 through 1960: *Connecticut State Medical Journal, New York State Medical Journal, Wisconsin Medical Journal, California Medicine, Medical Annals of the District of Columbia* (1955–60), and *Journal of the Medical Association of the State of Alabama*.

95. See, among many others, DeBakey et al., "Surgical Considerations of Occlusive Disease of the Abdominal Aorta and Iliac and Femoral Arteries," 306–24.

96. Barker, "A History of Endarterectomy," 1–12; Dos Santos, "From Embolectomy to Endarterectomy, or The Fall of a Myth," 113–28.

97. For the importance of arteriograms in peripheral vascular surgery, see, among others, Gilfillan, "Thromboendarterectomy," 2986–90.

98. Smith, Rush, and Evans, "The Technique of Translumbar Arteriography," 255–58.

99. Wallingford, "The Development of Organic Iodine Compounds as X-Ray Contrast Media," 721–28; Derrick, Logan, and Howard, "Pitfalls of Translumbar Aortography and Peripheral Arteriography," 517–20.

100. Seldginer, "Catheter Replacement of the Needle in Percutaneous Arteriography," 368–76. Initially developed to facilitate arteriograms, the Seldinger technique quickly spread to enable percutaneous procedures as diverse as tracheostomies to feeding tubes to central venous catheters.

101. Annual reports of the Department of Surgery, Baylor University College of Medicine, Houston, TX, 1949–1950, NLM Archives, DeBakey Collection, Box 9, Folder 43.

102. "Dr. DeBakey Discusses Advances in Vascular Surgery," *Medical News*, 28 January 1959, 6–8.

103. List of operations, DeBakey Collection, NLM Archives, Box 44, Folder 3.

104. R. Jasper Smith to Clyde R. Welman, 6 June 1961, NLM Archives, DeBakey Collection, Box 44, folder 5.

105. Haseltine, "Soldier Given Dead Man's Artery in Rare Operation," 15; Haseltine, "Blood Vessel Cures Save Lives of GIs," 6; Tuckman, "Marine Surgeon, 27, Saves Limbs at Front Through New Operation," 22; Haseltine, "Limb-Saving Surgery Successful in Korea," B2; "More G.I. Limbs Saved," *New York Times*, 14 March 1953, 4; "New Surgery Reduces Korea Amputations," *Los Angeles, California Examiner*, 7 June 1953; "Texas Surgeon Perfect Arterial Graft to Prevent Amputation," *Houston Chronicle*, 7 June 1953.

106. Michael E. DeBakey, interview with Don Schanche, 15–16 August 1972, NLM Archives, DeBakey Papers, Box 2, Folder 21.

107. Molner, "Clogged Arteries Remediable," 9; "Dead Man's Artery Used in Surgery Here," *Atlanta Constitution*, 6 February 1954, 1; Gibbons, "New Artery for Old Put Victim on Feet," 1, 16.

108. Barr, "Battle of the Bulge," 291–96.

109. National data prior to 1943, when the CDC began collecting data, are difficult to acquire or verify, but in World War I, about 30 percent of soldiers had syphilis, indicating its prevalence. Parran, *Shadow on the Land*; Brandt, *No Magic Bullet*, 54; Doroshow, "Wassermann before Wedding Bells."

110. Synopsis of statistics of operations performed for aneurisms at the Charity Hospital from August 1905 to July 1934, Rudolph Matas Papers, Box 2, Folder 32. See also Kampmeier, "Aneurysm of the Abdominal Aorta," 97–109; H. G. Garland, "The Pathology of Aneurysms," 334–50; Lucke and Rea, "Studies on Aneurysms," 935–40; Scott, "Abdominal Aneurysms," 682–710; Hubeny and Pollack, "Saccular Abdominal Aortic Aneurysm," 385–93; Gage, "Mycotic Aneurysm of the Common Iliac Artery," 667–91; Bryant, "Two Clinical Lectures on Aneurysms of the Abdominal Aorta," 71–80.

111. Estes, "Abdominal Aortic Aneurysm," 258–64; Gifford, Hines, and Janes, "An Analysis and Follow-up Study of One Hundred Popliteal Aneurysms," 284–93.

112. See, among many others, Bahnson, "Considerations in the Excision of Aortic Aneurysms," 377–86.

113. Barr, "Battle of the Bulge."

114. Dubost, Allary, and Oeconomos, "Resections of an Aneurysm of the Abdominal Aorta," 405–8. A year earlier, Jacques Oudat had performed a nearly identical procedure but for atherosclerotic occlusion of the distal aorta. Oudot, "La greffe vasculaire dans les thromboses du carrefour aortique," 234–36.

115. DeBakey and Cooley, "Surgical Treatment of Aneurysm of Abdominal Aorta by Resection and Restoration of Continuity with Homograft," 257–66.

116. Michael E. DeBakey, interview with Don Schanche, 10–11 September 1972, DeBakey Collection, NLM Archives, Box 2, Folder 24, p. 58.

117. Moore and Wantz, "Abdominal Aortic Aneurysm," 497–509.

118. DeBakey, interview with Schanche, 82, 83.

119. Voorhees, Jaretzki, and Blakemore, "The Use of Tubes Constructed from Vinyon 'N' Cloth in Bridging Arterial Defects," 332–36; Voorhees, "The Development of Arterial Prostheses," 289–95.

120. Creech et al., "Vascular Prosthesis," 62–75. For an environmental history of polymers like vinyon, see Blanc, *Fake Silk*.

121. Barr, "Battle of the Bulge"; Creech, "Endo-aneurysmorrhaphy and the Treatment of Aortic Aneurysm," 935–46. For extension to community hospitals, see Nolen, *The Making of a Surgeon*.

122. Rudolph Matas to Michael E. DeBakey, 2 October 1954, DeBakey Collection, NLM Archives, Box 5, Folder 27. Unintentionally continuing the mountain metaphor, surgeon historian Mark Ravitch labeled aortic aneurysm repair the "peak" of surgery in the 1950s. "The American Surgical Association," 282–87.

123. Molner, "Surgeons Can Correct Aneurysms," 6; "Rare Surgery Saves Life of Man," *Odessa American*, 11 July 1955, 3; "Carlisle Pastor Owes His Life to Heart Surgery Miracle," *Terra Haute Tribune-Star*, 9 June 1957, 76.

124. "Duke of Windsor in Happy Mood after Operation," *Maryview Daily Forum*, 17 December 1964, 14; Schmeck, "Windsor's Surgery," E7; Clayton, "Patch Sewn into Artery of Windsor," C11.

125. Blaisdell et al., "Aorto-Iliac Arterial Substitutions Utilizing Subcutaneous Grafts," 775–80.

126. Wylie, "Vascular Surgery," 645–48; Evans, "Presidential Address to the Midwestern Vascular Surgery Society," 161–68; Mills, "Vascular Surgery Training in the United States," 90s–97s.

127. Parodi, Palmaz, and Barone, "Transfemoral Intraluminal Graft Implantation for Abdominal Aortic Aneurysms," 491–99; interview with Juan Carlos Parodi, Society for Vascular Surgery Archives, available online: https://vascular.org/about-svs/history (accessed 17 July 2018).

128. While some recent literature explores the history of laparoscopic surgery in the setting of intra-abdominal operations, nothing yet analyzes this broader movement toward minimally invasive techniques that extends beyond general surgery to

vascular (endovascular), orthopedic (arthroscopic), cardiac (TAVR), urologic, gynecologic, and other specialties as well. For the laparoscopic literature, see Whitfield, "A Revolution through the Keyhole," 525–48; and Tang and Schlich, "Surgical Innovation and the Multiple Meanings of Randomized Controlled Trials," 117–41. Frampton and Kneebone, "John Wickham's New Surgery," 544–66.

Conclusion

1. As per Stigler's law of eponymy, almost nothing is actually named after its true inventor. See Holt, *When Einstein Walked with Gödel*, 291–93.

2. Lawrence, "Review of *Technological Change in Modern Surgery*," 380–82.

3. Beth Linker has explored this issue when analyzing the evolution of Harrington's rod treatment, invented for polio scoliosis but far more frequently used for idiopathic scoliosis. See her article "Spines of Steel," 222–49.

4. D. C. Smith, "Appendicitis, Appendectomy, and the Surgeon," 414–41; D. S. Jones, *Broken Hearts*.

5. Temkin, "The Scientific Approach to Disease," 441–55, see especially p. 453; and D. S. Jones, *Broken Hearts*.

6. Garvus, "'Making Bad Boys Good,'" 71–99; Pressman, *Last Resort*; Longo, "The Rise and Fall of Battey's Operation," 244–67; Moss, "Floating Kidneys," 92–104.

7. Barnes, "Discarded Operations," 109–23.

8. Wennberg, among others, demonstrated seemingly arbitrary but highly variable rates of surgery by county in the United States; see *Tracking Medicine*.

9. Crenner, "Placebos and the Progress of Surgery," 156–84; D. S. Jones, *Broken Hearts*; D. S. Jones, "Surgical Practice and the Reconstruction of the Therapeutic Niche," 184–215; D. S. Jones, "Surgery and Clinical Trials," 479–502.

10. Schlich, "Degrees of Control," 106–25.

11. Rifkin et al., "Achievements and Challenges in Facial Transplantation," 260–70. At the time of this writing, only forty face transplants have been performed in the world.

Bibliography

Archival Material

American Board of Surgery Archives, Philadelphia, Pennsylvania
American College of Surgeons Archives, Chicago, Illinois
American Medical Association Archives, Chicago, Illinois
Betty H. Carter Woman Veterans Historical Project, Jackson Library, University of North Carolina at Greensboro
Brigham and Women's Hospital Archives, Boston, Massachusetts
Francis A. Countway Library of Medicine, Boston, Massachusetts
George Washington University Archives, Washington, DC
Georgetown University Special Collections Center, Washington, DC
Medical College of Virginia Archives, Richmond, Virginia
Massachusetts General Hospital Archives, Boston, Massachusetts
National Archives and Records Administration at College Park, Maryland. Documents are cited as follows: author, "title," date, record group/stack area/compartment/row/shelf/box/folder.
National Library of Medicine, History of Medicine Division, Bethesda, Maryland
National Museum of Health and Medicine Archives, Silver Spring, Maryland
Northwestern University Medical School Archives, Chicago, Illinois
Rush Medical College Archives, Chicago, Illinois
Society for Vascular Surgery Archives, Chicago Illinois
Tulane University Archives (Louisiana Historical Society Collection), New Orleans, Louisiana
United States Army Heritage and Education Center, Military History Institute, Carlisle, Pennsylvania
United States Army Medical Department Center of History and Heritage Historical Research Collection, Fort Sam Houston, Texas
United States Navy Bureau of Medicine and Surgery Library and Archives, Washington, DC
University of Pennsylvania Archives, Philadelphia, Pennsylvania
University of Minnesota AHC Oral History Project, Minneapolis, Minnesota

University of Virginia Historical Collections of the Claude B. Moore Medical Library, Charlottesville, Virginia

Veterans' History Project, Library of Congress American Folklife Center, Online

Washington University in St. Louis Becker Medical Library Archives, St. Louis, Missouri

W. Bruce Fye History of Medicine Library at the Mayo Clinic in Rochester, Minnesota

Published Material

Abbe, Robert. "The Surgery of the Hand." *New York Medical Journal* 59 (13 January 1894): 33–40.

Ackerknecht, Erwin H. "A Plea for a 'Behaviorist' Approach in Writing the History of Medicine." *Journal of the History of Medicine and Allied Sciences* (July 1967): 211–14.

———. *Rudolf Virchow: Doctor, Statesman, Anthropologist.* Madison: University of Wisconsin Press, 1953.

Activities of Surgical Consultants. Washington, DC: Office of the Surgeon General, 1962.

Adamson, P. B. "A Comparison of Ancient and Modern Weapons in the Effectiveness of Producing Battle Casualties." *Journal of the Royal Army Medical Corps* 123 (1997): 93–103.

Adkins, Robinson E. *Medical Care of Veterans.* Washington, DC: US Government Printing Office, 1967.

Adler, Jessica. *Burdens of War: Creating the United States Veterans Health System.* Baltimore: Johns Hopkins University Press, 2017.

Akerman, J. "Award Ceremony Speech: The Nobel Prize in Physiology or Medicine, 1912." http://nobelprize.org/nobel_prizes/medicine/laureates/1912/press.html (accessed 1 August 2011).

Albert, Janice. "Air Evacuation from Korea—a Typical Flight." *Military Surgeon* 112, no. 4 (1953): 256–59.

Albright, Hollis L., and Laurence A. Van Hale. "Traumatic Aneurysms: A Study of Forty-Three Cases in an Overseas General Hospital." *Surgery* 20 (1946): 452–77.

Albucasis. *On Surgery and Instruments.* Translated by M. S. Spink and G. L. Lewis. London: Wellcome Institute of the History of Medicine, 1973.

Allen, E. V., and J. D. Camp. "Roentgenography of the Arteries of the Extremities with Thorotrast." *Proceedings of the Staff Meetings of the Mayo Clinic* 8 (1933): 61–63.

Allen, Edgar V., Nelson W. Barker, and Edgar A. Hines Jr., eds. *Peripheral Vascular Diseases.* Philadelphia: W. B. Sanders, 1946.

———. *Peripheral Vascular Diseases*, 2nd ed. Philadelphia: W. B. Sanders, 1955.

Altemeir, William A., and Edwin J. Pulaski. "The Occurrence of Wound Infection in Korean War Battle Casualties during May–June 1953." In *Recent Advances in Medicine and Surgery (19–30 April 1954) Based on Professional Medical Experiences in Japan and Korea, 1950–1953*, vol. 1, 334–63. Washington, DC: Army Medical Service Graduate School, 1955.

Altschuler, Lenn C. *The GI Bill: A New Deal for Veterans*. New York: Oxford University Press, 2009.

Alving, A. S., J. Arnold, and D. H. Robinson. "Status of Primaquine: I. Mass Therapy of Subclinical vivax Malaria with Primaquine." *JAMA* 149 (1952): 1558–62.

Alving, A. S., et al. "Korean vivax Malaria: II. Curative Treatment with Pamaquine and Primaquine." *American Journal of Tropical Medicine and Hygiene* 2 (1953): 970–76.

American Medical Association. *A History of the Council on Medical Education and Hospitals of the American Medical Association*. Chicago: American Medical Association, 1957.

Anderson, Julie, Francis Neary, and John V. Pickstone. *Surgeons, Manufacturers, and Patients: A Transatlantic History of Total Hip Replacement*. New York: Palgrave MacMillan, 2007.

Anderson, Odin W. *Blue Cross since 1929: Accountability and the Public Trust*. Cambridge, MA: Ballinger, 1975.

Anderson, Ronald, and John F. Newman. "Societal and Individual Determinants of Medical Care Utilization in the United States." *Milbank Quarterly* (1973): 95–124.

Apel, Otto, and Pat Apel. *MASH: An Army Surgeon in Korea*. Lexington: University of Kentucky Press, 1998.

Appelman, Roy E. *South to the Naktong, North to the Yalu*. Washington, DC: Office of Military History, 1961.

Apple, Rima D. *Vitamania: Vitamins in American Culture*. New Brunswick, NJ: Rutgers University Press, 1996.

Archibald, Edward W. "Higher Degrees in the Profession of Surgery." *Annals of Surgery* 102 (1935): 481–95.

Arnott, James M. "The Hunterian Oration." London: John Scott, 1843.

Artz, Curtis P., ed. *The Battle Wound: Clinical Experiences*. Vol. 3 of *Battle Casualties in Korea: Studies of the Surgical Research Team*. Washington, DC: Army Medical Service Graduate School, 1954.

———. "Massive Transfusions, Blood Derivatives, and Plasma Expanders." In *Recent Advances in Medicine and Surgery (19–30 April 1954) Based on Professional Medical Experiences in Japan and Korea, 1950–1953*, vol. 1, 202–13. Washington, DC: Army Medical Service Graduate School, 1955.

Artz, Curtis P., Yoshio Sako, and Alvin W. Brownell. "Massive Transfusion in the Severely Wounded." In *The Battle Wound: Clinical Experiences*, vol. 3 of *Battle Casualties in Korea: Studies of the Surgical Research Team*, edited by Curtis P. Artz, 66–71. Washington, DC: Army Medical Service Graduate School, 1954.

Asman, Conradus. "De aneurysmate." PhD diss., Groningue University, 1773.

Atwater, Edward C. "Of Grande Dames, Surgeons, and Hospitals: Batavia, New York, 1900–1940." *Journal of the History of Medicine and Allied Sciences* 45 (1990): 414–51.

Austen, Gerald, et al. "Hermes C. Grillo." *Harvard Gazette*, 15 November 2007. http://news.harvard.edu/gazette/story/2007/11/hermes-c-grillo/ (accessed 5 November 2013).

Baader, William, and Lloyd M. Nyhus. "The Life of Carl Beck and an Important Interval with Alexis Carrel." *SGO* 163, no. 1 (1986): 85–88.

Bahnson, Henry T. "Considerations in the Excision of Aortic Aneurysms." *Annals of Surgery* 138 (1953): 377–86.

Balch, Henry H., William H. Meroney, and Yoshio Sako. "Observations on the Surgical Care of Patients with Post-traumatic Renal Insufficiency." In *Post-traumatic Renal Insufficiency*, vol. 4 of *Battle Casualties in Korea: Studies of the Surgical Research Team*, edited by William H. Meroney, 71–95. Washington, DC: Army Medical Service Graduate School, 1954.

Bamberger, Peter Kurt. "The Adoption of Laparotomy for the Treatment of Penetrating Abdominal Wounds in War." *Military Medicine* 161, no. 4 (1996): 189–96.

Barker, Nelson W. "Diagnosis and Treatment of Chronic Occlusive Disease of the Peripheral Arteries." *Wisconsin Medical Journal* 49 (1950): 470–74.

Barker, Wiley F. *Clio: The Arteries.* Austin, TX: R. G. Landes, 1992.

———. "A History of Endarterectomy." *Perspectives in Vascular Surgery* 4 (1991): 1–12.

Barnes, Benjamin. "Discarded Operations: Surgical Innovation by Trial and Error." In *Cost, Risks, and Benefits of Surgery*, edited by John P. Bunker, Benjamin A. Barnes and Frederick Mosteller, 109–23. New York: Oxford University Press, 1977.

Barnes, J. M., and J. Trueta. "Arterial Spasm: An Experimental Study." *British Journal of Surgery* 30 (1942–43): 74–79.

Barr, Justin. "Battle of the Bulge: Aortic Aneurysm Management from Early Modernity to the Present." *Annals of Internal Medicine* 166 (2017): 291–96.

———. "The Education of American Surgeons and the Rise of Surgical Residencies, 1930–1960." *Journal of the History of Medicine and Allied Sciences* 73 (2018): 274–302.

———. "Military Medicine of the Russo-Japanese War and Its Influence on the Modernization of the US Army Medical Department." *US Army Medical Department Journal*, October–December 2016, 118–28.

———. "A Short History of Dapsone, or An Alternative Model of Drug Development." *Journal of the History of Medicine and Allied Sciences* 66, no. 5 (2011): 425–67.

Barr, Justin, Kenneth J. Cherry, and Norman M. Rich. "Vascular Surgery in the Pacific Theaters of World War II: The Persistence of Ligation Amid Unique Military Medical Conditions," *Annals of Surgery* 269, no. 6 (2019): 1054–58.

Barr, Justin, and Sean Montgomery. "Helicopter MEDEVAC in the Korean War: Did it Matter?" *Journal of Trauma and Acute Care Surgery* 87, no. 1 (2019): s10–s13.

Barr, Justin, and Theodore N. Pappas. "The Role of the American Board of Surgery on the Development of Surgical Residences in Post–World War II America." *American Surgeon* 85, no. 3 (2019): 245–51.

Barr, Justin, and Dale C. Smith. "The History of Trauma Care," in *Skeletal Trauma*, 6th ed., edited by Bruce Browner. (Philadelphia: Elsevier, 2019 forthcoming).

Bartrip, Peter. *Mirror of Medicine: A History of the BMJ*. Cambridge: Cambridge University Press, 1990.

Battle Circus. Directed by Richard Brooks, Metro-Goldwyn-Meyer, 1953.

Beck, Carl, and Alexis Carrel. "A Demonstration of Specimens Illustrating a Method of Formation of a Prethoracic Esophagus." *Illinois Medical Journal* 7 (1905): 463–64.

Beebe, Gilbert W., and Michael E. DeBakey. *Battle Casualties: Incidence, Mortality, and Logistic Considerations*. Springfield, IL: Charles C. Thomas, 1952.

Beecher, Henry K., Henrik H. Bendixen, Phillips Hallowell, Henning Pontoppidan, and Donald P. Todd. "The Anesthetist as a Physician." *JAMA* 188 (April 1964): 49–55.

Beger, Hans C. "John M. Howard, MD." *Langenbecks Archives of Surgery* 388 (2003): 140.

Berberish, J., and S. Hirsch. "Die Röntgenographische Darstellung der Arterien und Venen am Lebenden Menschen." *Klinische Wochenschrift* 2, no. 49 (December 1923): 2226–28.

Berman, Harry L. "The X-Ray Service in an Army Area Surgical Hospital." In *Recent Advances in Medicine and Surgery (19–30 April 1954) Based on Professional Medical Experiences in Japan and Korea, 1950–1953*, vol. 1, 135–44. Washington, DC: Army Medical Service Graduate School, 1955.

Bernheim, Bertrand M. "Blood-Vessel Surgery in the War." *SGO* 30 (1920): 564–67.

———. "The Ideal Operation for Aneurysm of the Extremity: Report of a Case." *Bulletin of the Johns Hopkins Hospital* 27, no. 302 (April 1916): 93–95.

———. *Surgery of the Vascular System*. Philadelphia: J. B. Lippincott, 1913.

Best, Charles H. "Preparation of Heparin and Its Use in the First Clinical Cases." *Circulation* 19 (1959): 79–86.

Betcher, Albert M., Benjamin J. Ciliberti, Paul M. Wood, and Lewis H. Wright. "The Jubilee Year of Organized Anesthesia." *Anesthesia* 17 (1956): 226–64.

Bevan, Arthur D. "The Carrel-Dakin Treatment." *JAMA* 69, no. 20 (17 November 1917): 1727–28.

———. "The Study and Teaching and the Practice of Surgery." *Annals of Surgery* 98 (1933): 481–94.

Beyer, James C, William F. Enos, and Robert H. Holmes. "Personnel Protective Armor." In *Wound Ballistics*, edited by James C. Beyer, 641–89. Washington, DC: Office of the Surgeon General, 1962.

Bickham, Warren Stone. "Arteriovenous Aneurisms." *Annals of Surgery* 39, no. 5 (May 1904): 767–75.

Bigger, I. A. "Treatment of Traumatic Aneurysms and Arteriovenous Fistula." *Archives of Surgery* 49, no. 3 (September 1944): 170–79.

Billings, John S. *The History and Literature of Surgery*. 1895. New York City: Argosy-Antiquarian, 1970.

Bird, Clarence E. "Sympathectomy as a Preliminary to the Obliteration of Popliteal Aneurisms, with a Suggestion as to Sympathetic Block in Cases of Ligature, Suture, or Thrombosis of Large Arteries." *SGO* 60 (May 1935): 926–29.

Blair, B. M. "Winslow and the Sympathetic System." *British Medical Journal* 2, no. 3756 (31 December 1932): 1200.

Blaisdell, F. William, Albert B. Hall, Robert C. Lim Jr., and Wesley C. Moore. "Aorto-Iliac Arterial Substitutions Utilizing Subcutaneous Grafts." *Annals of Surgery* 172 (1970): 775–80.

Blakemore, Arthur H. "Restorative Endoaneurysmorrhaphy by Vein Graft Inlay." *Transactions of the American Surgical Association* 65 (1947): 461–69.

Blakemore, Arthur H., and Jere W. Lord Jr. "A Nonsuture Method of Blood Vessel Anastomosis." *JAMA* 127, no. 12 (24 March 1945): 685–91; no. 13 (31 March 1945): 748–53.

———. "A Nonsuture Method of Blood Vessel Anastomosis: Review of Experimental Study, Report of Clinical Cases." *Annals of Surgery* 121, no. 4 (April 1945): 435–51.

Blakemore, Arthur H., Jere W. Lord Jr., and Paul L. Stefko. "Restoration of Blood Flow in Damaged Arteries: Further Studies on a Nonsuture Method of Blood Vessel Anastamosis." *Annals of Surgery* 117, no. 4 (April 1943): 481–97.

———. "The Severed Primary Artery in the War Wounded: A Nonsuture Method of Bridging Arterial Defects." *Surgery* 12 (1942): 488–508.

Blakemore, Arthur H., and Arthur B. Voorhees Jr. "The Use of Tubes Constructed from Vinyon 'N' Cloth in Bridging Arterial Defects—Experimental and Clinical." *Annals of Surgery* 140 (1954): 324–33.

Blanc, David. *Fake Silk: The Lethal History of Viscose Rayon*. New Haven, CT: Yale University Press, 2016.

Blight, David W. *Race and Reunion: The Civil War in American Memory*. Cambridge, MA: Harvard University Press, 2001.

Bliss, Michael. *The Discovery of Insulin*. Chicago: University of Chicago Press, 1982.

Blume, Stewart S. *Insight and Industry: On the Dynamics of Technological Change in Medicine*. Cambridge, MA: MIT Press, 1992.

Bollet, Alfred Jay. *Civil War Medicine: Challenges and Triumphs*. Tucson, AZ: Galen Press, 2002.

Bonner, Thomas N. *American Doctors and German Universities: A Chapter in International Intellectual Relations, 1870–1914*. Lincoln: University of Nebraska Press, 1963.

———. *Becoming a Physician: Medical Education in Britain, France, Germany, and the United States, 1750–1945*. Baltimore: Johns Hopkins University Press, 1995.

Bostetter, Mary. "The Journalism of Thomas Wakley." In *Innovators and Preachers: The Role of the Editor in Victorian England*, edited by J. H. Wiener, 275–92. Westport, CT: Greenwood Press, 1985.

Bourke, Joanna. *Dismembering the Male: Men's Bodies, Britain, and the Great War*. Chicago: University of Chicago Press, 1996.

Bourne, A. W. "Traumatic Aneurysm: A Series of Eight Cases from General Hospital Egypt." *Journal of the Royal Army Medical Corps* 28 (1917): 276–83.

Bowers, Raymond V. "Differential Intensity of Intra-societal Diffusion." *American Sociological Review* 3 (1938): 21–31.

Bowlby, Anthony, and Cuthbert Wallace. "The Development of British Surgery at the Front." *British Medical Journal* 1, no. 2944 (2 June 1917): 705–21.

Bradford, Bert J., Jr. "Vascular Injuries in Battle Casualties." *West Virginia Medical Journal* 42 (May 1946): 105–8.

Bradford, Bert J., Jr., and M. J. Moore. "Vascular Injuries in War." *SGO* 83 (1946): 667–73.

Brandt, Allan M. *The Cigarette Century: The Rise, Fall, and Deadly Persistence of the Product That Defined America*. New York: Basic Books, 2007.

———. *No Magic Bullet: A Social History of Venereal Disease in the United States Since 1880*. Expanded ed. New York: Oxford University Press, 1987.

Bresalier, Michael. "Fighting Flu: Military Pathology, Vaccines, and the Conflicted Identity of the 1918–19 Pandemic in Britain." *Journal of the History of Medicine and Allied Sciences* 68, no. 1 (January 2013): 87–128.

Brewer, George Emerson. "Some Experiments with a New Method of Closing Wounds of the Larger Arteries." *Annals of Surgery* 40, no. 6 (December 1904): 856–64.

Brewer, L. A. "The Contributions of the Second Auxiliary Surgical Group to Military Surgery During World War II with Special Reference to Thoracic Surgery." *Annals of Surgery* 197, no. 3 (1987): 318–26.

Briau, Eugène, and Mathieu Jaboulay. "Recherches expérimentales sur la suture et la greffe artérielles." *Lyon Medicale* 81 (1896): 97–99.

Bricker, Eugene, Frank Gerbode, and David Habif. "The Effect of Health Insurance Programs on Residency Training in Surgery." *Surgery* 32 (1952): 333–40.

Brieger, Gert H. "From Conservative to Radical Surgery in Late Nineteenth-Century America." In *Medical Theory, Surgical Practice: Studies in the History of Surgery*, edited by Christopher Lawrence, 216–31. New York: Routledge, 1992.

———. "A Portrait of Surgery: Surgery in America, 1875–1889." *Surgical Clinics of North America* 67 (December 1987): 1181–216.

Brock, Claire. "Women in Surgery: Patients and Practitioners." In *The Palgrave Handbook of the History of Surgery*, edited by Thomas Schlich, 133–52. London: Palgrave Macmillan, 2018.

Brock, R. C. *Life and Work of Astley Cooper*. London: E & S Livingstone, 1952.

Brooks, Barney. "Intra-arterial Injection of Sodium Iodid." *JAMA* 82, no. 13 (1924): 1016–19.

———. "Pathological Changes in Muscle as a Result of Disturbances of Circulation: An Experimental Study of Volkmann's Ischemic Paralysis." *Archives of Surgery* 5 (1922): 188–216.

———. "Surgical Application of Therapeutic Venous Obstruction." *Archives of Surgery* 19, no. 1 (1929): 1–23.

Brooks, Barney, et al. "Simultaneous Vein Ligation: An Experimental Study of the Effect of Ligation of the Concomitant Vein on the Incidence of Gangrene Following Arterial Obstruction." *SGO* 59 (1934): 496–500.

Brougham, E. J. "Arterial Anastamosis by Invagination." *SGO* 2, no. 4 (April 1906): 410–12.

Brown, George E., and Alfred W. Adson. "Calorimetric Studies of the Extremities Following Lumbar Sympathetic Ramisection and Ganglionectomy." *American Journal of Medical Science* 170 (August 1925): 232–40.

———. "Physiological Effects of Thoracic and of Lumbar Sympathetic Ganglionectomy or Section of Trunk." *Archives of Neurology and Psychiatry* 22 (August 1929): 322–57.

Bruce-Chwatt, L. J. "Changing Tides of Chemotherapy of Malaria." *British Medical Journal*, 7 (1964): 581.

Bryant, J. H. "Two Clinical Lectures on Aneurysms of the Abdominal Aorta." *Clinical Journal* 23 (1903): 71–80.

Bud, Robert. *Penicillin: Triumph and Tragedy*. New York: Oxford University Press, 2007.

Buderi, Robert. *The Invention That Changed the World: How a Small Groups of Radar Pioneers Won the Second World War and Launched a Technological Revolution*. New York: Simon and Schuster, 1996.

Buerger, Paul T. "Medical Support for Mountain Fighting in Korea." *Military Surgeon* 109, no. 6 (December 1951): 694–700.

Bull, James W., and Herman Fischgold. *A Short History of Neuroradiology*. N.p.: Schering, 1967.

Bundesen, Herman. "Artery Banks Now Aid Patients with Aneurysms." *Anderson Daily Bulletin*, 23 July 1954, 4.

Burci, Enrico. "Ricerche sperimentali sul processo di riparazione delle ferite longitudinali delle arterie." *Atti della Società Toscana di Scienze Natural* 11 (1890): 50–66.

Burns, Shock, Wound Healing, and Vascular Injuries. Philadelphia: W. B. Saunders, 1943.

Bush, Edward. "Doctor's Idea Leads to Firm and Success." *Chicago Daily Tribune,* 9 February 1953, F5.

Byerly, Carol R. *Fever of War: The Influenza Epidemic in the U.S. Army during World War I.* New York: New York University Press, 2005.

Bynum, William F., and Janice C. Wilson. "Periodical Knowledge: Medical Journals and Their Editors in Nineteenth Century Britain." In *Medical Journals and Medical Knowledge,* edited by William F. Bynum, Stephan Lock, and Roy Porter, 29–48. New York: Routledge, 1992.

Callow, Allan D., and C. Stuart Welch. "Arterial Anastomosis in Experimental Arterial Injury." *SGO* 90 (1950): 77–85.

Caplow, Theodore. *The First Measured Century: An Illustrated Guide to Trends in America, 1900–2000.* Washington, DC: AEI Press, 2001.

Carle, Donald E. "Medical Experiences in Korea." *U.S. Armed Forces Medical Journal* 2, no. 11 (1951): 1623–30.

Carrel, Alexis. "Heterotransplantation of Blood Vessels Preserved in Cold Storage." *Journal of Experimental Medicine* 9 (1907): 226–28.

———. "Latent Life of Arteries." *Journal of Experimental Medicine* 12 (1910): 460–90.

———. *Man, the Unknown.* New York: Harper & Brothers, 1935.

———. "The Preservation of Tissues and Its Application in Surgery." *JAMA* 59 (1912): 523–27.

———. "The Results of Transplantation of Blood Vessels, Organs, and Limbs." *JAMA* 51, no. 20 (1908): 1662–67.

———. "La technique opératoire des anastomeses vasculaires et la transplantation des viscères." *Lyon Medical* 98 (1902): 859–64.

———. "Traitement abortif de l'infection des plaies." *Bulletin Academie Medicine Paris* 74 (1915): 361–68.

———. "The Transplantation of Organs. A Preliminary Communication." *JAMA* 45, no. 22 (25 November 1905): 1645–46.

———. *The Voyage to Lourdes.* Translated by Virgilia Peterson. New York: Harper and Brothers, 1950.

Carrel, Alexis, and Georges Dehelly. *Le traitement des plaies infectées.* Paris: Masson et Cie, 1917.

———. *Treatment of Infected Wounds.* Translated by Herbert Child. New York: Paul B. Hoeber, 1917.

Carrel, Alexis, and Charles C. Guthrie. "Anastomosis of Blood Vessels by the Patching Method and Transplantation of the Kidney." *JAMA* 47, no. 20 (17 November 1906): 1648–51.

———. "Extirpation and Replantation of the Thyroid Gland with Reversal of the Circulation." *Science* 22, no. 565 (27 October 1905): 535.

———. "Functions of a Transplanted Kidney." *Science* 22, no. 563 (13 October 1905): 473.

———. "A New Method for the Homoplastic Transplantation of the Ovary." *Science* 23, no. 589 (13 April 1906): 591.

———. "Results of a Replantation of the Thigh." *Science* 23, no. 584 (9 March 1906): 393–94.

———. "The Transplantation of Vein and Other Organs." *American Medicine* 10 (December 1905): 1101.

Carter, B. Noland. "The Fruition of Halsted's Concept of Surgical Training." *Surgery* 32 (1952): 518–27.

Carter, B. Noland, and Michael E. DeBakey. "Special Reports and Statistical Data." In *Thoracic Surgery*, vol. 2, edited by Frank Berry, 529–53. Washington, DC: Office of the Surgeon General, 1965.

Centers for Disease Control and Prevention. "National Hospital Discharge Survey: 2010, Table: Number by Procedure Category and Age." https://www.cdc.gov/nchs/data/nhds/4procedures/2010pro4_numberprocedureage.pdf. Available 23 December 2018.

Chandler, James G., et al. "Ben Eiseman, MD (1917–2012)." *Journal of Trauma and Acute Care Surgery* 75, no. 3 (2013): 529–35.

Charles, Arthur F., and David A. Scott. "Studies on Heparin I: The Preparation of Heparin." *Journal of Biological Chemistry* 102 (1933): 425–29.

———. "Studies on Heparin II: Heparin in Various Tissues." *Journal of Biological Chemistry* 102 (1933): 431–35.

———. "Studies on Heparin III: The Purification of Heparin." *Journal of Biological Chemistry* 102 (1933): 437–48.

———. "Studies on Heparin IV: Observations on the Chemistry of Heparin, the Purification of Heparin." *Biochemical Journal* 30, no 10 (1936): 1927–33.

Chauliac, Guy. *The Major Surgery of Guy de Chauliac Surgeon and Master in Medicine of the University of Montpellier*. Translated by E. Nicase. Retranslated by Leonard D. Grossman. San Francisco: Xlibris, 2007.

Chesney, Alan M. *The Johns Hopkins Hospital and the Johns Hopkins University School of Medicine: A Chronicle*. Vols. 1–3. Baltimore: Johns Hopkins University Press, 1943–63.

Child, Charles G., III. "Eck's Fistula." *SGO* 96 (1953): 375–76.

Christopher, Frederick, ed. *A Textbook of Surgery by American Authors*. Philadelphia: W. B. Saunders, 1936.

Churchill, Edward D. "Graduate Training in Surgery at the Massachusetts General Hospital." *Harvard Medical Alumni Bulletin* 14 (1940): 28–36.

———. *Surgeon to Soldiers: Diary and Records of the Surgical Consultant Allied Force Headquarters, World War II*. Philadelphia: J. B. Lippincott, 1972.

Clayton, William. "Patch Sewn into Artery of Windsor." *Washington Post*, 17 December 1963, C11.

Cohn, Isidore, with Herman B. Deutsch. *Rudolph Matas: A Biography of One of the Great Pioneers in Surgery*. New York: Doubleday, 1960.

Cole, Frank R. "Results of Sympathectomy in Diabetic Arteriosclerotic Peripheral Vascular Disease." *New York State Medical Journal* 50 (1950): 1607–8.

Coleman, James S., Elihu Katz, and Herbert Menzel. *Medical Innovation: A Diffusion Study.* New York: Bobbs-Merrill, 1966.

Condie, Spencer J. *Russell M. Nelson: Father, Surgeon, Apostle.* Salt Lake City, UT: Deseret Book Company, 2013.

Condon-Rall, Mary Ellen, and Albert E. Cowdrey. *Medical Service in the War against Japan.* Washington, DC: Center of Military History, 1998.

Conklin, William S., and Elton Watkins Jr. "Use of the Potts-Smith-Gibson Clamp for Division of Patent Ductus Arteriosus." *Journal of Thoracic Surgery* 19 (1950): 361–70.

Conley, James, and C. M. Schroeder. "Session on Principles of Arterial Surgery." *Wisconsin Medical Journal* 50, no. 6 (1951).

Conway, Herbert, and George Plain. "Pulsating Hematoma, False Aneurysm, and Arteriovenous Fistula Due to War Injuries." *Surgery* 19 (1946): 383–406.

Cooke, Francis N., et al. "Blood Vessel Bank." *United States Armed Forces Medical Journal* 2, no. 1 (1951): 1779–85.

Cooke, Francis N., Carl W. Hughes, Edward J. Jahnke, and Sam F. Seeley. "Homologous Arterial Grafts and Autogenous Vein Grafts Used to Bridge Large Arterial Defects in Man." *Surgery* 33 (1953): 183–89.

Cooke, F. N., F. T. Kurzweg, and T. E. Starzl. "Blood Vessel Bank: Organization and Function." *Bulletin of the University of Miami School of Medicine and Jackson Memorial Hospital* 2 (1957): 26–31.

Cooper, Astley. "Case of Ligature on the Aorta." In *Surgical Essays*, 2nd ed, by Astley Cooper and Benjamin Travers, 111–41. London, 1818.

———. *The Lectures of Sir Astley Cooper on the Principles and Practice of Surgery.* Vol 3. London, 1827.

Cooper, David K. C. *Open Heart: The Radical Surgeons Who Revolutionized Medicine.* New York: Kaplan, 2010.

Cooper, Samuel. *A Dictionary of Practical Surgery: Containing a Complete Exhibition of the Present State of the Principles and Practices of Surgery.* 2nd ed. Philadelphia: B&T Kite, 1810.

Cooter, Roger. "Of War and Epidemics: Unnatural Couplings, Problematic Conceptions." *Journal for the Social History of Medicine* 16, no. 2 (2003): 283–302.

———. *Surgery and Society in Peace and War: Orthopaedics and the Organization of Modern Medicine, 1880–1948.* Houndsmill: MacMillan Press, 1993.

———. "War and Modern Medicine." In *Companion Encyclopedia of the History of Medicine*, vol. 2, edited by W. F. Bynum and Roy Porter, 1536–73. London: Routledge, 1993.

Cope, Zachary. *The Royal College of Surgeons of England: A History.* London: Anthony Blond, 1959.

Coppard, George. *With a Machinegun to Cambrai: The Tale of a Young Tommy in Kitchener's Army, 1914–1918.* London: Her Majesty's Stationery Office, 1969.

Corner, George W. *History of the Rockefeller Institute: Origin and Growth.* New York: Rockefeller Institute Press, 1964.

Cosmas, Graham A., and Albert E. Cowdrey. *Medical Service in the European Theater of Operations.* Washington, DC: Center of Military History, 1992.

Courington, Frederick W., and Roderick K. Calverley. "Anesthesia on the Western Front: The Anglo-American Experience of World War I." *Anesthesiology* 65 (1986): 642–53.

Cowdrey, Albert E. *Fighting for Life: American Military Medicine in World War II.* New York: Free Press, 1994.

———. "MASH vs. *M*A*S*H*: The Mobile Army Surgical Hospital." *Medical Heritage* 1 (1985): 4–11.

———. *The Medics' War.* Washington, DC: Center of Military History, 1987.

Cowell, E. M. "Simultaneous Ligation of Arterial and Venous Trunks in War Surgery." *British Medical Journal* 1 (1917): 577–78.

Crafoord, Clarence. "Preliminary Report on Post-operative Treatment with Heparin as a Preventive of Thrombosis." *Acta Chirurgica Scandinavia* 79 (1936): 407–26.

Crawford, E. Stanley, Michael E. DeBakey, and Denton A. Cooley. "Clinical Use of Synthetic Substitutes in Three Hundred Seventeen Patients." *Archives of Surgery* 76 (1958): 261–70.

Creager, Angela N. H. "Biotechnology and Blood: Edwin Cohn's Plasma Fractionation Project, 1940–1953." In *Private Science: Biotechnology and the Rise of the Molecular Sciences,* edited by Arnold Thackray, 39–62. Philadelphia: University of Pennsylvania Press, 1998.

———. *Life Atomic: A History of Radioisotopes in Science and Medicine.* Chicago: University of Chicago Press, 2013.

———. "Producing Molecular Therapeutics from Human Blood: Edwin Cohn's Wartime Enterprise." In *Molecularizing Biology and Medicine: New Practices and Alliances, 1910s–1970s,* edited by Sorraya de Chadarevian and Harmke Kamminga, 107–38. Amsterdam: Harwood Academic, 1998.

———. "'What Blood Told Dr. Cohn': World War II, Plasma Fractionation, and the Growth of Human Blood Research." *Studies for the History and Philosophy of Biology, Biomedicine, and Science* 30, no. 3 (1999): 377–405.

Creech, Oscar, Jr. "Endo-aneurysmorrhaphy and the Treatment of Aortic Aneurysm." *Annals of Surgery* 164 (1966): 935–46.

Creech, Oscar, Jr., Ralph A. Deterling Jr., Sterling Edwards, Ormand C. Julian, Robert R. Linton, and Harris Shumacker Jr. "Vascular Prosthesis: Report of the Committee for the Study of Vascular Prostheses of the Society for Vascular Surgery." *Surgery* 41 (1957): 62–75.

Crenner, Christopher. "Placebos and the Progress of Surgery." In *Technological Change in Modern Surgery: Historical Perspectives on Innovation,* edited by Christopher Crenner and Thomas Schlich, 156–84. Rochester, NY: University of Rochester Press, 2017.

Crewes, Emily M. "Colonel Edward Churchill's Transformation of Wound Care in the Mediterranean Theater of the Second World War." MA thesis, Valdosta State University, 2009.

Crile, George Washington. "Direct Transfusion of Blood in the Treatment of Hemorrhage: Preliminary Clinical Note." *JAMA* 47, no. 18 (1906): 1482–84.

―――. *Hemorrhage and Transfusion: An Experimental and Clinical Research*. New York: D. Appleton, 1909.

Crile, George Washington, and Grace Crile. *George Crile: An Autobiography*. New York: J. B. Lippincott, 1947.

Crosby, William H., ed. *Tools for Resuscitation*. Vol. 2 of *Battle Casualties in Korea: Studies of the Surgical Research Team*. Washington, DC: Army Medical Service Graduate School, 1954.

Crowe, Samuel J. *Halsted of Johns Hopkins: The Man and His Men*. Springfield, IL: Charles C. Thomas, 1957.

Crowther, M. Anne, and Marguerite W. Dupree. *Medical Lives in the Age of Surgical Revolution*. Cambridge: Cambridge University Press, 2007.

Cullen, Karen A., Margaret J. Hall, and Alexander Golosinskiy. "Ambulatory Surgery in the United States." *National Health Statistics Report* 11 (2009): 1–25.

Cushing, Harvey. "The Society of Clinical Surgery in Retrospect." *Annals of Surgery* 169 (January 1969): 1–9.

Cutler, Elliot C. "Military Surgery, United States Army, European Theater of Operations, 1944–1945." *SGO* 82 (1946): 261–74.

Dale, W. Andrew. "The Beginnings of Vascular Surgery." *Surgery* 76, no. 6 (December 1974): 849–66.

Dale, W. Andrew, ed., with George Johnson Jr., and James A. DeWeese. *Band of Brothers: Creators of Vascular Surgery*. Chapel Hill, NC: Self-published, 1996.

Dally, Ann. *Women under the Knife: A History of Surgery*. New York: Routledge, 1991.

Daunton, M. J. *Royal Mail: The Post Office since 1840*. London: Athlone Press, 1985.

Davis, Loyal. *Fellowship of Surgeons: A History of the American College of Surgeons*. Chicago: American College of Surgeons, 1988.

―――. *J. B. Murphy, Stormy Petrel of Surgery*. New York: G. P. Putnam's Sons, 1938.

Davis, Loyal, and Allen B. Kanavel. "The Effect of Sympathectomy on Spastic Paralysis of the Extremities." *JAMA* 86 (19 June 1926): 1890–93.

―――. "Sympathectomy in Raynaud's Disease, Erythromelalgia, and other Vascular Diseases of the Extremities." *SGO* 42 (1926): 729–42.

Davy, Henry, and Mabel Gates. "A Case of Dissecting Aneurysm of the Aorta." *British Medical Journal* 1, no. 3195 (25 March 1922): 471–72.

de Moulin, D. "Aneurysms in Antiquity." *Archivum Chirurgicum Neerlandicum* 13 (1961): 49–63.

―――. "Dominique Anel and His Operation for Aneurysm." *Bulletin of the History of Medicine* 34 (1960): 498–507.

————. "Historical Notes on Vascular Surgery II: Development of Vascular Suture in the 19th Century, after the Introduction of Antisepsis." *Archivum Chirurgicum Neerlandicum* 7 (1955): 321–30.

de Takáts, Gezá. "Vascular Surgery in the War." *War Medicine* 3 (1943): 291–96.

DeAnda, Abe, Jr., and Leora B. Balsam. "Historical Perspectives of the American Association for Thoracic Surgery: Keith Reemtsma (1925–2000)." *Journal of Thoracic and Cardiovascular Surgery* 150, no. 4 (2015): 762–64.

Deandra, Abe, Jr., and Aubrey C. Galloway. "Historical Perspectives of the American Association for Thoracic Surgery." *Journal of Thoracic and Cardiovascular Surgery* 145, no. 4 (2013): 906–8.

DeBakey, Michael E. "The Development of Vascular Surgery." *American Journal of Surgery* 137, no. 6 (June 1979): 697–738.

————. "Traumatic Vasospasm." *Bulletin of the U.S. Army Medical Department* (October 1944): 23–28.

DeBakey, Michael E., and William H. Amspacher. "Acute Arterial Injuries." *Surgical Clinics of North America* 29, no. 4 (1949): 1513–22.

DeBakey, Michael E., and Denton Cooley. "Surgical Treatment of Aneurysm of Abdominal Aorta by Resection and Restoration of Continuity with Homograft." *SGO* 97 (1953): 257–66.

DeBakey, Michael E., E. Stanley Crawford, Denton A. Cooley, and George C. Morris Jr. "Surgical Considerations of Occlusive Disease of the Abdominal Aorta and Iliac and Femoral Arteries: Analysis of 803 Cases." *Annals of Surgery* 14 (1958): 306–24.

DeBakey, Michael E., and Fiorindo Simeone. "Acute Battle-Incurred Arterial Injuries." In *Vascular Surgery in World War II*, edited by Daniel C. Elkin and Michael E. DeBakey, 60–148. Washington, DC: Office of the Surgeon General, 1955.

————. "Battle Injuries of the Arteries in World War II: An Analysis of 2,471 Cases." *Annals of Surgery* 123 (1946): 534–79.

"Delay Advised in Treatment of Aneurysm." *Bulletin of the U.S. Army Medical Department* 80 (September 1944): 3.

"Department of Surgery, Emory University School of Medicine, Atlanta, Georgia." *Archives of Surgery* 139 (2004): 359–61.

Derrick, John R., William D. Logan, and John M. Howard. "Pitfalls of Translumbar Aortography and Peripheral Arteriography." *Archives of Surgery* 76 (1958): 517–20.

Deterling, Ralph A. "Experience with Permanent By-pass Grafts in Treatment of Occlusive Arterial Disease." *Archives of Surgery* 76 (1958): 247–60.

Deterling, Ralph A., Jr., Claude C. Coleman Jr., and Mary S. Parshley. "Experimental Studies of the Frozen Homologous Aortic Graft." *Surgery* 29 (1951): 419–40.

Deterling, Ralph A., Jr., and Hiram E. Essex. "An Instrument Designed Primarily for Use in Surgical Procedures on the Aorta." *American Journal of Surgery* 77 (1949): 132–33.

Deterling, Ralph A., Jr., Mary S. Parshley, and J. Wallace Blunt. "A Critical Study of Present Criteria Governing Selection and Use of Blood Vessel Grafts." *Surgery* 33 (1953): 213–32.

Devine, Shauna. *Learning from the Wounded: The Civil War and the Rise of American Medical Science.* Chapel Hill: University of North Carolina Press, 2014.

Diamond, Louis K. "A History of Blood Transfusion." In *Blood, Pure and Eloquent: A Story of Discovery, of People, and of Ideas.* Edited by Maxwell M. Wintrobe, 659–90. New York: McGraw-Hill, 1980.

Dickinson, Everett H., Thomas E. Ashley, and Frank Gerbode. "The Definitive Treatment of Injuries to Major Blood Vessels Incurred in the Korean War." *Western Journal of Surgery, Obstetrics, and Gynecology* 59, no. 12 (1951): 625–34.

Diffrient, David Scott. *M*A*S*H.* Detroit: Wayne State University Press, 2008.

Dillard, Burl M., David L. Nelson, and Harold G. Norman Jr. "Review of 85 Major Traumatic Arterial Injuries." *Surgery* 63 (1968): 391–94.

Donovan, Thomas J. "The Uses of Plastic Tubes in the Reparative Surgery of Battle Injuries to Arteries with and without Intra-arterial Heparin Administration." *Annals of Surgery* 130 (1940): 1024–43.

Dörfler, Julius. "Ueber Arteriennaht." *Beiträge zur Klinischen Chirurgie* 25 (1899): 781.

Dorland, Peter, and James Nanney. *Dustoff: Army Aeromedical Evacuation in Vietnam.* Washington, DC: Center of Military History, 1982.

Doroshow, Deborah B. "Wassermann before Wedding Bells: Premarital Examination Laws in the United States, 1937–1950." *Social History of Medicine* (in press).

Dorrance, George Morris. "An Experimental Study of Suture of Arteries with a Description of a New Suture." *Annals of Surgery* 44, no. 3 (Sept 1906): 409–24.

"Dorsey's Operation for Inguinal Aneurism." *New England Journal of Medicine* 1 (1 January 1812): 106.

Dos Santos, Joao Cid. "From Embolectomy to Endarterectomy, or The Fall of a Myth." *Journal of Cardiovascular Surgery* 17 (1976): 113–28.

Doyon, M. "Rapport de foie avec la coagulation de sang: I. Conditions de l'incoagulabilité du sang circulant." *Journal de Physiologie et de Pathologie General* 14 (1912): 229–40.

"Dr. Mims Gage." *Bulletin of the Tulane Medical Faculty* 11, no. 3 (1952): 172–74.

Drachman, Virginia G. *Hospital with a Heart: Women Doctors and the Paradox of Separatism at the New England Hospital, 1862–1969.* Ithaca, NY: Cornell University Press, 1984.

Dripps, Robert D. "Anesthesia for Combat Casualties on the Basis of Experience in Korea." In *Tools for Resuscitation,* vol. 2 of *Battle Casualties in Korea: Studies of the Surgical Research Team,* edited by William H. Crosby, 241–55. Washington, DC: Army Medical Service Graduate School, 1954.

Driscoll, Robert S. "U.S. Army Medical Helicopters in the Korean War." *Military Medicine* 166, no. 4 (2001): 290–96.

Druml, W. "The Beginning of Organ Transplant: Emerich Ullmann (1861–1937)." *Wiener Klinische Wochenschrift* 114, no. 4 (2002): 128–37.

Dubost, Charles, Michel Allary, and Nicolas Oeconomos. "Resections of an Aneurysm of the Abdominal Aorta." *Archives of Surgery* 64, no. 3 (1952): 405–8.

Duffin, Jacalyn. "Religion and Medicine, Again: *JHMAS* Commentary on 'The Lourdes Medical Cures Revisited.'" *Journal of the History of Medicine and Allied Sciences* 69 (January 2014): 162–65.

Duffy, John, ed. *The Rudolph Matas History of Medicine in Louisiana.* Vol. 2. New Orleans: Louisiana State University Press, 1962.

Durkin, Joseph T. *Hope for Our Time: Alexis Carrel on Man and Society.* New York: Harper and Row, 1965.

Eastman, Joel W. *Styling vs. Safety: The American Automobile Industry and the Development of Automotive Safety, 1900–1966.* Lanham, MD: University Press of America, 1984.

Eccles, McAdam. "A Clinical Lecture on Aneurysms of War Wounds." *Journal of the Royal Army Medical Corps* 26 (1916): 405–15.

Eck, Nickolai V. "K voprosu o perevyazkie vorotnois veni: Predvaritelnoye soobshtshjenye." *Voenno-meditsinskiĭ Zhurnal* (St. Petersburg) 130, no. 2 (1877): 1–2.

Eckberg, Douglass Lee. "Crimes Known to Urban Police, by Type of Offense." In *Historical Statistics of the United States,* edited by Susan B. Carter et al., 5–225. Cambridge: Cambridge University Press, 2006.

———. "Estimates of Early Twentieth Century U.S. Homicide Rates: An Economic Forecasting Model." *Demography* 32 (1995): 1–16.

Edgcomb, J. H., et al. "Primaquine, SN 13272, a New Curative Agent in vivax Malaria: A Preliminary Report." *Journal of the Natural Malaria Society* 9 (1950): 285–92.

Edgerton, David. "From Innovation to Use: Ten Eclectic Theses on the Historiography of Technology." *History and Technology* 16 (1999): 111–36.

Edmonson, James E. "Asepsis and the Transformation of Surgical Instruments." *Transactions and Studies of the College of Physicians of Philadelphia* 13, no. 1 (1991): 75–91.

———. *American Surgical Instruments: The History of Their Manufacture and a Directory of Instrument Makers to 1900.* San Francisco: Norman, 1997.

Edwards, Jesse E. "A System for an Efficient Transfusion Service." *Bulletin of the US Army Medical Department* 4, no. 4 (1945): 481–85.

Ehrenfried, Alfred, and Walter Boothby. "The Technic of End-to-End Anastamosis." *Annals of Surgery* 54, no. 4 (1911): 485–95.

Elkin, Daniel C. "Aneurysm of the Aorta: Treatment by Ligation." *Annals of Surgery* 112 (1940): 895–908.

———. "Specialized Centers for the Management of Vascular Injuries and Diseases." In *Vascular Surgery,* edited by Daniel C. Elkin and Michael E. DeBakey, 1–16. Washington, DC: Office of the Surgeon General, 1955.

———. "Vascular Injuries of Warfare." *Annals of Surgery* 120 (1944): 284–306.

Elkin, Daniel C., and Harris B. Shumacker. "Arterial Aneurysms and Arteriovenous Fistulas—General Considerations." In *Vascular Surgery*, edited by Daniel C. Elkin and Michael E. DeBakey, 149–80. Washington, DC: Office of the Surgeon General, 1955.

Elliot, John, Walter L. Tatum, and George F. Busby. "Blood Plasma." *Military Surgeon* 88, no. 2 (February 1942): 118–28.

Ellis, Harold. "James Learmonth: Distinguished Academic Surgeon Who Operated on King George VI." *British Journal of Hospital Medicine* 78 (2017): 529.

Ellis, Terry A., II, Bradly J. Narr, and Douglas R. Bacon. "Developing a Specialty: J. S. Lundy's Three Major Contributions to Anesthesiology." *Journal of Clinical Anesthesia* 16 (2004): 226–29.

Engle, Eloise. *Medic: America's Medical Soldiers, Sailors, and Airmen from the Revolutionary War to Vietnam*. New York: John Day, 1967.

English, Peter C. *Shock, Physiological Surgery, and George Washington Crile: Medical Innovations in the Progressive Era*. Westport, CT: Greenwood Press, 1980.

Enos, William F., James C. Beyer, and Robert H. Holmes. "Pathogenesis of Coronary Disease in American Soldiers Killed in Korea." *JAMA* 158, no. 11 (1955): 912–14.

Enos, William F., Robert H. Holmes, and James Beyer. "Coronary Disease among United States Soldiers Killed in Action in Korea." *JAMA* 152, no. 12 (1953): 1091–93.

Erichsen, Johen E., ed. *Observations on Aneurism*. London: Sydenham Society, 1844.

Estes, J. Earle, Jr. "Abdominal Aortic Aneurysm: A Study of One Hundred and Two Cases." *Circulation* 2 (1950): 258–64.

Evans, William. "Presidential Address to the Midwestern Vascular Surgery Society, 1982." In *The Evolution of Modern Vascular Surgery: The Historical Perspective of the Midwestern Vascular Surgical Society, 1977–2001*, edited by John R. Pfeifer and John W. Hallet Jr., 161–68. Salem, MA: Midwestern Vascular Surgical Society: 2001.

"Extract of a letter from Mr. Lambert, surgeon at Newcastle upon Tyne, to Dr. Hunter; giving an account of a new method of treating an Aneurysm, Read June 15, 1761." In *Medical Observations and Inquiries*, vol. 2, edited by the Society of Physicians in London, 360–64. London: 1764.

Fehrenbach, T. R. *This Kind of War: A Study in Unpreparedness*. New York: MacMillan, 1963.

Fennell, Mary L. and Richard B. Warnecke. *The Diffusion of Medical Innovations: An Applied Network Analysis*. New York: Plenum Press, 1988.

Ferguson, Ira A., Sr., William B. Byrd, David K. McAfee. "Experience in the Management of Arterial Injuries." *Annals of Surgery* 153 (1961): 980–86.

Fernández-Zapico, Marín E. "'Keep at It!' Accept the Challenge of Your Critics." *Pancreatology* 9, no. 5 (2009): 551–53.

Feudtner, Christopher. *Bittersweet: Diabetes, Insulin, and the Transformation of an Illness*. Chapel Hill: University of North Carolina Press, 2003.

Fink, James J. *The Automobile Age.* Cambridge, MA: MIT Press, 1988.

Finney, J. M. T. *A Surgeon's Life: The Autobiography of J. M. T. Finney.* New York: G. P. Putnam's Sons, 1940.

Firor, Warfield M. "Residency Training in Surgery: Birth, Decay and Recovery." *Review of Surgery* 22 (1965): 153–57.

Floresco, M. N. "Conditions anatomique et technique de la transplantation du rein." *Journal de Physiologie et de Pathologie Generale* 7 (1905): 27–34.

Flothow, Paul G. "Diagnostic and Therapeutic Injections of the Sympathetic Nerves." *American Journal of Surgery* 14 (1931): 591–604, 625.

———. "Surgery of the Sympathetic Nervous System: A Report of Fourteen Sympathetic Ganglionectomies." *American Journal of Surgery* 10 (1930): 8–18.

———. "Sympathetic Alcoholic Injection for Relief of Arteriosclerotic Pain and Gangrene." *Northwest Medicine* 30 (1931): 408–12.

Fogelman, Morris J., and Elinor Reinmiller. "1880–1890: A Creative Decade in World Surgery." *American Journal of Surgery* 115 (1968): 812–24.

Fox, Daniel. "The Politics of the NIH Extramural Program, 1937–1950." *Journal of the History of Medicine and Allied Sciences* 42 (1987): 447–66.

Fox, Renée, and Judith P. Swazey. *Spare Parts: Organ Replacement in American Society.* New York: Oxford University Press, 1992.

Frampton, Sally, and Roger K. Kneebone. "John Wickham's New Surgery: 'Minimally Invasive Therapy,' Innovation, and Approaches to Medical Practice in Twentieth Century Britain." *Social History of Medicine* 30 (2016): 544–66.

Francis, Samuel W. *Biographical Sketches of Distinguished Living New York Surgeons.* New York: Bradburn, 1866.

François, Bernard, Esther M. Sternberg, and Elizabeth Fee. "The Lourdes Medical Cures Revisited." *Journal of the History of Medicine and Allied Sciences* 69 (January 2014): 135–62.

Freeman, Norman E., and Harris B. Shumacker Jr. "Arterial Aneurysms and Arteriovenous Fistulas: Maintenance of Arterial Continuity." In *Vascular Surgery*, edited by Daniel C. Elkin and Michael E. DeBakey, 264–301. Washington, DC: Office of the Surgeon General, 1955.

French, Roger D. *Antivivisection and Medical Science in Victorian Society.* Princeton, NJ: Princeton University Press, 1975.

Frieden, Nancy M. *Russian Physicians in an Era of Reform and Revolution: 1856–1905.* Princeton, NJ: Princeton University Press, 1981.

Friedman, David M. *The Immortalists: Charles Lindbergh, Dr. Alexis Carrel, and Their Daring Quest to Live Forever.* New York: Harper Collins, 2007.

Friedman, Steven G. *A History of Vascular Surgery.* 2nd ed. Mount Kisko, NY: Factura, 2005.

———. "Korea, M*A*S*H, and the Accidental Pioneers of Vascular Surgery." *Journal of Vascular Surgery* 66 (2017): 666–70.

Friedson, Eliot. *Profession of Medicine: A Study of the Sociology of Applied Knowledge.* Chicago: University of Chicago Press, 1988.

Fulton, John F. "Medicine, Warfare, and History." *JAMA* 135 no. 5 (1953): 482–88.

Fussel, Paul. *The Great War and Modern Memory*. New York: Oxford University Press, 2000.

Futrell, Robert F. *The United States Air Force in Korea*. Washington, DC: Government Printing Office, 2000 (1961).

Fye, W. Bruce. *American Cardiology: The History of a Specialty and Its College*. Baltimore: Johns Hopkins University Press, 1996.

———. *Caring for the Heart: Mayo Clinic and the Rise of Specialization*. New York: Oxford University Press, 2015.

———. "Heparin: The Contributions of William Henry Howell." *Circulation* 69 (1984): 1198–203.

———. "The Literature of Internal Medicine." In *Grand Rounds: One Hundred Years of Internal Medicine*, edited by Russell C. Maulitz and Diana E. Long, 55–84. Philadelphia: University of Pennsylvania Press, 1988.

Gage, Mims. "Editorial: The Development of the Collateral Circulation in Peripheral Arterial Aneurysms by Sympathetic Block." *Surgery* 7 (1940): 792–95.

———. "Mycotic Aneurysm of the Common Iliac Artery: Sympathetic Ganglion Block as an Aid in the Development of the Collateral Circulation in Arterial Aneurysms of Peripheral Arteries: Report of a Case." *American Journal of Surgery* 24, no. 3 (1934): 667–710.

Gage, Mims, and Alton Ochsner. "The Prevention of Ischemic Gangrene Following Surgical Operations upon the Major Peripheral Arteries by Chemical Section of the Cervicodorsal and Lumbar Sympathetics." *Annals of Surgery* 112 (1940): 938–59.

Gangloff, Amy B. "Medicalizing the Automobile: Public Health, Safety, and American Culture, 1920–1967." PhD diss., Stony Brook University, 2006.

Gariepy, Thomas P. "The Introduction and Acceptance of Listerian Antisepsis in the United States." *Journal of the History of Medicine and Allied Sciences*, 49 (1994): 167–206.

Garland, Hugh G. "The Pathology of Aneurysms: A Review of 167 Autopsies." *Journal of Pathology and Bacteriology* 35 (1932): 334–50.

Garland, Robert. "The Causation of Death in the *Iliad*: A Theological and Biological Investigation." *Bulletin of the Institute of Classical Studies* 28 (1981): 43–60.

Gavrus, Delia Elena. "'Making Bad Boys Good': Brain Surgery and the Juvenile Court in Progressive Era America." In *Technological Change in Modern Surgery: Historical Perspectives on Innovation*, edited by Thomas Schlich and Christopher Crenner, 71–99. Rochester, NY: University of Rochester Press, 2017.

———. "Men of Strong Opinion: Identity, Self-Representation, and the Performance of Neurosurgery, 1919–1950." PhD diss., University of Toronto, 2011.

General Principles Guiding the Treatment of Wounds of War: Conclusions Adopted by the Inter-Allied Surgical Conference Held in Paris, March and May, 1917. 2nd ed. London: His Majesty's Stationery Office, 1917.

Gibbons, Roy. "New Artery for Old Put Victim on Feet." *Chicago Daily Tribune*, 21 September 1953, 1, 16.

Gibson, Charles L. "The Carrel Method of Treating Wounds." *Annals of Surgery* 46 (1917): 262–79.

Gifford, Ray W., Edgar A. Hines, and Joseph M. Janes. "An Analysis and Follow-Up Study of One Hundred Popliteal Aneurysms." *Surgery* 33 (1953): 284–93.

Gilfillan, Rutherford S. "Thromboendarterectomy: Indication and Results in the Treatment of Localized Obstruction of Large Arteries." *New York State Medical Journal* 53 (1953): 2986–90.

Gillet, Mary C. *The Army Medical Department, 1917–1941*. Washington, DC: Center of Military History, 2009.

Ginn, L. Holmes, and H. Haskell Ziperman. "Surgery in Division Clearing Stations." *Military Surgeon* 113, no. 6 (December 1953): 443–47.

Gluck, Themosticles. "Über neuere Operationen an Blutgefäßen." *Archiv für Kinderheilkunde* 22 (1897): 374.

———. "Über zwei Fälle von Aortenaneurysmen nebst Bemerkungen über die Naht der Blutgefässe." *Chirurgie* 28 (1883): 548.

Goodman, Charles. "A Histological Study of the Circular Suture of the Blood-Vessels." *Annals of Surgery* 65 (1917): 693–703.

———. "Suture of Blood-Vessel Injuries from Projectiles of War." *SGO* 27 (1918): 528–29.

Gould, Alfred P. "Report to the Director-General Medical Services on Our Recent Visit to France to Study the Carrel-Dakin Treatment of Wounds." *Journal of the Royal Army Medical Corps* 29 (1917): 616–28.

Goyanes, José. "Nuevos trabajos de chirugia vascular." *El Siglo Medico* 2752 (September 1906): 561–64.

Grade, Carl J. "Vascular Anastomosis and Transplantation of Organs." MD thesis, Yale University, 1910.

Graduate Medical Education: Report of the Commission on Graduate Medical Education. Chicago: University of Chicago Press, 1940.

Graham, Evarts A. "Have the Armed Services Crippled Medical Education?" *Saturday Evening Post*, 27 January 1945, 34, 39, 41–42.

———. "What Kind of Medical Officers Do the Armed Services Want?" *SGO* 24 (August 1944): 217–19.

Grainger, Ronald G. "Development of Intravascular Contrast Agents: The First 100 Years." In *Advances in X-Ray Contrast: Collected Papers*, edited by P. Dawson and W. Clauss, 89–96. Springer eBook: 1997. http://link.springer.com/content/pdf/10.1007%2F978-94-011-3959-5.pdf (accessed 6 September 2013).

Grant, Ronald N. "Front Line Surgery in Korea." *Military Surgeon* 114, no. 4 (1954): 266–69.

Graves, Clifford L. *Front Line Surgeons: A History of the Third Auxiliary Surgical Group*. San Diego: Frye & Smith, 1950.

Greene, Jeremy. *Prescribing by Numbers: Drugs and the Definitions of Disease.* Baltimore: Johns Hopkins University Press, 2007.

Greenwood, John T., and Clifton Berry. *Medics at War.* Annapolis: Naval Institute Press, 2005.

Griffin, Ward O. "The American Board of Surgery in the 20th Century." Unpublished manuscript. American Board of Surgery, 2004.

Grillo, Hermes C. "Edward D. Churchill and the 'Rectangular' Surgical Residency." *Surgery* 136 (2004): 947–52.

Grob, Gerald. "The Rise and Decline of the Tonsillectomy in Twentieth-Century America." *Journal of the History of Medicine and Allied Sciences* 62, no. 2 (2007): 383–421.

Gross, Michael L. *Bioethics and Armed Conflict: Moral Dilemmas of Medicine and War.* Cambridge, MA: MIT Press, 2006.

Gross, Robert E. "Complete Surgical Division of the Patent Ductus Arteriosus." *SGO* 78 (1944): 36–43.

Gross, Robert E., A. H. Bill Jr., and E. C. Pierce. "Methods for Preservation and Transplantation of Arterial Grafts." *SGO* 88 (1949): 689–701.

Gross, Robert E., and John P. Hubbard. "Surgical Ligation of a Patent Ductus Arteriosus: Report of First Successful Case." *JAMA* 112, no. 8 (1939): 729–31.

Gross, Robert E., and Charles A. Hufnagel. "Coarctation of the Aorta: Experimental Studies Regarding Its Surgical Correction." *NEJM* 233, no. 10 (1945): 286–93.

Gross, Robert E., Elliot S. Hurwitt, Alexander H. Bill Jr., and E. Converse Peirce. "Preliminary Observations on the Use of Human Arterial Grafts in the Treatment of Certain Cardiovascular Defects." *NEJM* 239 (1948): 578–79.

Gross, Samuel D. *Valentine Mott, M.D., LL.D.* New York: D. Appleton, 1868.

Guinan, Patrick D., Kenneth J. Printen, James L. Stone, and James S. T. Yao. *A History of Surgery at Cook County Hospital.* Chicago: Amika Press, 2015.

Guthrie, Charles Claude. *Blood Vessel Surgery and Its Applications.* Pittsburgh: University of Pittsburgh Press, 1959.

———. "End Results of Arterial Restoration with Devitalized Tissue." *JAMA* 73 (1919): 186–87.

———. "On Misleading Statements." *Science* 29 (1909): 29–31.

———. "Transplantation of Formaldehyde-Fixed Blood Vessels." *Science* 27 (1908): 473.

Haiken, Elizabeth. *Venus Envy: A History of Cosmetic Surgery.* Baltimore: Johns Hopkins University Press, 1997.

Halberstam, David E. *The Coldest Winter: America and the Korean War.* New York: Hyperion, 2007.

———. *The Fifties.* New York: Villard Books, 1993.

Hall, Richard C. *The Balkan Wars, 1912–1913: Prelude to the First World War.* Florence, KY: Routledge, 2000.

Haller, John S. "Treatment of Infected Wounds During the Great War." *Southern Medical Journal* 85, no. 3 (March 1992): 303–15.

Halsted, William S. "Carrel-Dakin Method of the Treatment of Infected Wounds: Antiseptics in the Aseptic Period." In *The Treatment of War Wounds*, 2nd ed., edited by W. W. Keen, 252–59. Philadelphia: W. B. Saunders, 1918.

———. "Partial Occlusion of Large Arteries by Aluminum Bands." *Transactions of the American Surgical Association* 28 (1910): 49–52.

———. "A Striking Elevation of the Temperature of the Hand and Forearm Following the Excision of a Subclavian Aneurism and Ligations of the Left Subclavian and Axillary Arteries." *Johns Hopkins Hospital Bulletin* 31 (1920): 219–24.

———. "The Training of the Surgeon." In *The Surgical Papers of William Stewart Halsted*, edited by Walter C. Burket, vol. 2, 512–31. Baltimore: Johns Hopkins University Press, 1924.

Hamilton, David. *The First Transplant Surgeon: The Flawed Genius of Nobel Prize Winner Alexis Carrel.* London: World Scientific, 2017.

———. *A History of Organ Transplantation: From Ancient Legends to Modern Practice.* Pittsburgh: University of Pittsburgh Press, 2012.

Hansen, Bert. *Picturing Medical Progress from Pasteur to Polio: A History of Mass Media and Popular Images in America.* New Brunswick, NJ: Rutgers University Press, 2009.

Harbinson, Samuel P. "Experiences with Aneurysms in an Overseas General Hospital." *SGO* 81, no. 1 (July 1945): 128–37.

———. Introduction to *Blood Vessel Surgery and Its Applications.* By Charles C. Guthrie, v–xi. Pittsburgh: University of Pittsburgh Press, 1959.

———. "Origins of Vascular Surgery: The Carrel-Guthrie Letters." *Surgery* 52, no. 2 (August 1962): 406–18.

Harris, Ruth. *Lourdes: Body and Spirit in the Secular Age.* London: Allen Lane, 1990.

Harrison, Lynn. "Historical Aspects in the Development of Venous Autografts." *Annals of Surgery* 183, no. 2 (February 1976): 101–6.

Harrison, Mark. *The Medical War: British Military Medicine in World War I.* Oxford: Oxford University Press, 2010.

———. *Medicine and Victory: British Military Medicine in the Second World War.* Oxford: Oxford University Press, 2004.

Harvey, A. McGehee. "The Influence of William Stewart Halsted's Concepts of Surgical Training." *Johns Hopkins Medical Journal* 148 (1981): 215–36.

Haschek, E., and O. T. Lindenthal. "Ein Beitrag zur Praktischen Verwerthung der Photographie nach Röntgen." *Wiener Klinische Wochenschrift* 9 (January 1896): 63–64.

Haseltine, Nate. "Blood Vessel Cures Save Lives of GIs." *Washington Post*, 2 November 1951, 6.

———. "Limb-Saving Surgery Successful in Korea." *Washington Post*, 23 November 1952, B2.

———. "Soldier Given Dead Man's Artery in Rare Operation." *Washington Post*, 14 January 1951, 15.

"Health of Army Troops, FEC." *Surgeon General's Circular* 7, no. 1 (January 1952): 18.

Hedley-White, John, and Debra R. Milamed. "Our Blood, Your Money." *Ulster Medical Journal* 82 (2013): 114–20.

Helling, Thomas. *Desperate Surgery in the Pacific War: Doctors and Damage Control for Americans Wounded, 1941–1945*. Jefferson, NC: McFarland, 2017.

Helling, Thomas S., and Emmanuel Daon. "In Flanders Fields: The Great War, Antoine Depage, and the Resurgence of Debridement." *Annals of Surgery* 228 (1998): 173–81.

Herget, Carl M., George B. Coe, and James C. Breyer. "Wound Ballistics and Body Armor in Korea." In *Wound Ballistics*, edited by James C. Beyer, 691–767. Washington, DC: Office of the Surgeon General, 1962.

Heringman, Craig E., James D. Rives, and Harry A. Davis. "The Repair of Arteriovenous Fistulas: Evaluation of Operative Procedures and Analysis of Fifty-Three Cases." *JAMA* 133, no. 10 (8 March 1947): 663–68.

Herman, Jan K. *Frozen in Memory: U.S. Navy Medicine in the Korean War*. Washington, DC: Brassey's, 2004.

Hermes, Walter G. *Truce Tent and Fighting Front*. Washington, DC: Office of Military History, 1966.

Heuer, George. "Dr. Halsted." *Bulletin of the Johns Hopkins Hospital* 90, no. 2, suppl. (1952): 1–109.

———. "Graduate Teaching of Surgery." *SGO* 54 (1932): 729–32.

———. "Graduate Teaching of Surgery in University Clinics." *Annals of Surgery* 102 (1935): 507–15.

Heys, Steven D. "Abdominal Wounds: Evolution of Management and Establishment of Surgical Treatments." In *War Surgery 1914–18*, edited by Thomas Scotland and Steven Hays, 178–211. Solihull, England: Helion, 2012.

The History of the Medical Department of the United States Navy, 1945–1955. Washington, DC: US Government Printing Office, 1958.

A History of United States Army Base Hospital No. 36 (Detroit College Medicine and Surgery Unit). Detroit?: Self-published, 1922?

Hoepfner, E. "Ueber Gefaessnaht, Gefaesstransplantationen und replantation von amputirten extremitaeten." *Archiv Klinische Chirurgie* 70 (1903): 417.

Hogan, David G. *Selling 'em by the Sack: White Castle and the Creation of American Food*. New York: New York University Press, 1997.

Holman, Emile. "Diseases of the Arteries." In *A Textbook of Surgery by American Authors*, edited by Frederick Christopher, 147–64. Philadelphia: W. B. Saunders, 1936.

———. "Further Observations on Surgery of the Large Arteries." *SGO* 78, no. 3 (March 1944): 275–87.

———. *New Concepts in Surgery of the Vascular System*. Springfield, IL: Charles C. Thomas, 1955.

————. "Observations on the Surgery of the Large Arteries, with Report of Case of Ligation of the Innominate Artery for Varicose Aneurism of the Subclavian Vessels." *Annals of Surgery* 85, no. 2 (1927): 173–84.

————. "War Injuries to Arteries and Their Treatment." *SGO* 75 (1942): 183–92.

Holman, Emile, and Géza de Takáts. "The Vascular System." In *A Textbook of Surgery by American Authors*, 3rd ed. Edited by Frederick Christopher, 187–230. Philadelphia: W. B. Saunders, 1942.

————. "The Vascular System." In *A Textbook of Surgery by American Authors*, 5th ed., edited by Frederick Christopher, 620–55. Philadelphia: W. B. Saunders, 1949.

Holmes, Frederic L. *Claude Bernard and Animal Chemistry: The Emergence of a Scientist.* Cambridge, MA: Harvard University Press, 1974.

Holmes, Robert H. "Wound Ballistics and Body Armor." *JAMA* 150, no. 2 (13 September 1952): 73–78.

Holmes, Robert H., et al. "Medical Aspects of Body Armor Used in Korea." *JAMA* 155, no. 17 (21 August 1954): 1477–78.

Holt, Jim. *When Einstein Walked with Gödel: Excursions to the Edge of Thought.* New York: Farrar, Straus and Giroux, 2018.

Home, Everard. "An Account of Mr. Hunter's Methods of Performing the Operation for the Cure of the Popliteal Aneurysm." In *Transactions of a Society for the Improvement of Medical and Chirurgical Knowledge*, vol. 1, 143–44. London: 1793.

————. "A Short Account of the Life of the Author." In *A Treatise on the Blood, Inflammation, and Gun-Shot Wounds*, by John Hunter, xiii–lxvii. London: 1794, reprinted 1982.

Horsley, John Shelton. *Surgery of the Blood Vessels.* St. Louis, MO: C. V. Mosby, 1915.

Horton, Bayard T., and Winchell McK. Craig. "Evidence Shown in Roentgenograms of Changes in the Vascular Tree Following Experimental Sympathetic Ganglionectomy." *Archives of Surgery* 21 (1930): 698–701.

Horwitz, Dorothy G., ed. *We Will Not Be Strangers: Korean War Letters between a MASH Surgeon and His Wife.* Chicago: University of Illinois Press, 1997.

Howard, John M. "Dedication: Sam F. Seeley." *Journal of Trauma* 12, no. 13 (1973): 1009.

————. "Historical Vignettes of Arterial Repair: Recollections of Korea 1951–1953." *Annals of Surgery* 228 (1998): 716–18.

————. "Introduction—Historical Background and Development." In *The Systemic Response to Injury*, vol. 1 of *Battle Casualties in Korea: Studies of the Surgical Research Team*, edited by Carl W. Hughes, 1–12. Washington, DC: Army Medical Service Graduate School, 1954.

Howard, John M., and Frank K. Inui, "Clostridial Myositis—Gas Gangrene." In *The Battle Wound: Clinical Experiences*, vol. 3 of *Battle Casualties in Korea: Stud-*

ies of the Surgical Research Team, edited by Curtis P. Artz, 194–201. Washington, DC: Army Medical Service Graduate School, 1954.

Howard, John M., and Richard P. Mason. "The Value of a Field Research Project." In *The Systemic Response to Injury*, vol. 1 of *Battle Casualties in Korea: Studies of the Surgical Research Team*, edited by Carl W. Hughes, 16–23. Washington, DC: Army Medical Service Graduate School, 1954.

Howell, Joel D. *Technology in the Hospital: Transforming Patient Care in the Early Twentieth Century*. Baltimore: Johns Hopkins University Press, 1995.

Howell, William H. "The Purification of Heparin and Its Chemical and Physiological Reactions." *Bulletin of the Johns Hopkins Hospital* 42 (1928): 199.

———. "The Purification of Heparin and Its Presence in the Blood." *American Journal of Physiology*, 71, no. 3 (1925): 553–62.

Howell, W. H., and Emmett Holt. "Two New Factors in Blood Coagulation—Heparin and Pro-anti-thrombin." *American Journal of Physiology*, 47 (1918): 328–41.

Hoyt, Edwin P. *The Pusan Perimeter*. New York: Stein and Day, 1984.

Hubney, M. J., and Simon Pollack. "Saccular Abdominal Aortic Aneurysm." *American Journal of Roentgenology and Radium Therapy* 43 (1940): 385–93.

Hufnagel, Charles A. "The Use of Rigid and Flexible Plastic Prostheses for Arterial Replacement." *Surgery* 37, no. 2 (February 1955): 165–74.

Hufnagel, Charles A., and H. H. G. Eastcott. "The Preparation of Arterial Grafts by Freezing." *Lancet* 262 (March 1952): 531–37.

Hughes, Basil, and H. Stanley Banks. *War Surgery: From Firing Line to Base*. New York: William Wood, 1919.

Hughes, Carl W. "Acute Vascular Trauma in Korean War Casualties: An Analysis of 180 Cases." *SGO* 99 (1954): 91–100.

———. "Arterial Repair in the Korean War." *Annals of Surgery* 147 (April 1958): 555–61.

———. *Debridement*. Washington DC: Army Medical Service Graduate School, 1955.

———. "The Primary Repair of Wounds of Major Arteries." *Annals of Surgery* 141, no. 3 (March 1953): 297–303.

———. "Primary Surgery of Blood Vessels in Korea: An Analysis of Major Artery Repairs in Korea During 1953." In *Recent Advances in Medicine and Surgery (19–30 April 1954) Based on Professional Medical Experiences in Japan and Korea, 1950–1953*, vol. 1, 443–52. Washington, DC: Army Medical Service Graduate School, 1955.

———, ed. *The Systemic Response to Injury*. Vol. 1 of *Battle Casualties in Korea: Studies of the Surgical Research Team*. Washington, DC: Army Medical Service Graduate School, 1954.

———. "Vascular Surgery in the Armed Forces." *Military Medicine* 124, no. 1 (1959): 30–46.

Hughes, Carl W., and Warner F. Bowers. "Blood Vessel Surgery." *American Journal of Surgery* 85 (1953): 174–78.

Hughes, Thomas P. *American Genius: A Century of Invention and Technological Enthusiasm, 1870–1970.* New York: Viking Press, 1989.

Humphreys, Margaret. *Marrow of Tragedy: The Health Crisis of the American Civil War.* Baltimore: Johns Hopkins University Press, 2013.

Hunter, John. "Observations on the Inflammation of the Internal Coats of Veins." *Transactions of a Society for the Improvement of Medical and Chirurgical Knowledge,* vol. 1, 18–29. London: 1793.

———. *A Treatise on the Blood, Inflammation, and Gun-Shot Wounds.* London: 1794.

Hunter, John I. "The Postural Influence of the Sympathetic Innervation of Voluntary Muscle." *Medical Journal of Australia* 1, no. 4 (1924): 86–89.

———. "The Significance of the Double Innervation of Voluntary Muscle Illustrated by Reference to the Maintenance of the Posture of the Wing." *Medical Journal of Australia* 1, no. 24 (1924): 581–87.

Hunter, William. "The History of an Aneurysm of the Aorta, with Some Remarks on Aneurysms in General." *Medical Observations and Inquiries* 1 (1757): 323–57.

Hurwitt, Elliot S. "A Blood Vessel Bank under Military Conditions." *Military Surgeon* 106, no. 1 (1950): 19–27.

———. "Cardiovascular Surgery at Montefiore Hospital in 1957 as Compared to 1952." *New York State Medical Journal* 58 (1958): 1516–20.

Imber, Gerald. *Genius on the Edge: The Bizarre Double Life of Dr. William Stewart Halsted.* New York: Kaplan, 2010.

Imes, Pat R. "Suture of the Popliteal Artery: A Report of Three Cases." *Surgery* 18 (1945): 644–46.

Inui, Frank K., James Shannon, and John M. Howard. "Arterial Injuries in the Korean Conflict: Experiences with 111 Consecutive Injuries." *Surgery* 37, no. 5 (1955): 850–57.

Ireland, Merritt W. *Medical Department of the United States in World War I,* vol. 11, *Surgery,* part 1. Washington, DC: Government Printing Office, 1927.

Jaboulay, Mathieu. *Chirurgie du grand sympathique et du corps thyroïd.* Lyon: A. Storck and Cie, 1900.

Jackson, Kenneth T. *Crabgrass Frontier: The Suburbanization of the United States.* New York: Oxford University Press, 1985.

Jacyna, Stephen. "Images of John Hunter in the Nineteenth Century." *History of Science* 21 (1983): 85–108.

———. "The Laboratory and the Clinic: The Impact of Pathology on Surgical Diagnosis in the Glasgow Western Infirmary, 1875–1910." *Bulletin of the History of Medicine* 62 (1988): 384–406.

———. "Physiological Principles in the Surgical Writings of John Hunter." In *Medical Theory, Surgical Practice: Studies in the History of Surgery,* edited by Christopher Lawrence, 135–52. New York: Routledge, 1992.

Jaffin, Jonathan. "Medical Support for the American Expeditionary Forces in France during the First World War." MA thesis, Command and General Staff College, 1991.

Jahnke, Edward J. "Late Structural and Functional Results of Arterial Injuries Primarily Repaired." *Surgery* 43, no. 2 (February 1958): 175–83.

———. "The Surgery of Acute Vascular Injuries: A Report of 77 Cases." *Military Surgeon* 112, no. 4 (April 1953): 249–51.

Jahnke, Edward J., and John M. Howard. "Primary Repair of Major Arterial Injuries: A Report of Fifty-Eight Battle Casualties." *Archives of Surgery* 66, no. 5 (1953): 646–49.

Jahnke, Edward J., Carl W. Hughes, and John M. Howard. "The Rationale of Arterial Repair on the Battlefield." *American Journal of Surgery* 87, no. 3 (1954): 396–401.

Jahnke, Edward J., and Sam F. Seeley. "Acute Vascular Injuries in the Korean War: An Analysis of 77 Consecutive Cases." *Annals of Surgery* 138, no. 2 (August 1953): 158–77.

Janeway, T. C. "War and Medicine." *Johns Hopkins Alumni Magazine* 5 (1917): 215–33.

Jassinowsky, Alexander. "Die Arteriennhat." PhD diss., University of Dorpat, 1889.

———. "Ein Beitrag zur Lehre von der Gefässnaht." *Archiv für Klinische Chirurgie* 42 (1891): 816–41.

Jeger, Ernst. "Die Chirurgie der Blutgefäße und des Herzens." PhD diss, Hirschwald, 1913.

Jensen, Robert Travis. *Bloody Snow: A Doctor's Memoir of the Korean War.* Carmel, IN: Cork Hill Press, 2005.

John, Heather Varughese. "Practicing Physicians: The Intern and Resident Experience in the Shaping of American Medical Education, 1945–2003." PhD diss., Yale University, 2013.

Johnson, Julian, Charles K. Kirby, F. E. Greifenstein, and A. Castillo. "The Experimental and Clinical Use of Vein Grafts to Replace Defects of Large Arteries." *Surgery* 26 (1949): 945–56.

Jones, Claire L. *The Medical Trade Catalogue in Britain: 1870–1914.* London: Pickering & Chatto, 2013.

Jones, David S. *Broken Hearts: The Tangled History of Cardiac Care.* Baltimore: Johns Hopkins University Press, 2013.

———. "Surgery and Clinical Trials: The History and Controversies of Surgical Evidence." In *The Palgrave Handbook of the History of Surgery*, edited by Thomas Schlich, 479–502. London: Palgrave Macmillan, 2018.

———. "Surgical Practice and the Reconstruction of the Therapeutic Niche: The Case of Myocardial Revascularization." In *Technological Change in Modern Surgery: Historical Perspectives on Innovation*, edited by Christopher Crenner and Thomas Schlich, 184–215. Rochester, NY: University of Rochester Press, 2017.

Jones, Edgar, and Simon Wessely. *Shell Shock to PTSD: Military Psychiatry from 1900 to the Gulf War*. New York: Psychology Press, 2005.

Joy, Robert J. T. "Historical Aspects of Medical Defense against Chemical Warfare." In *Medical Aspects of Chemical and Biological Warfare*, edited by Zygmunt F. Dembek, 87–109. Washington, DC: Borden Institute, 2007.

———. "Malaria in American Troops in the South and Southwest Pacific in World War II." *Medical History* 43 (1999): 192–207.

Julian, Ormand C., William S. Dye, John H. Olwin, and Paul H. Jordan. "Direct Surgery of Arteriosclerosis." *Annals of Surgery* 136 (1952): 459–73.

Jung, Aldolphe. "Review of the Forty-Sixth French Congress of Surgery, Oct. 49, 1937, Paris." Translated by Michael E. DeBakey. *Surgery* 3 (1938): 306–16.

Kampmeir, R. H. "Aneurysm of the Abdominal Aorta: A Study of 73 Cases." *American Journal of Medical Science* 192 (1936): 97–109.

Katz, Sidney. "Hemorrhagic Fever of the Far Eastern Type." In *Recent Advances in Medicine and Surgery (19–30 April 1954) Based on Professional Medical Experiences in Japan and Korea, 1950–1953*, vol. 1, 109–17. Washington, DC: Army Medical Service Graduate School, 1955.

Kay, Jane H. *Asphalt Nation: How the Automobile Took Over America, and How We Can Take It Back*. New York: Crown, 1997.

Keefer, Edward B., et al. "The Blood Vessel Bank." *JAMA* 145 (1951): 888–93.

Keen, W. W. *Surgery: Its Practices and Principles*. Philadelphia: W. B. Saunders, 1911.

Kendrick, Douglass B. *Blood Program in World War II*. Washington, DC: Office of the Surgeon General, 1964.

———. "Operation of Blood Bank Systems." In *Recent Advances in Medicine and Surgery (19–30 April 1954) Based on Professional Medical Experiences in Japan and Korea, 1950–1953*, vol. 1, 145–54. Washington, DC: Army Medical Service Graduate School, 1955.

———. "Prevention and Treatment of Shock in the Combat Zone." *Military Surgeon* 88, no. 2 (February 1941): 97–113.

Kernahan, Peter J. "Franklin Martin and the Standardization of American Surgery, 1890–1940." PhD diss., University of Minnesota, 2010.

Keshishian, John M., and Andrew G. Prandoni. "The Surgical Management of Occlusive Vascular Disease." *Medical Annals of the District of Columbia* 29 (1960): 1–12.

Kevles, Bettyann Holtzmann. *Naked to the Bone: Medical Imaging in the Twentieth Century*. New Brunswick, NJ: Rutgers University Press, 1987.

Kevles, Daniel J. "K1, S2: Korea, Science, and the State." In *Big Science: The Growth of Large Scale Research*, edited by Peter Galison and Bruce Hevly, 312–33. Stanford, CA: Stanford University Press, 1992.

———. *The Physicists: The History of a Scientific Community in Modern America*. Cambridge, MA: Harvard University Press, 1995.

Kirk, Jeffery. *Machine in Our Hearts: The Cardiac Pacemaker, the Implantable Defibrillator, and American Health Care*. Baltimore: Johns Hopkins University Press, 2001.

Kirkland, Richard C. *MASH Angels: Tales of an Air-Evac Helicopter Pilot in the Korean War*. Short Hills, NJ: Buford Books, 2009.

Kirkup, John. *The Evolution of Surgical Instruments: An Illustrated History from Ancient Times to the Twentieth Century*. Novato, CA: historyofscience, 2005.

Kirtley, James A., Jr. "Arterial Injuries in a Theater of Operations." *Annals of Surgery* 122, no. 2 (July 1945): 223–34.

Kisacky, Jeanna. *Rise of the Modern Hospital: An Architectural History of Health and Healing, 1870–1940*. Pittsburg, PA: University of Pittsburg Press, 2017.

Klasen, Henk J. *History of Burns*. Rotterdam: Erasmus, 2004.

Klotz, Oskar, Howard H. Permar, and Charles C. Guthrie. "End Results of Arterial Transplants." *Annals of Surgery* 78 (1923): 305–20.

Kobler, John. *The Reluctant Surgeon: A Biography of John Hunter, Medical Genius and Great Inquirer of Johnson's England*. New York: Doubleday, 1960.

Kolsti, Nancy. "Beat of a Different Drummer." *North Texan Online* (Winter 2004) http://www.unt.edu/northtexan/archives/p05/differentdrummer.htm (accessed 6 November 2013).

Kronick, David A. *A History of Scientific and Technical Periodicals: The Origins and Development of the Scientific and Technological Press, 1665–1790*. New York: Scarecrow Press, 1962.

Kuttner, Herman. "Gefässplastiken." *Münchener Medizinische Wochenschrift* 20 (1916): 721–23.

———. "Kriegschirurgie der grossen Gefässstämme." *Deutsche Medizinische Wochenschrift* 41 (1916): 741.

Kvitting, John-Peder Escobar, and Christian L. Olin. "Clarence Crafoord: A Giant in Cardiothoracic Surgery, the First to Repair Aortic Coarctation." *Annals of Thoracic Surgery* 87 (2009): 342–46.

Lafollette, Marcel C. *Making Science Our Own: Public Images of Science, 1910–1955*. Chicago: University of Chicago Press, 1990.

Lancisi, Giovanni Maria. *De aneurysmatibus: Opus posthumum*. 1745. Translated by Wilmer Cave Wright. New York: Macmillan, 1952.

Landecker, Hannah L. "Technologies of Living Substance: Tissue Culture and Cellular Life in Twentieth Century Biomedicine." PhD diss., MIT, 1999.

Langely, G. F. "Repair of Ruptured Popliteal Artery, with Note on Heparin Therapy after Arterial Suture." *British Journal of Surgery* 31, no. 122 (October 1943): 161–65.

Lawrence, Christopher. "Democratic, Divine, and Heroic: The History and Historiography of Surgery." In *Medical Theory, Surgical Practice: Studies in the History of Surgery*, edited by Christopher Lawrence, 1–47. New York: Routledge, 1992.

———. "Review of *Technological Change in Modern Surgery*." *Bulletin of the History of Medicine* 92 (2018): 380–82.

————. "Surgery and Its Histories: Purposes and Contexts." In *The Palgrave Handbook of the History of Surgery*, edited by Thomas Schlich, 1–26. London: Palgrave Macmillan, 2018.

Lawrence, Christopher, and Richard Dixey. "Practising on Principle: Joseph Lister and the Germ Theories of Disease." In *Medical Theory, Surgical Practice: Studies in the History of Surgery*, edited by Christopher Lawrence, 153–214. New York: Routledge, 1992.

Lawrence, Ghislaine. "The Ambiguous Artifact: Surgical Instruments and the Surgical Past." In *Medical Theory, Surgical Practice: Studies in the History of Surgery*, edited by Christopher Lawrence, 295–311. New York: Routledge, 1992.

Leavell, Byrd Stuart. *The 8th Evac: A History of the University of Virginia Hospital Unit in World War II.* Richmond: Dietz Press, 1970.

Lederer, Susan E. *Flesh and Blood: Organ Transplantation and Blood Transfusion in Twentieth Century America.* New York: Oxford University Press, 2008.

————. *Frankenstein: Penetrating the Secrets of Nature.* New Brunswick, NJ: Rutgers University Press, 2002.

Leese, Peter. *Shell Shock: Traumatic Neurosis and the British Soldiers of the First World War.* New York: Palgrave Macmillan, 2002.

Leriche, René. "De la sympathectomie perí-artérielle et de ses résaltats." *Presse Médicine* 25 (1919): 513–15.

————. "De l'elongation et de la section des nerfs périvasculaires dans certains syndromes douloureux d'origine artérielle et dans quelques troubles trophiques." *Lyons Chirurgerie* 10 (1913): 378–82.

————. "Experimental and Clinical Contribution to the Question of the Innervation of the Vessels." *SGO* 47 (1928): 631–43.

————. "Surgery of the Sympathetic System: Indications and Results." *Annals of Surgery* 88 (1920): 449–69.

Lerner, Baron H. *The Breast Cancer Wars: Hope, Fear, and the Pursuit of a Cure in Twentieth-Century America.* New York: Oxford University Press, 2001.

————. *One for the Road: Drunk Driving since 1900.* Baltimore: John Hopkins University Press, 2011.

Lesch, John E. *The First Miracle Drugs: How the Sulfa Drugs Transformed Medicine.* New York: Oxford University Press, 2007.

————. *Science and Medicine in France: The Emergence of Experimental Physiology, 1790–1855.* Cambridge, MA: Harvard University Press, 1984.

LeVeen, Harry H. "Nonsuture Method for Vascular Anastomosis Utilizing the Murphy Button Principle." *Archives of Surgery* 58 (1949): 504–10.

Lewis, Tom. *Divided Highways: Building the Interstate Highways, Transforming American Life.* Ithaca, NY: Cornell University Press, 2013.

Lexer, Erich. "Die ideale Operation des Arteriellen und des arteriellvenösen Aneurysma." *Archiv Klinische Chirurgie* 83 (1907): 459–63.

Lilly, George D. "The First Ten Years of the Society for Vascular Surgery." *Surgery* 41 (January 1957): 1–5.

Lindberg, Robert B. "The Bacterial Flora of Wounds in the Korean War." In *Recent Advances in Medicine and Surgery (19–30 April 1954) Based on Professional Medical Experiences in Japan and Korea, 1950–1953*, vol. 1, 311–21. Washington, DC: Army Medical Service Graduate School, 1955.

Lindsey, Douglass. "Evacuation and Specialty Centers." In *Recent Advances in Medicine and Surgery (19–30 April 1954) Based on Professional Medical Experiences in Japan and Korea, 1950–1953*, vol. 1, 24–40. Washington, DC: Army Medical Service Graduate School, 1955.

———. "Professional Considerations of Patient Evacuation." In *Recent Advances in Medicine and Surgery (19–30 April 1954) Based on Professional Medical Experiences in Japan and Korea, 1950–1953*, vol. 1, 60–99. Washington, DC: Army Medical Service Graduate School, 1955.

Link, Mae M. "Development of the Armed Services Blood, Blood Derivatives, and Plasma Expanders Program." *United States Armed Forces Medical Journal* 4, no, 1 (January 1953): 1221–25.

Link, Mae M., and Hubert A. Coleman. *Medical Support of the Army Air Forces in World War II*. Washington, DC: Department of the Air Force, 1955.

Linker, Beth. "Spines of Steel: A Case of Surgical Enthusiasm in Cold War America." *Bulletin of the History of Medicine* 90 (2016): 222–49.

———. *War's Waste: Rehabilitation in World War I America*. Chicago: University of Chicago Press, 2011.

Linton, Derek S. "'War Dysentery' and the Limitations of German Military Hygiene during World War I." *Bulletin of the History of Medicine* 84, no. 4 (2010): 607–39.

Loewy, G. "Carrel's Method of Treatment of Infected Wounds." *New York Medical Journal* 106 (1917): 798–802.

Longo, Lawrence D. "The Rise and Fall of Battey's Operation: A Fashion in Surgery." *Bulletin of the History of Medicine* 53 (1979): 244–67.

Loudon, Irvine. *Medical Care and the General Practitioner, 1750–1850*. Oxford: Clarendon Press, 1986.

Loudon, Jean, and Irvine Loudon. "Medicine, Politics and the Medical Periodical, 1800–1850." In *Medical Journals and Medical Knowledge*, edited by William F. Bynum, Stephan Lock, and Roy Porter, 49–69. New York: Routledge, 1992.

Lowenberg, Robert T. "Treatment of Peripheral Arterial Insufficiency." *Connecticut State Medical Journal* 15 (1951): 809–14.

Lucke, Baldwin, and Marion H. Rea. "Studies on Aneurysms." *JAMA* 77, no. 12 (1921): 935–40.

Ludmerer, Kenneth M. *Learning to Heal: The Development of American Medical Education*. New York: Basic Books, 1985.

———. *Let Me Heal: The Opportunity to Preserve Excellence in American Medicine*. New York: Oxford University Press, 2015.

———. *Time to Heal: American Medical Education from the Turn of the Century to the Era of Managed Care*. New York: Oxford University Press, 1999.

Lundy, John S. "Factors That Influenced the Development of Anesthesiology." *Anesthesia and Analgesia* 25 (January/February 1946): 38–43.

MacCallum, W. G. *William Stewart Halsted: Surgeon.* Baltimore: Johns Hopkins University Press, 1930.

MacEachern, Malcolm T. "The Expanded Program of the American College of Surgeons for Graduate Training in Surgery." *Special Bulletin of the American College of Surgeons* (September 1945): 9.

MacFee, William F. "Arterial Anastomosis in War Wounds of the Extremities." *Surgical Clinics of North America* 28 (1948): 381–89.

MacPherson, W. G. *Medical Services: General History.* Vol. 3. London: His Majesty's Stationery Office, 1924.

———. *Medical Services: Surgery of the War.* Vols. 1–2. London: His Majesty's Stationery Office, 1922.

Magnuson, Paul B. *Ring the Night Bell: The Autobiography of a Surgeon.* 1960. Edited by Finley Peter Dunne Jr. Birmingham: University of Alabama Press, 1986.

Majno, Guido. *The Healing Hand: Man and His Wound in the Ancient World.* Cambridge, MA: Harvard University Press, 1975.

Makins, George H. *On Gunshot Injuries to the Blood-Vessels, Founded on Experience Gained in France during the Great War, 1914–1918.* Bristol: J. Wright and Sons, 1919.

———. *Surgical Experiences in South Africa, 1899–1900; Being Mainly a Clinical Study of the Nature and Effects of Injuries Produced by Bullets of Small Calibre.* London: Smith, Elder, 1901.

Malinin, Theodore I. *Surgery and Life: The Extraordinary Career of Alexis Carrel.* New York: Harcourt Brace Jovanovich, 1979.

Marble, W. Sanders. "The Evolution and Demise of the MASH, 1946–2006: Organizing to Perform Forward Surgery as Medicine and the Military Change." *Army History* 92 (2014): 22–39.

———. "Forward Surgery and Combat Hospitals: The Origins of MASH." *Journal of the History of Medicine and Allied Sciences* 69, no. 1 (January 2014): 68–100.

———, ed. *King of Battle: Artillery in World War I.* Leiden: Ashgate, 2013.

Marcum, James A. "The Development of Heparin in Toronto." *Journal of the History of Medicine and Allied Sciences* 52 (1997): 310–37.

———. "The Origins of the Dispute over the Discovery of Heparin." *Journal of the History of Medicine and Allied Sciences* 55 (2000): 37–66.

Markel, Howard A. *An Anatomy of Addiction: Sigmund Freud, William Halsted, and the Miracle Drug Cocaine.* New York: Pantheon, 2011.

Marks, Harry M. *The Progress of Experiment: Science and Therapeutic Reform in the United States, 1900–1990.* Cambridge: Cambridge University Press, 2000.

Martin, Arthur Anderson. *A Surgeon in Khaki: Through France and Flanders in World War I.* Lincoln: University of Nebraska Press, 2011.

Martin, David P., Christopher M. Burke, Brian P. McGlinch, Mary E. Warner, Alan D. Seesler, and Douglass R. Bacon. "The Mayo Clinic World War II Short Course and Its Effect on Anesthesiology." *Anesthesiology* 105 (2006): 209–13.

Martin, Franklin H. *Fifty Years of Medicine and Surgery: An Autobiographical Sketch.* Chicago: Surgical, 1934.

Martin, John D., Jr. "Pulsating Hematoma: Report of Cases." *Bulletin of the US Army Medical Department* 4, no. 2 (1945): 219–24.

Masini, Queirolo u. "Ueber die Funktion des Leber." *Moleschott: Untersuchungen zur Naturlehre des Mensch* 15 (1895): 225.

Mason, E. C. "A Note on the Use of Heparin in Blood Transfusion." *Journal of Laboratory Clinical Medicine* 10 (1924): 203–6.

Matas, Rudolph. "An Operation for the Radical Cure of Aneurism Based upon Arteriorrhaphy." *Annals of Surgery* 37, no. 2 (February 1903): 161–96.

———. "Traumatic Aneurism of the Left Brachial Artery." *Medical News* 53 (1888): 462–70.

Maulitz, Russel C. *Morbid Appearances: The Anatomy of Pathology in the Early Nineteenth Century.* Cambridge: Cambridge University Press, 1987.

Mayhew, Emily. *Wounded: A New History of the Western Front in World War I.* New York: Oxford University Press, 2014.

Mayo, Charles H. "Surgery of the Sympathetic Nervous System." *Annals of Surgery* 96, no. 4 (October 1932): 481–87.

Mayo, William J. "Observations on the Sympathetic Nervous System." *British Medical Journal* 2 (18 October 1930): 627–28.

McKellar, Shelley. *Artificial Hearts: The Allure and Ambivalence of a Controversial Medical Technology.* Baltimore: Johns Hopkins University Press, 2018.

———. *Surgical Limits: The Life of Gordon Murray.* Toronto: University of Toronto Press, 2003.

McLean, Jay. "The Discovery of Heparin." *Circulation* 19 (1959): 75–78.

———. "The Thromboplastic Action of Cephalin." *American Journal of Physiology* 41 (1916): 250–57.

Meillier, Andrew, Crescent Edwards, Heather K. Feld, and Kenneth G. Swan, "Arthur Hendley Blakemore's Life and Contributions to Vascular Surgery." *Journal of Vascular Surgery* 61 (2015): 1094–97.

Memorandum on the Treatment of Injuries in War Based on the Experience of the Present Campaign: July 1915. London: His Majesty's Stationery Office, 1915.

Meroney, William H. Introduction to *Post-traumatic Renal Insufficiency,* vol. 4 of *Battle Casualties in Korea: Studies of the Surgical Research Team,* edited by William H. Meroney, 1–5. Washington, DC: Army Medical Service Graduate School, 1954.

Meroney, William H., and R. F. Herndon. "The Management of Acute Renal Insufficiency." In *Post-traumatic Renal Insufficiency,* vol. 4 of *Battle Casualties in Korea: Studies of the Surgical Research Team,* edited by William H. Meroney, 51–70. Washington, DC: Army Medical Service Graduate School, 1954.

MGH News 133 (April 1954), 2.

Michel, Jean-Baptiste, et al. "Quantitative Analysis of Culture Using Millions of Digitized Books." *Science* 331 (2011): 176–82.

Miller, G. Wayne. *King of Hearts: The True Story of the Maverick Who Pioneered Open Heart Surgery.* New York: Random House, 2000.

Miller, Harry H., Allan D. Callow, C. Stuart Welch, and H. Edward MacMahon. "The Fate of Arterial Grafts in Small Arteries." *SGO* 92 (1951): 581–88.

Miller, Harry H., and C. Stuart Welch. "Quantitative Studies on the Time Factor in Arterial Injuries." *Annals of Surgery* 130, no. 3 (1949): 428–38.

Millett, Allan R. *The War for Korea, 1945–1950: A House Burning.* Lawrence: University of Kansas Press, 2005.

———. *The War for Korea, 1950–1951: They Came from the North.* Lawrence: University of Kansas, 2010.

Mills, Joseph L. "Vascular Surgery Training in the United States: A Half-Century of Evolution." *Journal of Vascular Surgery* 48 (2008): 90s–97s.

Mitchiner, Philip H. "Injuries of Blood Vessels and their Treatment." *St. Thomas Hospital Gazette* 38 (1940): 92–96.

Molner, Joseph G. "Clogged Arteries Remediable." *Atlanta Constitution* (11 August 1964): 9.

———. "Surgeons Can Correct Aneurysms." *Atlanta Constitution* (4 August 1963): 6.

Monti, Achille. *Antonia Scarpa in Scientific History and His Role in the Fortunes of the University of Pavia.* Translated by Frank L. Loria. New York: Vigo Press, 1957.

Moore, Maurice R. "Endocrine Therapy of Arteriosclerosis: A Preliminary Report of 100 Cases." *Connecticut State Medical Journal* 18 (1954): 26–30.

Moore, Robert M., J. Harris Williams, and Albert O. Singleton. "Vasoconstrictor Fibers: Peripheral Course as Revealed by Roentgenographic Method." *Archives of Surgery* 26 (1933): 308–22.

Moore, S. W., and George Wantz. "Abdominal Aortic Aneurysms." *Surgical Clinics of North America* 41 (1961): 497–509.

Moore, Wendy. *The Knife Man: Blood, Body-Snatching, and the Birth of Modern Surgery.* New York: Broadway Books, 2005.

Moniz, Egas. "Arterial Encephalography: Importance in the Localization of Cerebral Tumors." *Société de Neurologie* 34 (1927): 72–90.

Montgomery, Albert H., and Jay Ireland. "Traumatic Segmental Arterial Spasm." *JAMA* 105 (1935): 1741–46.

Morantz-Sanchez, Regina. *Conduct Unbecoming a Woman: Medicine on Trial in Turn-of-the-Century Brooklyn.* New York: Oxford University Press, 1999.

Morino, Mario. "The Impact of Technology on Surgery: The Future Is Unwritten." *Annals of Surgery* 258 (2018): 709–11.

Morris, George C., Jr., Oscar Creech Jr., and Michael E. DeBakey. "Acute Arterial Injuries in Civilian Practice." *American Journal of Surgery* 93 (1957): 565–72.

Moss, Sandra W. "Floating Kidneys." In *Clio in the Clinic: History in Medical Practice*, edited by Jacalyn Duffin, 92–104. New York: Oxford University Press, 2005.

Mossman, Billy C. *Ebb and Flow: November 1950–July 1951.* Washington, DC: Center for Military History, 1990.

Mott, Valentine. *Reflections on Securing in a Ligature the Arteria Innominata.* New York: 1819.

Moure, Paul. "Etude des greffes vasculaires et particulièrement de leurs applications chirurgicales au rétablissement de la continuité des vaisseaux et des conduits musculo-membraneux." PhD diss., Octave Doin et Fils, 1914.

Mueller, C. Barber. *Evarts A. Graham: The Life, Lives, and Times of the Surgical Spirit of St. Louis.* London: BC Decker, 2002.

Mufson, Isidor, et al. "An Evaluation of Priscoline by Artery in the Treatment of Peripheral Arterial Obliterative Disease." *New York Journal of Medicine* 52 (1952): 2651–54.

Mullins, Richard. "Albert Starr." *The Oregon Encyclopedia.* https://oregonencyclopedia.org/articles/starr_albert_1926_/ (accessed 5 November 2013).

Mulvihill, Daniel A., and Samuel C. Harvey. "Studies on Collateral Circulation: I. Thermic Changes after Arterial Ligation and Ganglionectomy." *Journal of Clinical Investigation* 10 (1931): 423–29.

Munson, Edward L. "The Needs of Medial Education as Revealed by War." *JAMA* 72, no. 15 (1919): 1050–55.

Murphy, J. B. "Resection of Arteries and Veins Injured in Continuity—End-to-End Suture—Experimental and Clinical Research." *Medical Record* 51, no. 3 (January 1897): 73–88.

Murray, Gordon. "Embolism in the Peripheral Arteries." *Canadian Medical Association Journal* 35 (1935): 61–66.

———. "Heparin in Surgical Treatment of Blood Vessels." *Archives of Surgery* 40, no. 2 (1940): 307–25.

———. "Heparin in Thrombosis and Embolism." *British Journal of Surgery* 27, no. 107 (1940): 567–98.

Murray, Gordon, et al. "Heparin and Vascular Occlusion." *Canadian Medical Association Journal* 35 (December 1936): 621–22.

Musson, A. E. "Newspaper Printing in the Industrial Revolution." *Economic History Review* 10, no. 3 (1958): 411–26.

Mustard, W. T. "The Technic of Immediate Restoration of Vascular Continuity after Arterial Wounds: Indications and Results." *Annals of Surgery* 124, no. 1 (1946): 46–59.

Nahrwold, David L., and Peter J. Kernahan. *A Century of Surgeons and Surgery: The American College of Surgeons, 1913–2013.* Chicago: American College of Surgeons, 2012.

Neff, James M., and John G. O'Malley. "Some Observations on Military Surgery during One Year's Service in the 23rd General Hospital, B.E.F., France." *SGO* 26, no. 1 (January 1918): 60.

Negri, Gloria. "Hermes C. Grillo, 83, Thoracic Surgeon at MGH." *Boston Globe*, 24 October 2006.

Nelson, Russel M. *From Heart to Heart: An Autobiography.* N.p.: Quality Press, 1979.

Nelson, William P. "Treatment of Acute Vascular Catastrophes: A Two-Way Radio Discussion." *New York State Medical Journal* 58 (1957): 3487–92.

Newhauser, L. R., and D. B. Kendrick. "Blood Substitutes: Their Development and Use in the Armed Services." *U.S. Naval Medical Bulletin* 40 (January 1942): 1–13.

Nicholson, Debbie. "The Effects of Local Context on the Development of Obstetric Ultrasound Scanning in Two Scottish Hospitals." In *Innovations in Health and Medicine: Diffusion and Resistance in the Twentieth Century*, edited by Jennifer Stanton, 21–36. New York: Routledge, 2002.

Nimier, H. "The War in Manchuria and the Wounded by Small Arms Bullets." *Military Medicine* 17 (1905–6): 460–61.

"The 1945 Graduate Training in Surgery." *Special Bulletin of the American College of Surgeons* (September 1945): 38.

Nolen, William. *The Making of a Surgeon.* New York: Random House, 1968.

Nunn, Daniel B., Hartwig Bunzendahl, and John R. Handy. "Ernst Jeger: A Forgotten Pioneer in Cardiovascular Surgery." *Surgery* 116, no. 3 (1994): 569–75.

Odom, Charles B. "Causes of Amputations in Battle Casualties with Emphasis on Vascular Injuries." *Surgery* 19 (1946): 562–69.

Ogilvie, W. H. "War Surgery in Africa." *British Journal of Surgery* 31, no. 124 (April 1944): 313–24.

Olch, Peter D. "Evarts A. Graham, the American College of Surgeons, and the American Board of Surgery." *Journal of the History of Medicine and Allied Sciences* 27, no. 3 (1972): 247–61.

Olry, Régis. "Winslow's Contribution to Our Understanding of the Cervical Portion of the Sympathetic Nervous System." *Journal of the History of the Neurosciences* 5, no. 2 (1996): 190–96.

Olszewski, Todd. "Cholesterol: A Scientific, Medical, and Social History, 1908–1962." PhD diss, Yale University, 2008.

Omori, Frances. *Quiet Heroes: Navy Nurses of the Korean War, 1950–1953, Far East Command.* St. Paul, MN: Smith House Press, 2000.

Osbourne, Earl D., et al. "Roentgenography of Urinary Tract during Excretion of Sodium Iodid." *JAMA* 80, no. 6 (February 1923): 368–73.

Oshinsky, David M. *Polio: An American Story.* New York: Oxford University Press, 2005.

Osler, William. "Sir Astley Cooper's Case of Ligature of the Abdominal Aorta." *Guy's Hospital Gazette* (8 July 1911): 277.

Oudat, Jacques. "La greffe vasculaire dans les thromboses du carrefour aortique." *Presse Medicale* 59 (1951): 234–36.

"Our New Nobel Prize." *Literary Digest* 45, no. 21 (23 November 1912): 233–34.

Packard, Randall M. *The Making of a Tropical Disease: A Short History of Malaria*. Baltimore: Johns Hopkins University Press, 2007.

Parascandola, John. "The Introduction of Antibiotics into Therapeutics." In *Sickness and Health in America*, edited by Judith Walzer Leavitt and Ronald L. Numbers, 102–12. Madison: University of Wisconsin Press, 1997.

Parks, Robert J. *Medical Training in World War II*. Washington, DC: Center for Military History, 1974.

Parodi, Juan C., J. C. Palmaz, H. D. Barone. "Transfemoral Intraluminal Graft Implantation for Abdominal Aortic Aneurysms." *Annals of Vascular Surgery* 5 (1991): 491–99.

Parran, Thomas. *Shadow on the Land: Syphilis*. New York: American Social Hygiene Association, 1937.

Payne, Lynda. *The Best Surgeon in England: Percivall Pott, 1713–88*. New York: Peter Lang, 2017.

Peitzman, Steven J. *Dropsy, Dialysis, Transplant: A Short History of Failing Kidneys*. Baltimore: Johns Hopkins University Press, 2007.

———. "Science, Inventors, and the Introduction of the Artificial Kidney in the United States." *Seminars in Dialysis* 9, no. 3 (1996): 276–81.

———. "'Thoroughly Practical': America's Polyclinic Medical Schools." *Bulletin of the History of Medicine* 54 (1980): 166–87.

Pelis, Kim. "Taking Credit: The Canadian Army Medical Corps and the British Conversion to Blood Transfusion in WWI." *Journal for the History of Medicine and Allied Sciences* 56 (July 2001): 238–77.

Pernick, Martin S. *A Calculus of Suffering: Pain, Professionalism, and Anesthesia in Nineteenth-Century America*. New York: Columbia University Press, 1985.

Peterson, Jeanne M. *The Medical Profession in Mid-Victorian London*. Berkeley: University of California Press, 1978.

Phelan, John T. "A New Method of Artery Graft Anastomosis: An Experimental Study." *Surgery* 44 (1958): 990–93.

———. "Newer Aspects of Peripheral Vascular Surgery." *Wisconsin Medical Journal* 58 (1959): 691–93.

Phelan, John T., Richard J. Botham, William P. Young, and Erwin Schmidt. "The Effect of Suture Material in Determining the Patency of Small Artery Grafts: A Comparison Study Using Silk, Nylons, and Dacron Arterial Suture Material." *Surgery* 43 (1958): 969–73.

Phelan, John T., and William P. Young, "The Recognition and Management of Disease of the Aorta and Great Vessels." *Wisconsin Medical Journal* 57 (1958): 373–78.

Phelan, John T., William P. Young, Richard Botham, et al. "The Development of the Artery Bank at the University Hospitals." *Wisconsin Medical Journal* 57 (1958): 232–34, 248.

Phelan, John T., William P. Young, and Joseph W. Gale. "The Effect of Suture Material on Small Artery Anastomoses." *Surgery, Gynecology, and Obstetrics* 1077 (1958): 79–83.

Pickstone, John V. Introduction to *Medical Innovations in Historical Perspective*, edited by John V. Pickstone, 1–15. London: MacMillan, 1992.

Pierce, E. Converse, Robert E. Gross, Alexander H. Bill Jr., and Keith Merrill Jr. "Tissue-Culture Evaluation of Viability of Blood Vessels Stored by Refrigeration." *Annals of Surgery* 129 (1949): 333–48.

Pierce, John R., and Jim Writer, *Yellow Jack: How Yellow Fever Ravaged America and Walter Reed Discovered Its Deadly Secret*. Hoboken, NJ: John Wiley & Sons, 2005.

Podolsky, Scott. *The Antibiotic Era: Reform, Resistance, and the Pursuit of Rational Therapeutics*. Baltimore: Johns Hopkins University Press, 2015.

Power, D'Arcy. *Wounds in War: Their Treatment and Results*. London: Oxford University Press, 1915.

Post, Alfred C. *Eulogy on the Late Valentine Mott, M.D., LL.D*. New York: Messrs/ Bailliére Brothers, 1866.

Pott, Percivall. *The Chirurgical Works of Percivall Pott, FRS and Surgeon to St. Bartholomew's Hospital: A New Edition*. Vol. 3. London, 1779.

Potts, Willis. "A New Clamp for Surgical Division of the Patent Ductus Arteriosus." *Quarterly Bulletin of Northwestern University Medical School* 22, no. 4 (1948): 321–24.

Potts, Willis, et al. "Diagnosis and Surgical Treatment of Patent Ductus Arteriosus." *Archives of Surgery* 58, no. 5 (1949): 612–22.

A Practitioner of Many Years Standing. "The Fellowship Examinations in Lincoln's-Inn-Fields." *Lancet* 45, no. 1114 (January 1845): 16–17.

Pratt, Gerald H. "Surgical Sympathectomy for Obliterative Vascular Disease." *New York State Medical Journal* 54 (1954): 3357–61.

———. "Vascular Wounds." In *Surgery of Trauma*, edited by Warner F. Bowers, 261–94. Philadelphia: Lippincott, 1953.

Pressman, Jack. *Last Resort: Psychosurgery and the Limits of Medicine*. New York: Cambridge University Press, 1998.

Principles of War Surgery, Based on the Conclusions Adopted at the Various Interallied Surgical Conferences. Washington, DC: Government Printing Office, 1918.

Pringle, J. Hogart. "Two Cases of Vein-Grafting for the Maintenance of a Direct Arterial Circulation." *Lancet* (28 June 1913): 1795–96.

Province, Charles M., ed. *I Was Patton's Doctor: The Reminiscences of Colonel Charles B. Odom, Third Army Surgical Consultant and General Patton's Personal Physician*. 2nd ed. N.p.: CMP Productions, 2010.

Radin, Joanna. *Life on Ice: A History of New Uses for Cold Blood*. Chicago: Chicago University Press, 2017.

Rather, L. J. *Addison and the White Corpuscles: An Aspect of Nineteenth Century Biology*. Berkeley: University of California Press, 1972.

Ravitch, Mark M. "The American Surgical Association: The Peaks of Excitement." *Annals of Surgery* 192 (1980): 282–87.

———. *A Century of Surgery: The History of the American Surgical Association.* Philadelphia: Lippincott, 1981.

———. "The Surgical Residency: Then, Now, and Future." *Pharos* (Winter 1987): 11–16.

Recent Advances in Medicine and Surgery (19–30 April 1954) Based on Professional Medical Experiences in Japan and Korea, 1950–1953. Vol. 1. Washington, DC: Army Medical Service Graduate School, 1955.

Reggiani, Andres. "Alexis Carrel, the Unknown: Eugenics and Population Research under Vichy." *French Historical Studies* 25 (2002): 331–56.

Reichert, Frederick L. "The Importance of Circulatory Balance in the Survival of Replanted Limbs." *Johns Hopkins Hospital Bulletin* 49 (1931): 86–93.

Reis, Almiro dos, Jr. "Eulogy to August Karl Gustav Bier on the 100th Anniversary of Intravenous Regional Block and the 110th Anniversary of the Spinal Block." *Revista Brasileira de Anestesiologia* 58, no. 4 (2008): 409–24.

Reiser, Stanley Joel. "The Machine at the Bedside: Technological Transformations of Practices and Values." In *The Machine at the Bedside: Strategies for Using Technology in Patient Care,* edited by Stanley Joel Reiser and Michael Anbar, 3–19. New York: Cambridge University Press, 1984.

Reiser, Joel, and Michael Anbar, eds. *The Machine at the Bedside: Strategies for Using Technology in Patient Care.* New York: Cambridge University Press, 1984.

Reister, Frank. *Battle Casualties and Medical Statistics: U.S. Army Experience in the Korean War.* Washington, DC: Office of the Surgeon General, 1973.

Report of the U.S. Surgeon General's Office, U.S. Army for Fiscal Year 1920. Washington, DC: Government Printing Office, 1920.

Reverby, Susan M. *Ordered to Care: The Dilemma of American Nursing, 1850–1945.* New York: Cambridge University Press, 1987.

Review of War Surgery and Medicine 1, no. 1 (March 1918): 60–62.

Rhodes, Richard. *The Making of the Atomic Bomb.* New York: Simon and Schuster, 1986.

Rich, Norman M. "Historical and Military Aspects of Vascular Trauma (with Lifetime Reflections of Doctor Norman Rich)." In *Vascular Trauma,* 2nd ed., edited by Norman M. Rich, Kenneth L. Mattox, and Asher Hirshberg, 3–72. Philadelphia: Elsevier Science, 2004.

Rich, Norman M., et al. "The Matas/Soubbotitch Connection." *Surgery* 93, no. 1 (1983): 17–19.

Rich, Norman M., Joseph H. Baugh, and Carl W. Hughes. "Acute Arterial Injuries in Vietnam: 1000 Cases." *Journal of Trauma* 10, no. 5 (1970): 359–69.

Rich, Norman M., and Peter Rhee. "An Historical Tour of Vascular Injury Management: From Its Inception to the New Millennium." *Surgical Clinics of North America* 81, no. 6 (December 2001): 1199–215.

Rich, Norman M., and Franck C. Spencer, eds. *Vascular Trauma*. Philadelphia: W. B. Saunders, 1978.

Richardson, Ruth, ed. *Vintage Papers from the Lancet*. New York: Elsevier Press, 2006.

Richter, Brüno. "Surgical Forceps." US patent no. US2478595, filed 24 August 1948, granted 9 August 1949.

Ricketts, Edward A. "Report of the Clinical and Physiological Research at Hemorrhagic Fever Center, Korea, Fall of 1953." *Medical Bulletin of the U.S. Army Far East* 2, no. 2 (1954): 2931.

Rifkin, William J., et al. "Achievements and Challenges in Facial Transplantation." *Annals of Surgery* 268 (2018): 260–70.

Riker, William L., A. Nielson, and Willis J. Potts. "A Technic of Portacaval Anastomosis." *Annals of Surgery* 132, no. 5 (November 1950): 937–43.

Riskin, Daniel J., Michael T. Longbaker, Michael Gertner, and Thomas M. Krummel. "Innovation in Surgery," *Annals of Surgery* 244 (2006): 686–93.

Roberston, E. Ann. "Anesthesia, Shock, and Resuscitation." In *War Surgery 1914–1918*, edited by Thomas Scotland and Steven Heys, 85–115. West Midland: Helion, 2013.

Rodman, J. Stewart. *History of the American Board of Surgery, 1937–1952*. Philadelphia: J. B. Lippincott, 1956.

Rogers, Everett M. *Diffusion of Innovations*. 1963. 5th ed. New York: Free Press, 2003.

Romanelli, Thomas, and Douglass Bacon. "The Origins of Modern Anesthesia throughout the American Experience Spanning the World Wars." *Bulletin of Anesthesia History* 17 (1999): 1, 4–7.

Rose, Charles A., Orvan W. Hess, and Charles S. Welch. "Vascular Injuries of the Extremities in Battle Casualties." *Annals of Surgery* 123 (1946): 161–79.

Rosen, George. *A History of Public Health*. Expanded ed. Baltimore: Johns Hopkins University Press, 1993.

———. *The Specialization of Medicine, with Particular Reference to Ophthalmology*. New York: Froben Press, 1944.

Rosenberg, Charles. *The Care of Strangers: The Rise of America's Hospital System*. New York: Basic Books, 2007.

Ross, Patterson J. "Sympathectomy as an Experiment in Human Physiology." *British Journal of Surgery* 21 (1933): 5–19.

Rowe, R. M. "A Note on the Carrel-Dakin-Daufresne Treatment." *British Medical Journal* 2 (22 September 1917): 387.

Rowland, Sidney. "Report on the Application of the New Photography to Medicine and Surgery." *British Medical Journal* (22 February 1896): 492–96.

Rowntree, Leonard G. "Result of Bilateral Lumbar Sympathetic Ganglionectomy and Ramisectomy for Polyarthritis of the Lower Extremities." *Proceedings of the Weekly Staff Meeting of the Mayo Clinic* 3 (1928): 333–34.

Royale, Norman D. "A New Operative Procedure in the Treatment of Spastic Paralysis and Its Experimental Basis." *Medical Journal of Australia* 1, no. 4 (1924): 77–86.

———. "The Operations of Sympathetic Ramisection." *Medical Journal of Australia* 1, no. 24 (1924): 587–91.

———. "The Treatment of Spastic Paralysis by Sympathetic Ramisection." *SGO* 39 (December 1924): 701–20.

Russell, Edmund. *War and Nature: Fighting Humans and Insects with Chemicals from World War I to Silent Spring.* New York: Cambridge University Press, 2001.

Rutkow, Ira. "The Education, Training, and Specialization of Surgeons: Turn-of-the-Century America and Its Postgraduate Medical Schools." *Annals of Surgery* 258 (2013): 1130–36.

Sako, Yoshio, et al. "A Survey of Evacuation, Resuscitation, and Mortality in a Forward Surgical Hospital." In *The Battle Wound: Clinical Experiences*, vol. 3 of *Battle Casualties in Korea: Studies of the Surgical Research Team*, edited by Curtis P. Artz, 9–21. Washington, DC: Army Medical Service Graduate School, 1954.

Salomoni, Annibale. "Sutura circolare delle arterie con l'affrontamento dell'endotelio." *La Clinica Chirurgica* 8 (1900): 241.

Salyer, John M. "The Training of Medical Officers." In *Recent Advances in Medicine and Surgery (19–30 April 1954) Based on Professional Medical Experiences in Japan and Korea, 1950–1953*, vol. 2, 83–94. Washington, DC: Army Medical Service Graduate School, 1955.

Schafer, James A., Jr. Fighting for Business: The Limits of Professional Cooperation among American Doctors during the First World War." *Journal of the History of Medicine and Allied Sciences* 70 (2015): 165–94.

Schede, Max. "Einige Bemerkungen über die Naht von Venenwunden, nebst Mittheilung eines Falles von geheilter Naht der Vena caver inferior." *Archiv für Klinische Chirurgie* 43 (1893): 338–45.

Schlich, Thomas. "'The Days of Brilliancy Are Past': Skill, Style and the Changing Rules of Surgical Performance, ca. 1820–1920." *Medical History* 59 (2015): 379–403.

———. "Degrees of Control: The Spread of Operative Fracture Treatment with Metal Implants, a Comparative Perspective on Switzerland, East Germany and the USA, 1950s to 1990s." In *Innovations in Health and Medicine: Diffusion and Resistance in the Twentieth Century*, edited by Jennifer Stanton, 106–25. New York: Routledge, 2002.

———. "The Emergence of Modern Surgery." In *Medicine Transformed: Health, Disease and Society in Europe, 1800–1930*, edited by Deborah Brunton, 61–91. Manchester: Manchester University Press, 2004.

———. "How Gods and Saints Became Transplant Surgeons." *History of Science* 33, no. 101 (1995): 311–31.

———. "Negotiating Technologies in Surgery: The Controversy about Surgical Gloves in the 1890s." *Bulletin of the History of Medicine* 87, no. 2 (2013): 170–97.

————. "'One and the Same the World Over': The International Culture of Surgical Exchange in an Age of Globalization, 1870–1914." *Journal of the History of Medicine and Allied Sciences* 71 (2016): 247–70.

————. *The Origins of Organ Transplantation: Surgery and Laboratory Science, 1880–1930.* Rochester, NY: University of Rochester Press, 2010.

————. *Surgery, Science and Industry: A Revolution in Fracture Care, 1950s–1990s.* New York: Palgrave, 2002.

————. "Surgery, Science and Modernity: Operating Rooms and Laboratories as Spaces of Control." *History of Science* 45, no. 3 (2007): 231–56.

Schlich, Thomas, and Christopher Crenner, eds. *Technological Change in Modern Surgery: Historical Perspectives on Innovation.* Rochester, NY: University of Rochester Press, 2017.

Schlich, Thomas, and Audrey Hasegawa. "Order and Cleanliness: The Gendered Role of Operating Room Nurses in the United States (1870s–1930s)." *Social History of Medicine* 31 (2017): 106–21.

Schloss, Gerd, and Harris B. Shumacker Jr. "Studies in Vascular Repair: IV. The Use of Free Vascular Transplants for Bridging Arterial Defects; An Historical Review with Particular Reference to Histological Observations." *Yale Journal of Biology and Medicine* 22 (1950): 273–90.

Schmeck, Harold M., Jr. "Windsor's Surgery." *New York Times,* 20 December 1964, E7.

Schmitz, Everett J., Edmund A. Kanar, Lester R. Sauvage, Edward H. Storer, and Henry N. Harkins. "The Influence of Diameter Disproportion and of Length on the Incidence of Complications in Autogenous Venous Grafts in the Abdominal Aorta." *Surgery* 33 (1953): 190–206.

Scotland, Thomas R. "Evacuation Pathway for the Wounded." In *War Surgery 1914–1918,* edited by Thomas Scotland and Steven Heys, 51–84. West Midland: Helion, 2013.

Scott, Virgil. "Abdominal Aneurysms." *American Journal of Syphilis, Gonorrhea, and Venereal Disease* 28 (1944): 682–710.

Seaman, Louis Livingstone. "Observations in the Russo-Japanese War." *Military Surgeon* 16 (1904–5): 6–7.

Seeley, Sam F. "Vascular Surgery at Walter Reed Army Hospital." *United States Armed Forces Medical Journal* 5 (1954): 8–9.

Seeley, Sam F., Carl W. Hughes, Francis N. Cook, and Daniel C. Elkin. "Traumatic Arteriovenous Fistulas and Aneurysms in War Wounds: A Study of 101 Cases." *American Journal of Surgery* 83 (March 1952): 471–79.

Seeley, Sam F., Carl W. Hughes, and Edward J. Jahnke Jr. "Surgery of the Popliteal Artery." *Annals of Surgery* 138, no. 5 (1953): 712–17.

Seidenberg, Bernard, Elliot S. Hurwitt, and Charles A. Carton. "The Technique of Anastomosing Small Arteries." *SGO* 106 (1958): 743–46.

Seldinger, Sven. "Catheter Replacement of the Needle in Percutaneous Arteriography: A New Technique." *Acta Radiologica* 39 (1953): 368–76.

Serlin, David. *Replaceable You: Engineering the Body in Postwar America.* Chicago: University of Chicago Press, 2004.

Shepherd, Ben. *A War of Nerves: Soldiers and Psychiatrists in the Twentieth Century.* Cambridge, MA: Harvard University Press, 2001.

Shephard, David. *From Craft to Specialty: A Medical and Social History of Anesthesia and Its Changing Role in Health Care.* Thunder Bay, ON: York Point, 2009.

Sherman, William O. "The Abortive Treatment of Wound Infection: Carrel's Method—Dakin's Solution." *JAMA* 69, no. 3 (21 July 1917): 185–92.

Shilcutt, Tracy. "First Link in the Chain: Infantry Combat Medics in Europe, 1944–1945." PhD diss., Texas Christian University, 2003.

"Shipment of Whole Blood to Pacific Theaters of Operation." *Bulletin of the US Army Medical Department*, no. 87 (April 1945): 45.

Shumacker, Harris B., Jr. "Arterial Aneurysms and Arteriovenous Fistulas: Sympathectomy as an Adjunct Measure in Operative Treatment." In *Vascular Surgery*, edited by Daniel C. Elkin and Michael E. DeBakey, 318–60. Washington, DC: Office of the Surgeon General, 1955.

———. "Ramuald Weglowski: Neglected Pioneer in Vascular Surgery." *Annals of Vascular Surgery* 6, no. 1 (1987): 95–97.

———. "The Arteries." In *A Textbook of Surgery by American Authors*, 6th ed., edited by Loyal Davis, 1298–315. Philadelphia: W. B. Saunders, 1956.

———. *The Society for Vascular Surgery: A History; 1945–1983.* Manchester, MA: Society for Vascular Surgery, 1984.

———. "Vascular Injuries." In *Early Care of Acute Soft Tissue Injuries*, edited by American College of Surgeons Committee on Trauma, 144–53. Chicago: n.p., 1954.

———. "Vascular Injuries." In *Early Care of Acute Soft Tissue Injuries*, edited by American College of Surgeons Committee on Trauma, 88–96. Chicago, 1960.

Shumacker, Harris B., Jr., David L. Abramson, and Herbert H. Lambert. "Arterial Aneurysms and Arteriovenous Fistulas: Anticoagulant Therapy in Reparative Surgery." In *Vascular Surgery*, edited by Daniel C. Elkin and Michael E. DeBakey, 310–17. Washington, DC: Office of the Surgeon General, 1955.

Shumacker, Harris B., Jr., and Robert I. Lowenberg. "Experimental Studies in Vascular Repair: I. Comparison of Reliability of Various Methods End-to-End Arterial Sutures." *Surgery* 24 (1948): 79–89.

Shumacker, Harris B., Jr., G. Schloss, L. W. Freeman, E. E. Wayson, and N. H. Stahl. "Studies in Vascular Repair: V. Experiments with the Use of Free Venous Transplants for Bridging Aortal Defects." *Yale Journal of Biology and Medicine* 23 (1950): 81–93.

Sicard, A., and J. Forestier. "L'huile idoée en clinique: Applications thérapeutiques et diagnostiques." *Bulletins et Mémoires de la Société Médicale des Hôpitaux de Paris* 47 (1923): 309–17.

Silbert, Samuel. "Surgical Consideration in the Treatment of Infection and Gangrene in the Diabetic." *Connecticut State Medical Journal* 17 (1953): 895–903.

Simeone, Fiorindo. "The Anastomosis of Severed Arteries by a Nonsuture Method." *Surgical Clinics of North America* 27 (1947): 1088–99.

———. "Notes of the Treatment of Wounds of the Arteries." In *Symposium on Military Medicine in the Far East Command,* 72–73. Tokyo(?): United States Army Far East Command, 1951.

Simpson, Andrew. "Transporting Lazarus: Physicians, the State, and the Creation of the Modern Paramedic and Ambulance, 1955–1973." *Journal of the History of Medicine and Allied Sciences* 68 (2013): 163–97.

Sinkler, William H., and Andrew D. Spencer. "The Importance of Early Exploration of Vascular Injuries." *SGO* 107 (1958): 228–34.

Slater, Leo B. *War and Disease: Biomedical Research on Malaria in the Twentieth Century.* New Brunswick, NJ: Rutgers University Press, 2009.

Smadel, Joseph E. "Epidemic Hemorrhagic Fever." *American Journal of Public Health and Nations Health* 43, no. 10 (1953): 1327–30.

Smith, Allen D. "Medical Air Evacuation in Korea and Its Influence on the Future." *Military Surgeon* 110, no. 5 (1952): 323–32.

Smith, Dale C. "Appendicitis, Appendectomy, and the Surgeon." *Bulletin of the History of Medicine* 70, no. 3 (1996): 414–41.

———. "Austin Flint and Auscultation in America." *Journal of the History of Medicine and Allied Sciences* 33 (1978): 129–49.

———. "A Historical Overview of the Recognition of Appendicitis." *New York State Medical Journal* 86 (1986): 571–83 and 639–47.

———. "Surgery: It's Not Random Therapy." *Caduceus* 12 (1996): 19–38.

Smith, Morris K. "Arterial Injuries." *Annals of Surgery* 126 (1947): 866–72.

Smith, Parke G., T. W. Rush, and Arthur T. Evans. "The Technique of Translumbar Arteriography." *JAMA* 148 (1952): 255–58.

Snowden, Frank. *The Conquest of Malaria: Italy, 1900–1962.* New Haven, CT: Yale University Press, 2006.

Snyder, John M. "Vascular Wounds: Report of a Series of 108 Cases Encountered in a Forward Evacuation Hospital." *Surgery* 21, no. 1 (1947): 77–85.

Soper, Frederick Lowe. *Ventures in World Health: The Memoirs of Fred Lowe Soper,* edited by John Duffy. Washington, DC: Pan American Health Organization, 1977.

Soubbotitch, Vojislav. "Military Experiences of Traumatic Aneurysms." *Lancet* 182, no. 4697 (6 September 1913): 720–21.

Spencer, Frank C. "Historical Vignette: The Introduction of Arterial Repair into the US Marine Corps, US Naval Hospital, in July–August 1952." *Journal of Trauma* 60 (2006): 906–9.

Spencer, Frank C., and Ray V. Grewe. "The Management of Arterial Injuries in Battle Casualties." *Annals of Surgery* 141, no. 3 (March 1955): 304–13.

Standlee, Mary W. *Borden's Dream: The Walter Reed Army Medical Center in Washington D.C.* Washington, DC: Borden Institute, 2009.

Stanley, Peter. *For Fear of Pain: British Surgery, 1790–1850.* Amsterdam, NY: Rodopi, 2003.

Stanton, Jennifer Stanton, ed. *Innovations in Health and Medicine: Diffusion and Resistance in the Twentieth Century.* New York: Routledge University Press, 2002.

Starr, Paul. *The Social Transformation of American Medicine: The Rise of a Sovereign Profession and the Making of a Vast Industry.* New York: Basic Books, 1982.

Starzl, Thomas E. *The Puzzle People: Memoirs of a Transplant Surgeon.* Pittsburgh: University of Pittsburgh Press, 1992.

Steckel, Richard H. "Persons with Hospital and Surgical Benefits, by Type of Private Health Insurance Plan: 1939–1992." In *Historical Statistics of the United States,* edited by Susan B. Carter et al. Cambridge: Cambridge University Press, 2006.

Steer, Arthur, Robert L. Hullinghorst, and Richard P. Mason. "The Blood Program in the Korean War." In *The Battle Wound: Clinical Experiences,* vol. 3 of *Battle Casualties in Korea: Studies of the Surgical Research Team,* edited by Curtis P. Artz, 150–65. Washington, DC: Army Medical Service Graduate School, 1954.

Stephenson, George W. "American College of Surgeons and Graduate Education in Surgery: A Chronicle of Surgical Advancement." *Special Edition Bulletin of the American College of Surgeons* 56, no. 5 (May 1971).

———. *American College of Surgeons at 75.* Chicago: American College of Surgeons, 1990.

Stephenson, Hugh, Jr. "A Brief Biography of Charles Claude Guthrie." In *The Evolution of Modern Vascular Surgery: The Historical Perspective of the Midwestern Vascular Surgical Society, 1977–2001,* edited by John R. Pfeifer and John W. Hallet Jr., 450–57. Salem, MA: Midwestern Vascular Surgical Society: 2001.

Stevens, Alden. "Spare Parts for People." *Harper's Magazine,* July 1955, 74–76.

Stevens, Rosemary. *American Medicine and the Public Interest.* New Haven, CT: Yale University Press, 1971.

———. *In Sickness and in Wealth: American Hospitals in the Twentieth Century.* Baltimore: Johns Hopkins University Press, 1989.

———. *A Time of Scandal: Charles R. Forbes, Warren G. Harding, and the Making of the Veterans Bureau.* Baltimore: Johns Hopkins University Press, 2016.

Stevenson, Lloyd. "A Further Note on John Hunter and Aneurism." *Bulletin of the History of Medicine* 26 (1952): 162–67.

———. "The Stag of Richmond Park: A Note on John Hunter's Most Famous Animal Experiment." *Bulletin of History of Medicine* 22 (1948): 467–75.

Steward, Charles. "War Experiences with Nonsuture Technic of Anastomosis in Primary Arterial Injuries." *Annals of Surgery* 125 (1947): 157–70.

Stimson, Lewis A. "An Inquiry into the Origin of the Use of the Ligature in the Treatment of Aneurysm." *Annals of Surgery* 1 (1885): 13–25.

Storck, Ambrose H. "Evaluation of the Vascular Status in Traumatic and Nontraumatic Lesions of the Blood Vessels." In *Vascular Surgery,* edited by Daniel C. Elkin and Michael E. DeBakey, 17–59. Washington, DC: Office of the Surgeon General, 1955.

Strong, D. Michael. "The US Navy Tissue Bank: 50 Years on the Cutting Edge." *Cell and Tissue Banking* 1 (2000): 9–16.

Stueck, William. *Rethinking the Korean War: A New Diplomatic and Strategic History.* Princeton, NJ: Princeton University Press, 2002.

Summerfield, Arthur E. *U.S. Mail: The Story of the United States Postal Service.* New York: Holt, Rinehart, and Winston, 1960.

Surgery in the United States: A Summary Report of the Study on Surgical Services for the United States. Executive Report. American College of Surgeons and American Surgical Association, 1975.

"Surgical Treatment of War Wounds of the Abdomen." *Review of War Surgery and Medicine* 1, no. 2 (April 1918): 20–26.

Swan, Henry. "Arterial Grafts," *SGO* 94 (1952): 115–17.

Swanson, Kara W. *Banking on the Body: The Market in Blood, Milk, and Sperm in Modern America.* Cambridge, MA: Harvard University Press, 2014.

Swick, Moses. "Intravenous Urography by Means of Uroselectan." *American Journal of Surgery* 8, no. 2 (1930): 405–14.

Taffel, Max. "Samuel Clark Harvey, 1886–1953." *Yale Journal of Biology and Medicine* 26, no. 1 (1953): 1–7.

Tang, Cynthia, and Thomas Schlich. "Surgical Innovation and the Multiple Meanings of Randomized Controlled Trials: The First RCT on Minimally Invasive Cholecystectomy (1980–2000)." *Journal of the History of Medicine and Allied Sciences* 72, no. 2 (2016): 117–41.

Tarizzo, Richard A., Robert W. Alexander, E. J. Beattie Jr., Steven G. Economou. "Atherosclerosis in Synthetic Vascular Grafts: Studies in Humans and Experimental Animals." *Archives of Surgery* 8 (1961): 826–32.

Temkin, Oswei. "The Role of Surgery in the Rise of Modern Medical Thought." *Bulletin of the History of Medicine* 25 (1951): 248–59.

———. "The Scientific Approach to Disease: Specific Entity and Individual Sickness." In *The Double Face of Janus and Other Essays in the History of Medicine,* edited by Oswei Temkin, 441–55. Baltimore: Johns Hopkins University Press, 1977.

TerHorst, J. F. "Auto Safety Devices Gain Public Favor." *Detroit Michigan News,* 18 March 1956.

Terraine, John. *White Heat: The New Warfare, 1914–1918.* London: Sidgwick & Jackson, 1982.

Theirs, Frank V. "Effect of Neurectomy on the Collateral Arteriole Circulation of the Extremities." *SGO* 42 (1933): 737–44.

Thomas, David E. "Continuous Lumbar Sympathetic Block by the Catheter Technique." *Medical Bulletin of the U.S. Army Far East* 1, no. 3 (1953): 47–48.

Thomaselli, Giovanni. "Esiti lontani della sutura col metodo dell'affrontamento dell'endotelio et sui processi di guarigione delle ferite arteriose." *Clinica Chirurgia* 11, no. 5 (1903): 36–379.

———. "Sutura circolare delle arterie coll'affrontamento dell'endoletio." *Clinica Chirurgia*, 6 (1902): 497–511.

Thompson, Jesse E. "The Founding Fathers." *Surgery* 82 (December 1977): 801–8.

Thompson, W. "Simultaneous Double Distal Ligature of the Carotid and Subclavian Arteries for High Innominate Aneurysm." *Annals of Surgery* 1 (1885): 582.

Tilney, Nicolas L. *Transplant: From Myth to Reality*. New Haven, CT: Yale University Press, 2003.

Timmerman, Stefan. "A Black Technician and Blue Babies." *Social Studies of Science* 33 (1997): 197–228.

Toland, John. *Battle: The Story of the Bulge*. New York: Random House, 1958.

Trendelenburg, F. *Die ersten 25 Jahre der Deutschen Gesellschaft für Chirurgie: Ein Beitrag zur Geschichte der Chirurgie*. Berlin: Springer; 1923.

Tribble, William D. *Doctor Draft Justified? A Management Diagnosis*. San Antonio: National Medical Laboratories, 1968.

Tuckman, Robert. "Marine Surgeon, 27, Saves Limbs at Front Through New Operation." *Hartford Courant*, 7 June 1953, 22.

Turney, Jon. *Frankenstein's Footsteps: Science, Genetics and Popular Culture*. New Haven, CT: Yale University Press, 1998.

Turow, Joseph, and Rachel Gans-Boriskin. "From Expert in Action to Existential Angst: A Half Century of Television Doctors." In *Medicine's Moving Pictures: Medicine, Health, and Bodies in American Film and Television*, edited by Leslie Reagan, Nancy Tomes, and Paula A. Treichler, 263–81. Rochester, NY: University of Rochester Press, 2007.

US Postal Service. *The United States Postal Service: An American History, 1775–2006*. Washington, DC: eBook, 2006.

van Bergen, Leo. *Before My Helpless Sight: Suffering, Dying, and Military Medicine on the Western Front*. Translated by Liz Walters. Burlington: Ashgate, 2009.

———. "Surgery and War: The Discussions about the Usefulness of War for Medical Progress." In *The Palgrave Handbook of the History of Surgery*, edited by Thomas Schlich, 389–410. London: Palgrave Macmillan, 2018.

van Horoch, Cajetan. "Die Gefässnaht." *Allgemeine Wiener Medizin Zeitung*, 22 (1888): 263–64.

"Vascular Injuries." In *Early Care of Acute Soft Tissue Injuries*, 2nd ed., edited by American College of Surgeons Committee on Trauma, 88–96. Philadelphia: W. B. Saunders, 1960.

"Vascular Injuries in War." *Review of War Surgery and Medicine* 1, no. 7 (September 1918): 1–26.

Veal, J. Ross. "The Value of Sympathetic Interruption Following the Surgical Repair of Peripheral Aneurysms." *Medical Annals of the District of Columbia* 9, no. 7 (July 1940): 227–30.

Voorhees, Arthur B. "The Development of Arterial Prostheses: A Personal View." *Archives of Surgery* 120, no. 3 (1985): 289–95.

―――. "The Origin of the Permeable Arterial Prosthesis: A Personal Reminiscence." *Surgery Rounds* 2 (1988): 79–84.

Voorhees, Arthur B., Alfred. Jaretzki, and Arthur H. Blakemore. "The Use of Tubes Constructed from Vinyon 'N' Cloth in Bridging Arterial Defects: A Preliminary Report." *Annals of Surgery* 135 (1952): 332–36.

Waisel, David B. "Norman's War: Norman B. Kornfield, M.D., World War II Physician-Anesthetist." *Anesthesiology* 98 (April 2003): 995–1003.

―――. "The Role of World War II and the European Theater of Operations in the Development of Anesthesiology as a Physician Specialty in the USA." *Anesthesiology* 94 (2001): 907–14.

Wallace, Cuthbert S. "Gas Gangrene as Seen at the Casualty Clearing Stations." *Journal of the Royal Army Medical Corps* 28 (1917): 528–38.

Wallingford, V. H. "The Development of Organic Iodine Compounds as X-Ray Contrast Media." *Journal of Pharmaceutical Sciences* 42 (1953): 721–28.

Walsh, J. J. "Post-graduate Medical School and Hospital." *History of Medicine in New York* 2 (1919): 573–93.

Wangensteen, Owen D., and Sarah A. Wangensteen. *The Rise of Surgery: From Empiric Craft to Scientific Discipline*. Minneapolis: University of Minnesota Press, 1978.

Ward, W. "Blood Vessel Anastamosis by Means of Rubber Tubing." *New York Medical Record* 74 (1908): 671.

Warner, John Harley. *Against the Spirit of System: The French Impulse in Nineteenth Century American Medicine*. Baltimore: Johns Hopkins University Press, 1998.

―――. "Science in Medicine," *Osiris*, 2nd ser., 1 (1985): 37–58.

Warren, Richard. "War Wounds of Arteries." *Archives of Surgery* 53 (1946): 86–99.

Warthmüller, Hans. "Über die bisherigen Erfolge der Gefässtransplantation am Menschen: Inaugural-Dissertation der medizinischen Fakultät der Universität Jena; Zur Erlangung der Doktorwürde in der Medizin, Chirurgie und Geburtshilfe." Druck von G. Neuenhahn, Universitäts-Buchdruckerei, 1917.

Warwick, Andrew. "X-Rays as Evidence in German Orthopedic Surgery." *Isis* 96 (2005): 1–24.

Watts, Stephen H. "The Suture of Blood Vessels and Direct Transfusion of Blood by Vascular Anastomoses." *Virginia Medical Semi-monthly* 13, no. 10 (21 August 1908): 217–22.

―――. "The Suture of the Blood Vessels: Implantation and Transplantation of Vessels and Organs; An Historical and Experimental Study." *Bulletin of the Johns Hopkins Hospital* 18, no. 194 (May 1907): 153–79.

Welch, Claude E. *A Twentieth Century Surgeon: My Life in the Massachusetts General Hospital*. Boston: Massachusetts General Hospital, 1992.

Welch, William H. "Thrombosis." In *Papers and Addresses by William Henry Welch*, edited by Walter C. Burket, 110–92. Baltimore: Johns Hopkins University Press, 1920.

Weisz, George. *Divide and Conquer: A Comparative History of Medical Specialization.* New York: Oxford University Press, 2006.

Wennberg, John E. *Tracking Medicine: A Researcher's Quest to Understand Health Care.* New York: Oxford, 2010.

Wertenbaker, Lael. *To Mend the Heart: The Dramatic Story of Cardiac Surgery and Its Pioneers.* New York: Viking Press, 1980.

Westover, John G. *Combat Support in Korea.* Washington, DC: Combat Forces Press, 1955.

Whipple, Allen O. "Opportunities for Graduate Teaching of Surgery in Larger Qualified Hospitals." *Annals of Surgery* 102 (1935): 516–30.

Whitaker, William G., Jr., Walter Faust Durden, and Ira A. Ferguson. "Acute Arterial Injuries." *SGO* 99 (1954): 129–34.

Whitcomb, Darrel. *Call Sign—Dustoff: A History of U.S. Army Aeromedical Evacuation from Conception to Hurricane Katrina.* Washington, DC: Borden Institute Press, 2011.

White, James C. "Diagnostic Blocking of the Sympathetic Nerves to the Extremities with Procaine." *JAMA* 94 (1930): 1382–88.

———. "Progress in Surgery of the Autonomic Nervous System, 1940–1942." *Surgery* 15 (1944): 491–517.

White, Richard. *Railroaded: The Transcontinentals and the Making of Modern America.* New York: Norton, 2011.

White, William L. *Back Down the Ridge.* New York: Harcourt, Brace, 1953.

Whitehead, Ian R. *Doctors in the Great War.* Barnsley, England: Leo Cooper, 1989.

Whitfield, Nicolas. "A Revolution through the Keyhole: Technology, Innovation, and the Rise of Minimally Invasive Surgery." In *The Palgrave Handbook of the History of Surgery,* edited by Thomas Schlich, 525–48. London: Palgrave Macmillan, 2018.

Wilde, Sally Diana Howard. "Practising Surgery: A History of Surgical Training in Australia, 1927–1974." PhD diss., University of Melbourne, 2003.

Wilde, Sally, and Geoffrey Hirst. "Learning from Mistakes: Early Twentieth Century Surgical Practice." *Journal of the History of Medicine and Allied Sciences* 64, no. 1 (January 2009): 38–77.

Williams, G. Melville. "Bertram M. Bernheim: A Southern Vascular Surgeon." *Journal of Vascular Surgery* 16, no. 3 (1992): 311–18.

Wiltse, Charles M. *Medical Service in the Mediterranean and Minor Theaters.* Washington, DC: Office of the Chief of Military History, 1965.

Winslow, Jacques-Bénigne. *An Anatomical Exposition of the Structure of the Human Body.* 3rd ed. Translated by G. Douglass. London: 1749.

Winslow, Nathan, and W. Wallace Walker. "End-to-End Vascular Anastomosis: An Experimental Study." *Annals of Surgery* 103, no. 6 (June 1936): 959–63.

Wittebols, James H. *Watching "M*A*S*H," Watching America: A Social History of the 1972–1983 Television Series.* Jefferson, NC: McFarland, 1998.

Wolff, Luther H. *Forward Surgeon: The Diary of Luther H. Wolff, MD, Mediterranean Theater, World War II, 1943–45.* New York: Vantage Press, 1985.

Woodard, Scott. "The Story of the Mobile Army Surgical Hospital." *Military Medicine* 168, no. 7 (July 2003): 503–13.

Woods, Abigail. "From One Medicine to Two: The Evolving Relationship between Human and Veterinary Medicine in England, 1791–1835." *Bulletin of the History of Medicine* 91 (2017): 494–523.

"The Wounded from Alamein: Observations on Wound Shock and Its Treatment." *Army Medical Department Bulletin* no. 7 (September 1943): 11–19.

Wright, Almoth E. "Memorandum on the Treatment of Infected Wounds by Physiological Methods: (Drainage of Infected Tissues by Hypertonic Salt Solution and Utilization of the Antibacterial Powers of the Blood Fluids and White Blood Corpuscles)." *British Medicine Journal* 1, no. 2892 (1916): 793–97.

Wylie, E. Jack. "Vascular Surgery: A Quest for Excellence." *Archives of Surgery* 101 (1970): 645–48.

"A Yale Unit at the Front." *Yale Alumni Weekly* 37 (1918): 133–34.

Yao, James S. T. "First Textbook in Vascular Surgery." *Journal of Vascular Surgery* 54, no. 1 (July 2011): 269–72.

———. "Society for Vascular Surgery (SVS)—the Beginning." *Journal of Vascular Surgery* 51 (March 2010): 776–79.

Yater, Wallas M. "Coronary Artery Disease in Men Eighteen to Thirty-Nine Years of Age." *American Heart Journal* 36, no. 4 (1948): 481–526.

Ziman, John M. "Information, Communication, and Knowledge." *Nature* 224 (25 October 1969): 318–24.

———. *Public Knowledge: An Essay Concerning the Social Dimension of Science.* Cambridge: Cambridge University Press, 1968.

Zink, Brian J. *Anyone, Anything, Anytime: A History of Emergency Medicine.* Philadelphia: Mosby, 2006.

Ziperman, H. Haskell. "Acute Arterial Injuries in the Korean War: A Statistical Study." *Annals of Surgery* 139, no. 1 (January 1954): 1–8.

Zollinger, Richard W. "Traffic Injuries—a Surgical Problem." *Archives of Surgery* 70 (1955): 694–700.

Index